R. Jakesz H. Rainer (Eds.)

Progress in Regional Cancer Therapy

With 86 Figures and 111 Tables

Springer-Verlag
Berlin Heidelberg New York London
Paris Tokyo Hong Kong Barcelona

Professor Dr. Raimund Jakesz
Allgemeines Krankenhaus der Stadt Wien
I. Chirurgische Universitätsklinik
Alser Straße 4, 1090 Wien IX, Austria

Professor Dr. Hugo Rainer
Universitätsklinik für Chemotherapie
Lazarettgasse 14, 1090 Wien IX, Austria

ISBN-13: 978-3-642-74820-2 e-ISBN-13: 978-3-642-74818-9
DOI: 10.1007/978-3-642-74818-9

Library of Congress Cataloging-in-Publication Data
Progress in regional cancer therapy/R. Jakesz, H. Rainer (eds.).
p. cm. Based on a symposium held on Nov. 3-5, 1988 in Vienna.
ISBN 0-387-51259-4 (U.S.:alk. paper)
1. Cancer-Treatment-Congresses. 2. Antineoplastic agents-Administration-Congresses.
3. Drug targeting-Congresses. I. Jakesz, R. (Raimund), 1950-. II. Rainer, H. (Hugo)
[DNLM: 1. Antineoplastic Agents-administration & dosage-congresses.
2. Neoplasms-drug therapy-congresses. 3. Perfusion, Regional-congresses.
QZ 267 P9637 1988]
RC270.8.P75 1990 616.99'4061-dc20 DNLM/DLC 90-9521

Typesetting: Thomson Press (India) Ltd., New Delhi
2125/3140-543210 – Printed on acid-free paper.

Preface

Systemic chemotherapy has long been used as a supplement to the surgical resection of primary tumors. Its relative lack of selectivity and its severe side effects prompted the search for more specific therapeutic modalities. The techniques using tumor-specific antigen-binding antibodies to carry substances which kill cancer cells and the approaches that take advantage of specific metabolic characteristics or of the presence of hormone receptors are examples of such therapies. Cancer therapy can also be made more specific by administering drugs directly to the target lesions via completely implantable, well-tolerated systems. Knowledge of pharmacokinetics, metabolism, drug distribution, and tolerance in defined anatomic regions is exploited to minimize the concentration of the anticancer agent in those parts of the body believed to be at lesser cancer risk. For most cytotoxics, the higher their concentration the greater their activity in tumor tissue. Selective administration increases the target: nontarged relation up to 1000-fold.

The symposium "Progress in Regional Cancer Therapy", held on November 3–5, 1988 in Vienna, updated our knowledge of palliative and adjuvant therapies. It also showed us that much remains to be done in improving drug combinations, administration schedules and galenic forms for efficient treatment in the different anatomic regions, as well as in selection of cancer types and stages for regional therapy. Although many questions are far from being answered, improvements in tumor remission rates, tolerance of treatment and quality of life will undoubtedly stimulate further research in this young area of chemotherapy. We hope that these edited proceedings of the Vienna meeting will be helpful in that pursuit.

R. Jakesz
H. Rainer

Contents

List of Authors

Adler; S.
Abteilung für Radiotherapie, Westdeutsches Tumorzentrum
Hufelandstraße 55, 4300 Essen, FRG

Albrecht, W.
Abteilung für Urologie
Krankenanstalt Rudolfstiftung der Stadt Wien
Juchgasse 25, 1030 Wien, Austria

Anderson, J. R.
University Department of Surgery, Royal Infirmary
Glasgow G31 2ER, United Kingdom

Arian-Schad, K.
Chirurgische Abteilung, Medizinische Hochschule
Auenbruggerplatz 1, 8030 Graz, Austria

Arigoni, M.
Chirurgische Abteilung, Kantonsspital, Universität Basel
4031 Basel, Switzerland

Arma, S.
Chirurgische Abteilung, Kantonsspital, Universität Basel
4031 Basel, Switzerland

Armbruster, C.
I. Chirurgische Abteilung
Krankenanstalt Rudolfstiftung der Stadt Wien
Juchgasse 25, 1030 Wien, Austria

Athlin, L.
Surgical Clinic, University Hospital, 90185 Umea, Sweden

Avella, M.
Istituto Ortopedico Rizzoli, Via Puppili 1
40136 Bologna, Italy

Bacci, G.
Istituto Ortopedico Rizzoli, Via Puppili 1
40136 Bologna, Italy

Barras, J.
Chirurgische Abteilung, Kantonsspital, Universität Basel
4031 Basel, Switzerland

Barzan, L.
Division of Otolaryngology, Pordenone Hospital
Pordenone, Italy

Baum, R.P.
Klinik für Allgemeinchirurgie
Johann Wolfgang Goethe-Universität
Theodor-Stern-Kai 7, 6000 Frankfurt/Main, FRG

Baumgartner, G.
Abteilung für Onkologie, Krankenhaus Lainz
Wolkersbergenstraße 1, 1130 Wien, Austria

Beger, H. G.
Abteilung für Allgemeine Chirurgie, Universität Ulm
Steinhövelstraße 9, 7900 Ulm, FRG

Bencivenga, R.
Special Oncology Department, Regional Hospital Torette
60020 Ancona, Italy

Benckhuijsen, C.
Department of Surgery, The Netherlands Cancer Institute
(Antoni van Leeuwenhoek Huis)
Plesmanlaan 121, 1066 CX Amsterdam, The Netherlands

Bergemann, W.
Abteilung für Geriatrie, Krankenhaus Neukölln
Mariendorfer Weg 28/48, 1000 Berlin 44, FRG

Berger, A.
Chirurgische Abteilung, Medizinische Hochschule
Auenbruggerplatz 1, 8030 Graz, Austria

Berger, M. R.
Institut für Toxikologie und Chemotherapie
Deutsches Krebsforschungszentrum
Im Neuenheimer Feld 280, 6900 Heidelberg, FRG

Bihl, H.
Institut für Radiologie und Pathophysiologie
Deutsches Krebsforschungszentrum
Im Neuenheimer Feld 280, 6900 Heidelberg, FRG

Bitter, K.
Klinik für Mund-, Kiefer- und Gesichtschirurgie
Johann Wolfgang Goethe-Universität
Theodor-Stern-Kai 7, 6000 Frankfurt/Main, FRG

Bittner, R.
Abteilung für Allgemeine Chirurgie, Universität Ulm
Steinhövelstraße 9, 7900 Ulm FRG

Blackie, R.
Department of Vascular Surgery, Gartnavel General Hospital
1053 Great Western Road, Glasgow G12 OYN
United Kingdom

Blauensteiner, W.
I. Chirurgische Abteilung
Krankenanstalt Rudolfstiftung der Stadt Wien
Juchgasse 25, 1030 Wien, Austria

Bonsignori, M.
Special Oncology Department, Regional Hospital Torette
60020 Ancona, Italy

Brach del Prever, A.
Istituto Ortopedico Rizzoli, Via Puppili 1
40136 Bologna, Italy

Brücke, P.
I. Chirurgische Klinik, Allgemeines Krankenhaus Linz
Krankenhausstraße 9, 4020 Linz, Austria

Budihna, M.
Universitätsklinik für Radiotherapie und Radiologie
Alser Straße 4, 1090 Wien, Austria

Burk, J.
Abteilung für medizinische Onkologie
Farmitalia Carlo Erba GmbH
Merzhauser Straße 112, 7800 Freiburg, FRG

Burk, M.
Abteilung Hämatologie, Onkologie und klinische Immunologie
Medizinische Klinik und Poliklinik, Heinrich Heine-Universität
Moorenstraße 5, 4000 Düsseldorf 1, FRG

Caldora, P.
Istituto Ortopedico Rizzoli, Via Puppili 1
40136 Bologna, Italy

Campanacci, M.
Istituto Ortopedico Rizzoli, Via Puppili 1
40136 Bologna, Italy

Carbone, A.
Division of Pathology, Centro di Riferimento Oncologico
Via Pedemontana, Occidentale, 33081 Aviano, Italy

Caruso, G.
Division of Otolaryngology, Pordenone Hospital
Pordenone, Italy

Cavicchi, A.
Surgery Department, Regional Hospital Torrette
Ancona University, 60020 Ancona, Italy

Chang, A. E.
National Cancer Institute, Bethesda, MD 20892, USA

Chang, D.
University Department of Surgery, Royal Infirmary
Glasgow G40 SG, United Kingdom

Comoretto, R.
Division of Otolaryngology, Pordenone Hospital
Pordenone, Italy

Cooke, T.
University Department of Surgery, Royal Infirmary
Glasgow G40 SG, United Kingdom

Crippa, E.
Department of Medical Oncology, SMC Hospital
48000 Ravenna, Italy

Cruciani, G.
Division di Oncologia Medical
Ospedale S. Maria Delle Croci
Via Missiroli 8, 48100 Ravenna, Italy

Dinstl, K.
I. Chirurgische Abteilung
Krankenanstalt Rudolfstiftung der Stadt Wien
Juchgasse 25, 1030 Wien, Austria

Dobrowsky, W.
Klinik für Kiefer- und Gesichtschirurgie, Universität Wien
Alser Straße 4, 1090 Wien, Austria

Domellöf, L.
Department of Surgery, Örebro Medical Central Hospital
70185 Örebro, Sweden

Egeli, R.
Chirurgische Abteilung, Kantonsspital, Universität Basel
4031 Basel, Switzerland

Eilber, F. R.
Division of Surgical Oncology, University of California
Leconte Avenue, Los Angeles, CA 10833, USA

Encke, A.
Klinik für Allgemeinchirurgie
Johann Wolfgang Goethe-Universität
Theodor-Stern-Kai 7, 6000 Frankfurt/Main, FRG

Feliciotti, F.
Surgery Department, Regional Hospital Torrette
Ancona University, 60020 Ancona, Italy

Feldmann, H. J.
Abteilung für Radiotherapie, Westdeutsches Tumorzentrum
Hufelandstraße 55, 4300 Essen, FRG

Ferraro, A.
Istituto Ortopedico Rizzoli, Via Puppili 1
40136 Bologna, Italy

Ferruzzi, A.
Istituto Ortopedico Rizzoli, Via Puppili 1
40136 Bologna, Italy

Fontana, M.
Istituto Ortopedico Rizzoli, Via Puppili 1
40136 Bologna, Italy

Foth, H.
Institut für Pharmakologie und Toxikologie der Universität
Robert-Koch-Straße 40, 3400 Göttingen, FRG

Franklin, H. R.
Department of Surgery, The Netherlands Cancer Institute
(Antoni van Leeuwenhoek Huis)
Plesmanlaan 121, 1066 CX Amsterdam, The Netherlands

Friehs, G.
Department für Thoraxchirurgie
Universitätsklinik für Chirurgie,
Auenbruggerplatz 15, 8036 Graz, Austria

Frohwein, J.
Abteilung für Strahlentherapie und Nuklearmedizin
Universitätsklinikum Rudolf Virchow
Augustenburger Platz 1, 1000 Berlin, FRG

Frustaci, S.
Division of Medical Oncology, Centro di Riferimento
Oncologico, Via Pedemontana Occidentale
33081 Aviano, Italy

Garzon, F. T.
Institut für Toxikologie und Chemotherapie
Deutsches Krebsforschungszentrum
Im Neuenheimer Feld 280, 6900 Heidelberg, FRG

Germann, R.
Chirurgische Abteilung, Medizinische Hochschule
Auenbruggerplatz 1, 8030 Graz, Austria

Gherlinzoni, F.
Istituto Ortopedico Rizzoli, Via Puppili 1
40136 Bologna, Italy

Gnani, G.
Department of Medical Oncology, SMC Hospital
48100 Ravenna, Italy

Gramlich, F.
I. Innere Abteilung, Universitätsklinikum Rudolf Virchow
Augustenburger Platz 1, 1000 Berlin, FRG

Graziani, L.
Special Oncology Department, Regional Hospital Torette
60020 Ancona, Italy

Griffith, K. D.
National Cancer Institute, Bethesda, MD 20892, USA

Groeningen, C. J. van
Department of Medical Oncology, Free University Hospital
De Boelelaan 1117, 1081 HV Amsterdam, The Netherlands

Gross, C.
I. Chirurgische Klinik, Allgemeines Krankenhaus Linz
Krankenhausstraße 9, 4020 Linz, Austria

Gruenagel, H. H.
Chirurgische Abteilung, Evangelisches Krankenhaus
Kirchfeldstraße 40, 4000 Düsseldorf, FRG

Gustavsson, B.
Department of Surgery, Östra Hospital
41685 Göteborg, Sweden

Göhl, J.
Chirurgische Universitätsklinik
Maximiliansplatz, 8520 Erlangen, FRG

Hagberg, M.
Clinic of Pediatrics, University Hospital
90185 Umea, Sweden

Håkansson, L.
Department of Oncology, University Hospital of Linköping
581 85 Linköping, Sweden

Handl-Zeller, L.
Universitätsklinik für Radiotherapie und Radiologie
Alser Straße 4, 1090 Wien, Austria

Hasun, R.
Abteilung für Urologie
Krankenanstalt Rudolfstiftung der Stadt Wien
Juchgasse 25, 1030 Wien, Austria

Heinlein, W.
Medizinische Klinik III, Klinikum Großhadern
Ludwig Maximilian-Universität
Marchioninistraße 15, 8000 München 70, FRG

Herrhausen, T.
Chirurgische Abteilung
Johann Wolfgang Goethe-Universität
Theodor-Stern-Kai 7, 6000 Frankfurt/Main, FRG

Hoekstra, H. J.
Division of Surgical Oncology
Groningen University Hospital
P.O. Box 30001, 9700 RB Groningen, The Netherlands

Hohenberger, W.
Chirurgische Universitätsklinik
Maximiliansplatz, 8520 Erlangen, FRG

Hollmann, K.
Klinik für Kiefer- und Gesichtschirurgie, Universität Wien
Alser Straße 4, 1090 Wien, Austria

Horst, F.
Abteilung Allgemeinchirurgie, Zentrum Chirurgie
Universitätsklinikum, Robert-Koch-Straße 40
3400 Göttingen, FRG

Hottenrott, C.
Abteilung für Allgemein- und Abdominalchirurgie
Zentrum der Chirurgie,
Theodor-Stern-Kai 7, 6000 Frankfurt/Main, FRG

Howaldt, H. P.
Klinik für Mund-, Kiefer- und Gesichtschirurgie
Johann Wolfgang Goethe-Universität
Theodor-Stern-Kai 7, 6000 Frankfurt/Main, FRG

Huth, J. F.
Division of Surgical Oncology, University of California
Leconte Avenue, Los Angeles, CA 10833, USA

Höltl, W.
Abteilung für Urologie
Krankenanstalt Rudolfstiftung der Stadt Wien
Juchgasse 25, 1030 Wien, Austria

Inglis, R.
Chirurgische Abteilung, Johann Wolfgang Goethe-Universität
Theodor-Stern-Kai 7, 6000 Frankfurt/Main, FRG

Jakesz, R.
I. Chirurgische Universitätsklinik
Alser Straße 4, 1090 Wien, Austria

Jungblut, R. M.
Abteilung Hämatologie, Onkologie und klinische Immunologie
Medizinische Klinik und Poliklinik, Heinrich Heine-Universität
Moorenstraße 5, 4000 Düsseldorf 1, FRG

Kahl, G. F.
Institut für Pharmakologie und Toxikologie der Universität
Robert-Koch-Straße 40, 3400 Göttingen, FRG

Kastenbauer, E. R.
Hals-Nasen-Ohrenklinik, Klinikum Großhadern
Ludwig Maximilian-Universität
Marchioninistraße 70, 8000 München 70, FRG

Kaye, S. B.
Department of Vascular Surgery, Gartnavel General Hospital
1053 Great Western Road, Glasgow G12 OYN
United Kingdom

Kerr, D. J.
Department of Vascular Surgery, Gartnavel General Hospital
1053 Great Western Road, Glasgow G12 OYN
United Kingdom

Kessler, C.
Chirurgische Universitätsklinik
Maximiliansplatz, 8520 Erlangen, FRG

Kirkowa-Reimann, M.
Chirurgische Abteilung, Johann Wolfgang Goethe-Universität
Theodor-Stern-Kai 7, 6000 Frankfurt/Main, FRG

Klasse, J. M.
Department of Surgery, The Netherlands Cancer Institute
(Antoni van Leeuwenhoek Huis)
Plesmanlaan 121, 1066 CX Amsterdam, The Netherlands

Klimpfinger, M.
Chirurgische Abteilung, Medizinische Hochschule
Auenbruggerplatz 1, 8030 Graz, Austria

Koch, K.
Abteilung für Strahlentherapie und Nuklearmedizin
Universitätsklinikum Rudolf Virchow
Augustenburger Platz 1, 1000 Berlin 65, FRG

Kogelnik, H. D.
Institut für Radiotherapie und Radio-Onkologie
Landeskrankenanstalten Salzburg, Müllner Hauptstraße 48
5020 Salzburg, Austria

Kohek, P.
Department für Thorax-Hyperbare Chirurgie
Universitätsklinik für Chirurgie, Auenbruggerplatz 15
8036 Graz, Austria

Kokron, O.
5. Medizinische Abteilung, Lainz Krankenhaus
Wolkersbergenstraße 1, 1130 Wien, Austria

Kolb, R.
I. Chirurgische Abteilung,
Krankenhaus der Barmherzigen Schwestern
Stumpergasse 13, 1060 Wien, Austria

Kriwanek, S.
I. Chirurgische Abteilung
Krankenanstalt Rudolfstiftung der Stadt Wien
Juchgasse 25, 1030 Wien, Austria

Kroon, B. B. R.
Department of Surgery, The Netherlands Cancer Institute
(Antoni van Leeuwenhoek Huis)
Plesmanlaan 121, 1066 CX Amsterdam, The Netherlands

Kärcher, H.
Abteilung für Kiefer- und Gesichtschirurgie
Universitäts-Zahn-Klink
Auenbruggerplatz 12, 8010 Graz, Austria

Kärcher, K.-H.
Universitätsklinik für Strahlentherapie
Alser Straße 4, 1090 Wien, Austria

Kühböck, J.
II. Medizinische Universitätsklinik
Alser Straße 4, 1090 Wien, Austria

Laffer, U.
Chirurgische Abteilung, Kantonsspital, Universität Basel
4031 Basel, Switzerland

Lesnicar, H.
Universitätsklinik für Radiotherapie und Radiologie
Alser Straße 4, 1090 Wien, Austria

Leyh, H.
Urologische Klinik und Poliklinik der TU München
Klinikum rechts der Isar
Ismaningerstraße 22, 8000 München 80, FRG

Liermann, D.
Klinik für Allgemeinmedizin
Johann Wolfgang Goethe-Universität
Theodor-Stern-Kai 7, 6000 Frankfurt/Main, FRG

Link, K. H.
Abteilung für Allgemeine Chirurgie, Universität Ulm
Steinhövelstraße 9, 7900 Ulm, FRG

Loos, U.
Abteilung für Innere Medizin, Universitätsklinik Bonn
Sigmund-Freud-Straße 25, 5300 Bonn, FRG

Lorenz, M.
Klinik für Allgemeinchirurgie
Johann Wolfgang Goethe-Universität
Theodor-Stern-Kai 7, 6000 Frankfurt/Main, FRG

Mackie, R. M.
Department of Vascular Surgery, Gartnavel General Hospital
1053 Great Western Road, Glasgow G12 OYN
United Kingdom

Maier, U.
Urologische Universitätsklinik Wien
Alser Straße 4, 1090 Wien, Austria

Mair, R.
I. Chirurgische Klinik, Allgemeines Krankenhaus Linz
Krankenhausstraße 9, 4020 Linz, Austria

Mancini, A.
Istituto Ortopedico Rizzoli, Via Puppili 1
40136 Bologna, Italy

Marangolo, M.
Department of Medical Oncology, SMC Hospital
48100 Ravenna, Italy

Marberger, M.
Abteilung für Urologie
Krankenanstalt Rudolfstiftung der Stadt Wien
Juchgasse 25, 1030 Wien, Austria

Marsden, W.
Department of Surgery, University of Sydney
Sydney, Australia

Martinoli, S.
Chirurgische Abteilung, Kantonsspital, Universität Basel
4031 Basel, Switzerland

Matejka, M.
Klinik für Kiefer- und Gesichtschirurgie, Universität Wien
Alser Straße 4, 1090 Wien, Austria

Matzku, S.
Institut für Radiologie und Pathophysiologie
Deutsches Krebsforschungszentrum
Im Neuenheimer Feld 280, 6900 Heidelberg, FRG

McKay, A. J.
Department of Vascular Surgery, Gartnavel General Hospital
1053 Great Western Road, Glasgow G12 OYN
United Kingdom

Mehta, D. M.
Department of Radiotherapy, Groningen University Hospital
P.O. Box 30001, 9700 RB Groningen, The Netherlands

Mercuri, M.
Istituto Ortopedico Rizzoli, Via Puppili 1
40136 Bologna, Italy

Metzger, U.
Department für Chirurgie, Universitätsspital
8091 Zürich, Switzerland

Meyer, H.-J.
Abteilung für Chirurgie
Klinik für Abdominal- und Transplantationschirurgie
Zentrum Chirurgie, Medizinische Hochschule Hannover
Konstanty-Gutschow-Straße 8, 3000 Hannover 61, FRG

Michaelis, H. C.
Institut für Pharmakologie und Toxikologie der Universität
Robert-Koch-Straße 40, 3400 Göttingen, FRG

Micksche, M.
Klinik für Kiefer- und Gesichtschirurgie, Universität Wien
Alser Straße 4, 1090 Wien, Austria

Micksche, M.
Krebsforschungsinstitut, Borschkegasse 8a
1090 Wien, Austria

Miller, A. A.
Abteilung Hämatologie, Onkologie und klinische Immunologie
Medizinische Klinik und Poliklinik, Heinrich Heine-Universität
Moorenstraße 5, 4000 Düsseldorf 1, FRG

Minardi, D.
Special Oncology Department, Regional Hospital Torette
60020 Ancona, Italy

Mingolla, F.
Surgery Department, Regional Hospital Torrette
Ancona University, 60020 Ancona, Italy

Mischinger, H. J.
Chirurgische Abteilung, Medizinische Hochschule
Auenbruggerplatz 1 8030 Graz, Austria

Molenaar, W. M.
Department of Pathology, Groningen University Hospital
P.O. Box 30 001, 9700 RB Groningen, The Netherlands

Molls, M.
Abteilung für Radiotherapie, Westdeutsches Tumorzentrum,
Hufelandstraße 55, 4300 Essen, FRG

Molzahn, E.
Chirurgische Abteilung, Evangelisches Krankenhaus
Kirchfeldstraße 40, 4000 Düsseldorf, FRG

Monfardini, S.
Division of Medical Oncology, Centro di Riferimento
Oncologico, Via Pademontona Occidentale,
33081 Aviano, Italy

Montironi, R.
Special Oncology Department, Regional Hospital Torette,
60020 Ancona, Italy

Morelli, M.
Department of Medical Oncology, SMC Hospital,
48100 Ravenna, Italy

Morran, C. G.
University Department of Surgery, Royal Infirmary,
Glasgow G31 2ER, United Kingdom

Mueller, W.
Chirurgische Abteilung, Kantonsspital, Universität Basel,
4031 Basel, Switzerland

Musch, E.
Abteilung für Innere Medizin, Universitätklinik Bonn,
Sigmund-Freud-Straße 25, 5300 Bonn, FRG

Muzzonigro, G.
Special Oncology Department, Regional Hospital Torette,
60020 Ancona, Italy

Neuhold, N.
Klinik für Kiefer- und Gesichtschirurgie, Universität Wien,
Alser Straße 4, 1090 Wien, Austria

Neukamp, G.-U.
Chirurgische Abteilung, Evangelisches Krankenhaus
Kirchfeldstraße 40, 4000 Düsseldorf, FRG

Neumann, S.
Chirurgische Abteilung, Evangelisches Krankenhaus
Kirchfeldstraße 40, 4000 Düsseldorf, FRG

Novogrodsky, A.
The Rogosin Institut,
Cornell University Medical College Center,
505 East 70th Street, New York, NY 10021, USA

Occhipini, S.
Surgery Department, Regional Hospital Torrette,
Ancona University, 60020 Ancona, Italy

Olbert, F.
Jörgerstraße 52, 1170 Wien, Austria

Oldhoff, J.
Division of Surgical Oncology, Groningen University Hospital,
P.O. Box 30001, 9700 RB Groningen, The Netherlands

Paccapelo, A.
Oncology Department, Regional Hospital Torette,
60020 Ancona, Italy

Paccapelo, A.
Special Oncology Department, Regional Hospital Torrette,
60020 Ancona, Italy

Packard, B. S.
Division of Cytokine Biology,
Center for Biologics Evaluation and Research,
U.S. Food and Drug Administration,
8800 Rockville Pine, Bethesda, MD 20892, USA

Pakisch, B.
Department für Thoraxchirurgie,
Universitätsklinik für Chirurgie,
Auenbruggerplatz 15, 8036 Graz, Austria

Pavelka, R.
II. Universitätsklinik für Hals-Nasen-Ohrenheilkunde,
Alser Straße 4, 1090 Wien, Austria

Petru, E.
Klinik für Gynäkologie und Geburtshilfe, Universität Graz,
Auenbruggerplatz 14, 8036 Graz, Austria

Peyerl, G.
Medizinische Klinik III, Klinikum Großhadern
Ludwig Maximilian-Universität
Marchioninistraße 15, 8000 München 70, FRG

Picci, P.
Istituto Ortopedico Rizzoli, Via Pupilli 1
40136 Bologna, Italy

Pichlmayr, R.
Klinik für Abdominal- und Transplantationschirurgie,
Zentrum Chirurgie, Medizinische Hochschule Hannover,
Konstanty-Gutschow-Straße 8, 3000 Hannover 61, FRG

Polito, M.
Special Oncology Department, Regional Hospital Torette,
60020 Ancona, Italy

Porteder, H.
Klinik für Kiefer- und Gesichtschirurgie, Universität Wien,
Alser Straße 4, 1090 Wien, Austria

Possati, L.
Special Oncology Department, Regional Hospital Torette,
60020 Ancona, Italy

Ramirez, G.
Department of Human Oncology and Radiology,
University of Wisconsin School of Medicine,
600 Highland Avenue, Madison, WI 537923, USA

Rauschecker, H.
Abteilung Allgemeinchirurgie, Zentrum Chirurgie,
Universitätsklinikum, Robert-Koch-Straße 40,
3400 Göttingen, FRG

Rehak, P.
Department für Thoraxchirurgie, Auenbruggerplatz 1,
8036 Graz, Austria

Reiner, G.
I. Chirurgische Universitätsklinik, Alser Straße 4,
1090 Wien, Austria

Rodeck, G.
Urologische Universitätsklinik, Baldingerstraße,
3550 Marburg, FRG

Roscher, R.
Abteilung für Allgemeine Chirugie, Universität Ulm,
Steinhövelstraße 9, 7900 Ulm, FRG

Rosen, G.
Division of Surgical Oncology, University of California,
Leconte Avenue, Los Angeles, CA 10833, USA

Sack, H.
Abteilung für Radiotherapie, Westdeutsches Tumorzentrum
Hufelandstraße 55, 4300 Essen, FRG

Safi, F.
Abteilung für Allgemeine Chirurgie, Universität Ulm
Steinhövelstraße 9, 7900 Ulm, FRG

Salerno, V.
Department of Medical Oncology, SMC Hospital
48100 Ravenna, Italy

Schalhorn, A.
Medizinische Klinik III, Klinikum Großhadern
Ludwig Maximilian-Universität
Marchioninistraße 15, 8000 München 70, FRG

Scheel, J. von
Hals-Nasen-Ohrenabteilung
Allgemeines Krankenhaus Altona
Paul-Ehrlich-Straße 1, 2000 Hamburg 50, FRG

Schlegl, A.
1. Chirurgische Abteilung, Krankenhaus Lainz
1130 Wien, Austria

Schmid, A. P.
Universitätsklinik für Radiotherapie und Radiobiologie
Alser Straße 4, 1090 Wien, Austria

Schmähl, D.
Institut für Toxikologie und Chemotherapie
Deutsches Krebsforschungszentrum
Im Neuenheimer Feld 280, 6900 Heidelberg, FRG

Schneider, W.
Abteilung Hämatologie, Onkologie und klinische Immunologie
Medizinische Klinik und Poliklinik Heinrich Heine-Universität
Moorenstraße 5, 4000 Düsseldorf 1, FRG

Schober, C.
Universitätsklinik für Kieferchirurgie Wien
Alser Straße 4, 1090 Wien, Austria

Scholz, F.
Universitätsklinik für Kieferchirurgie Wien
Alser Straße 4, 1090 Wien, Austria

Scholz, R.
Klinik für Kiefer- und Gesichtschirurgie, Universität Wien
Alser Straße 4, 1090 Wien, Austria

Schoppe, W. D.
Abteilung Hämatologie, Onkologie und klinische Immunologie
Medizinische Klinik und Poliklinik Heinrich Heine-Universität
Moorenstraße 5, 4000 Düsseldorf 1, FRG

Schraffordt Koops, H.
Division of Surgical Oncology, Groningen University Hospital
P.O. Box 30001, 9700 RB Groningen, The Netherlands

Schreier, K.
Universitätsklinik für Radiotherapie und Radiologie
Alser Straße 4, 1090 Wien, Austria

Schultze-Seemann, W.
Abteilung Urologie, Chirurgische Universitätsklinik
Hugstetter Straße 55, 7800 Freiburg, FRG

Schweizer, W.
Chirurgische Abteilung, Kantonsspital, Universität Basel
4031 Basel, Switzerland

Scott, R. N.
Department of Vascular Surgery, Gartnavel General Hospital
1053 Great Western Road, Glasgow G12 OYN
United Kingdom

Seitz, W.
Universitätsklinik für Radiotherapie und Radiobiologie
Alser Straße 4, 1090 Wien, Austria

Selch, M.
Division of Surgical Oncology, University of California
Leconte Avenue, Los Angeles, CA 10833, USA

Semler, P.
I. Innere Abteilung, Wenckebach-Krankenhaus
Wenckebachstraße 23, 1000 Berlin 42, FRG

Silver, R. T.
The Rogosin Institut
Cornell University Medical College Center
505 East 70th Street, New York, NY 10021, USA

Sleijfer, D. T.
Department of Medical Oncology
Groningen University Hospital, P.O. Box 30001
9700 RB Groningen, The Netherlands

Smolle-Jüttner, F.-M.
Department für Thoraxchirurgie
Universitätsklinik für Chirurgie
Auenbruggerplatz 15, 8036 Graz, Austria

Sperlich, M.
I. Chirurgische Universitätsklinik, Alser Straße 4,
1090 Wien, Austria

Spona, J.
I. Universitäts-Frauenklinik, Spitalgasse 23,
1090 Wien, Austria

Starkhammar, H.
Department of Oncology, University Hospital of Linköping,
581 85 Linköping, Sweden

Steindorfer, P.
Universitäts-Klinik für Chirurgie, Auenbruggerplatz 15,
8036 Graz, Austria

Stenzel, K. H.
The Rogosin Institut,
Cornell University Medical College Center,
505 East 70th Street, New York, NY 10021, USA

Stephens, F. O.
Department of Surgery, University of Sydney,
Sydney, NSW 2066, Australia

Stephenson, J. A.
Department of Human Oncology and Radiology,
University of Wisconsin School of Medicine,
600 Highland Avenue, Madison, WI 537923, USA

Sturba, F.
Special Oncology Department, Regional Hospital Torette,
60020 Ancona, Italy

Stückelschweiger, G.
Department für Thoraxchirurgie,
Universitätsklinik für Chirurgie, Auenbruggerplatz 15,
8036 Graz, Austria

Sulfaro, S.
Division of Pathology, Centro di Riferimento Oncologico,
Via Pedemontana Occidentale, 33081 Aviano, Italy

Surgarbaker, P. H.
National Cancer Institute, Bethesda, MD 20892, USA

Suthanthiran, M.
The Rogosin Institut,
Cornell University Medical College Center,
505 East 70th Street, New York, NY 10021, USA

Tattersall, M. H. N.
Department of Surgery, University of Sydney,
Sydney, Australia

Tilgen, W.
Institut für Radiologie und Pathophysiologie,
Deutsches Krebsforschungszentrum,
Im Neuenheimer Feld 280, 6900 Heidelberg, FRG

Tuchmann, A.
I. Chirurgische Abteilung,
Krankenanstalt Rudolfstiftung der Stadt Wien,
Juchgasse 25, 1030 Wien, Austria

Uranus, S.
Chirurgische Abteilung, Medizinische Hochschule,
Auenbruggerplatz 1, 8030 Graz, Austria

van Geel, A. N.
Dr. Daniel den Hoed Cancer Center, Groene Hilldijk 301,
3075 EA Rotterdam, The Netherlands

Vinzenz, K. G.
Klinik für Kiefer- und Gesichtschirurgie, Universität Wien,
Alser Straße 4, 1090 Wien, Austria

Volpe, R.
Division of Pathology, Centro di Riferimento Oncologico,
Via Pedemontana Occidentale, 33081 Aviano, Italy

Voth, E.
Abteilung Nuklearmedizin, Zentrum Radiologie,
Universitätsklinikum, Robert-Koch-Straße 40,
3400 Göttingen, FRG

Wahlqvist, Y.
Clinic of Pediatrics, University Hospital,
90185 Umea, Sweden

Walle, A.
The Rogosin Institut,
Cornell University Medical College Center,
505 East 70th Street, New York, NY 10021, USA

Wang, J.
The Rogosin Institut,
Cornell University Medical College Center,
505 East 70th Street, New York, NY 10021, USA

Watzek, G.
Klinik für Kiefer- und Gesichtschirurgie, Universität Wien,
Alser Straße 4, 1090 Wien, Austria

Wheldon, T. E.
Department of Vascular Surgery, Gartnavel General Hospital,
1053 Great Western Road, Glasgow G12 OYN,
United Kingdom

Wiley, A. L., jr.
Cancer Center, East Carolina University,
Greenville, NC, USA

Willenbrock, C.
Abteilung Röntgendiagnostik I, Zentrum Radiologie,
Universitätsklinikum, Robert-Koch-Straße 40,
3400 Göttingen, FRG

Wilmanns, W.
Medizinische Klinik III, Klinikum Großhadern,
Ludwig Maximilian-Universität,
Marchioninistraße 15, 8000 München 70, FRG

Wirtanen, G. W.
Department of Human Oncology and Radiology,
University of Wisconsin School of Medicine,
600 Highland Avenue, Madison, WI 537923, USA

Wolf, G.
Chirurgische Abteilung, Medizinische Hochschule,
Auenbruggerplatz 1, 8030 Graz, Austria

Zepponi, L.
Special Oncology Department, Regional Hospital Torette,
60020 Ancona, Italy

Zschiederich, M.
Abteilung für Innere Medizin, Schlosspark-Klinik,
Heubnerweg 2, 1000 Berlin 19, FRG

ADVANCES IN DRUG DELIVERY

Advances in Drug Delivery to Cancer Patients: Introduction

L. Domellöf

Department of Surgery, Örebro Medical Central Hospital, 701 85 Örebro, Sweden

The targeted delivery of cytotoxic drugs to cancer patients is intended to optimize therapeutic efficacy and reduce side effects. Early results from pioneer work in Boston using a clockwork drive were positive and led to development of the Chronometric Infusor [2]. This external pump was linked to a percutaneous arterial or venous catheter. It was carried in a foam-rubber pouch to dampen the ticking of the clockwork and attached by straps around the patient's neck and chest. The plastic drug reservoir of the pump had a capacity of 25 ml, and the system allowed a delivery rate of 5 ml per 24 h. The clockwork required winding after 8–12 h.

Watkins reported on use of the Chronometric Infusor for continuous infusion chemotherapy for more than a year and for interrupted courses during a period of 3 years. This device was soon followed by the Sigma motor pump with rechargeable batteries and a drug reservoir of 50 ml. On the market today are a great variety of infusion systems for both extra- and intra-corporeal use [1].

Major improvements have been achieved in some of the latest, expensive implantable systems offering the capacity to alter the pump flow rate electronically via a programmable memory inside the device (Medtronics model 866 and Siemens DFA-1-S). Much cheaper alternatives are external, disposable pumps and subcutaneous access ports. Important considerations that should be more stressed are interactions between the drug and the materials used in the construction of the device, accuracy of flow, and alarms warning of weak battery load, flow occlusion, flow spills, etc. This section starts with a presentation of the new technical developments in drug administration systems. In the following chapter the rationales for different drug delivery regimens and targeted therapy are addressed. Systemic anticancer treatment is most frequently given in the form of intravenous bolus infusions. However, the pharmacodynamic and pharmacokinetic superiority of continuous infusion is well recognized, especially in the case of regional therapy. Recent advances in our knowledge of intracellular pharmacokinetics indicate that individual mechanisms of drug resistance may be identified. Consequently therapeutic efficacy may be increased by biochemical drug modulation.

The rationale for intra-arterial drug delivery is being evaluated. Pharmacokinetic analysis indicates the advantages of this treatment over systemic administration when drugs with high first-pass uptake are used for vascularized tumors with moderate or low blood flow at the infusion site. Primary and secondary liver cancer

R. Jakesz/H Rainer (Eds)
Progress in Regional Cancer Therapy

are common causes of cancer death. The treatment benefit conferred by intrahepatic drug delivery is being discussed in light of experimental and clinical data.

Intracavitary drug delivery has been tried with some promising results in patients with malignant effusions. At present, intraperitoneal drug delivery ("belly bath") is attracting increasing interest in ovarian carcinoma and certain cases of gastrointestinal adenocarcinoma. This is due to novel approaches improving the therapeutic index through intracavitary biochemical modulation.

Targeting with monoclonal antibodies (Mab) has been tried in early clinical studies in cancer of the large bowel, cancer of the pancreas, and melanoma, and clinical response has been observed in some cases. Simultaneously, targeting with labeled Mab or fragments of Mab has been used in modern immunoscintigraphy. The rapid penetration of labeled fragments of Mab or intact Mab may also have therapeutic potential by delivering a higher radiation dose to the tumor than to normal tissues. This has been studied in the nude mouse model and represents an entirely different therapeutic approach. Site-specific drug delivery may be achieved by either systemic or regional administration. This technique is still in the developmental stage.

References

1. Tucker EM (1987) Drug administration systems for infusion chemotherapy. In: Lokich JJ (ed) Cancer chemotherapy by infusion. Precept, Chicago, pp 41–58
2. Watkins E Jr (1963) Chronometric Infusor—an apparatus for protracted ambulatory infusion therapy. N Engl J Med 269:850–851

Technical Developments in the Delivery of Antineoplastic Agents

C.J. van Groeningen

Department of Medical Oncology, Free University Hospital, de Boelelaan 1117, 1081 HV Amsterdam, The Netherlands

Clinical cancer research has attracted much interest during recent years. Many new anticancer drugs and new treatment modalities are being developed. An important consequence is an increased need for reliable and safe methods of vascular access. Because most of the presently available anticancer drugs are administered intravenously, the greatest emphasis has been placed on venous access. However, intra-arterial and also intraperitoneal access are being investigated as a result of an increased interest in regional drug delivery.

Regarding venous access, older methods like simple venipuncture, arteriovenous grafts or fistula, standard central venous catheters, and Hickman-type catheters all have important drawbacks, making them not very reliable for long-term use.

A major improvement was the designing of totally implantable venous access devices: with a simple percutaneous puncture one has access to the venous system. Such devices have increasingly come into use in the past 5–7 years. Devices from different manufacturers are presently available. The intersystem differences are generally small. Those systems with the thickest septum, and thus the smallest chance of needle dislodgement, are to be preferred. The fact that maintenance is not necessary makes these devices convenient for the large majority of cancer patients. The implantation of a venous access device can be considered a simple surgical procedure to be performed under local anaesthesia. However, implantation by a surgeon experienced with the procedure is highly desired as this will reduce complications and problems with daily use. Implantable venous access devices may be used for bolus injections and prolonged infusions of anticancer drugs, for administration of blood products, for parenteral nutrition, and for drawing blood samples.

Several articles have been published reporting experience with totally implantable venous access devices. According to most of these, the average patient will benefit for a period of 6 months to 1 year. This length of time is determined not by limited patency of the device, but rather by the death of the patients from their underlying malignant disease. In many patients with a better prognosis the devices have been used for periods exceeding 1–4 years. Obviously, the incidence of complications in large groups of patients with these devices is important. The most common types of complication observed are infection and thrombosis; however, the incidence reported in most of the studies did not exceed 5% for either. Meticulously sterile handling of the systems will limit the number of infections. The occurrence of thrombosis may be related to continuous infusion; thrombosis seems hardly ever to be observed in patients treated with chemotherapy by bolus injection. One important observation has been that the incidence of thrombosis is significantly lower in patients on low doses of an oral anticoagulant. A variety of other, rarely occurring complications have been reported, but it is clear that these will not limit the widespread application of the devices. On the basis of in vitro and, to a lesser extent, in vivo experimental studies it has been suggested that the therapeutic index of several antineoplastic agents is better when these agents are administered by continuous infusion rather than by bolus injection. A limited number of clinical studies indicate the same. It is obvious that, for continuous infusion chemotherapy, reliable venous access is a prerequisite. Totally implantable venous access devices have been shown to fulfill this criterion. Infusion devices that can be used for ambulant treatment are another requirement, and great progress has also been made in this area during the past few years. Advances in materials technology and the miniaturization of complex mechanical and electronic components have led to major improvements in the accuracy, size, and safety of drug delivery pumps and systems. Both external portable and fully implantable infusion pumps are presently available. Portable devices seem to be preferred because they are more flexible, can be used in more than one patient, and are less expensive. On the other hand, the lack of interference with normal daily activities is an advantage of implantable pump systems. Thus far, the use of both these types of device has given rise to continuous infusion chemotherapy programs on an ambulant basis. Complications and problems in these programs have been limited. However, it has to be realized that departments conducting continuous infusion therapy should be well organized with respect to both patient education and management on this therapy on a 24-hour basis.

In summary, recent technical developments have made an important contribution to the possibilities for delivery of antineoplastic agents to cancer patients. Irrespective of these technical novelties, however, the development of new, more effective anticancer drugs and new treatment modalities remains urgently needed if we are to make significant progress in the treatment of neoplastic diseases.

Selected Reading

1. van Groeningen CJ (1987) New technical developments in antineoplastic drug delivery and their role in cancer treatment. In: Domellöf L (ed) Drug delivery in cancer treatment, ESO monograph. Springer, Berlin Heidelberg New York, pp 39–52
2. Lokich JJ (ed) (1987) Cancer chemotherapy by infusion. MTP, Lancaster

Is There a Pharmacologic Rationale for Continuous Cancer Chemotherapy?*

B. Gustavsson

Department of Surgery, Östra Hospital, 416 85 Göteborg, Sweden

Introduction

The ultimate goal of research into pharmacokinetics is to assist in the optimization of therapy. In the past decade our knowledge of the pharmacokinetics of the cytotoxic drugs used in cancer chemotherapy has expanded significantly. The primary goal of regional drug delivery in cancer chemotherapy is to achieve greater drug exposure in a tumor region with decreased systemic exposure in an attempt to improve the therapeutic index. The rationale for hepatic arterial infusion therapy rests on a number of observations suggesting that, for some drugs, a greater antitumor effect in the liver can be produced with less systemic toxicity than results from peripheral venous administration [1–3]. As recently reported by Wagner et al., steady-state systemic and intrinsic clearances and extraction ratios decrease progressively as the proportion of the dose reaching the target increases [4]. Extensive clinical experience with regional infusion chemotherapy of hepatic tumors has been reported since its introduction to clinical practice in 1964 [5, 6]. Although response rates ranging from 29% to 88% have been reported, it is not clear whether intra-arterial hepatic infusion is followed by prolonged survival.

It should be emphasized that most drug schedules used today are based mainly on empirical findings concerning side effects and measurements of plasma concentration of the parent drug. However, in order to ascertain optimal schedules pharmacodynamic studies are needed. 5-Fluorouracil (5-FU) is one of the most useful drugs in the treatment of neoplastic diseases, either as a single agent or in combination. The anabolic pathways of the fluorinated pyrimidines are complex (Fig. 1) [7]. Since the pathways of 5-FU activation used by tumors and normal tissues are a question of considerable relevance to the chemotherapeutic use of the fluorinated pyrimidines, enzyme activity must be taken into consideration in order to individualize and optimize cytotoxic treatment. The cytotoxic effect of 5-FU is mainly dependent on inhibition of thymidylate synthase (TS). Further, direct incorporation of drug into RNA and DNA has been described [8].

*This study was supported by Medical Research Council grant no. B88-04X-07155-04B, by Swedish Cancer Society grant no. 512-B89-01X, and by the Assar Gabrielsson Foundation.

R. Jakesz/H Rainer (Eds)
Progress in Regional Cancer Therapy

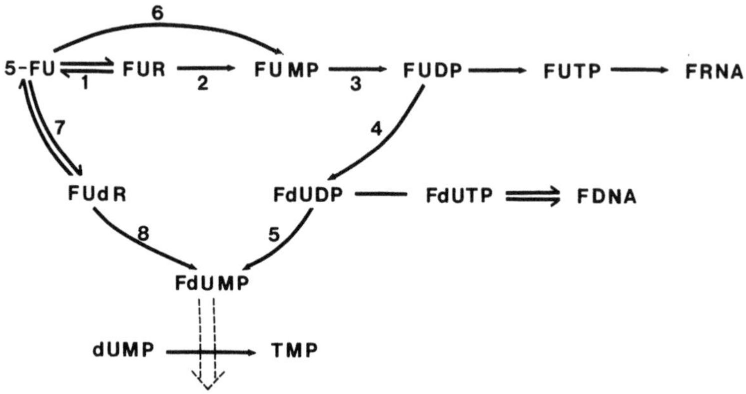

Fig. 1. Anabolic pathways of 5-FU. *1*, Uridine phosphorylase; *2*, uridine kinose; *3*, uridylate kinase; *4*, ribonucleotide reductase; *5*, phosphatases; *6*, uracil phosphoribyltransferase; *7*, thymidine phosphorylase; *8*, thymidine kinase

We have developed a practicable method for assay of several key biochemical determinants of TS inhibition following fluoropyrimidine therapy in vivo [9, 10]. The principal goal of these studies has been to demonstrate that individual mechanisms of resistance of tumors to 5-FU can be identified and potentially overcome by means of specific biochemical strategies.

Material and Methods

Patients

Fifty-four patients received IV 5-FU, 500 mg/m^2, given as a 1- to 2-min bolus prior to surgical biopsy of tumor. The primary site of original tumor was large bowel or rectum in 37, stomach in five, pancreas in four, and liver in three patients. In addition, five patients with metastatic breast cancer were studied. Biopsy sites were metastatic hepatic nodules in 37 cases.

Tissue Handling

Specimens, pared of fat and necrotic tissue, were frozen in liquid nitrogen or dry ice within 30 s of surgical removal. Free and total (FdUMP-bound + free) TS levels were assayed on the day of tissue processing by determination of ^{3}[H]FdUMP binding sites by the dextran-coated charcoal method that corrects for ^{3}[H]FdUMP labeling of endogenous cytosolic FdUMP-bound enzyme. The methods have recently been described in detail elsewhere [9, 10].

Results

The distribution of the various anabolic enzymes of fluorinated pyrimidines has been analyzed by taking biopsy specimens during surgery of patients operated upon for colorectal carcinoma. As demonstrated in Fig. 2, there are great differences even among tumors in the level of pyrimidine salvage enzymes.

FdUMP levels showed a general relationship to the degree of TS inhibition. Normal hepatic tissue and colonic mucosa are naturally highly resistant to the toxic effects of IV bolus 5-FU. The low degree of inhibition of TS, low FdUMP levels, and very low FdUMP/dUMP ratios in these tissues are consistent with the hypothesis that TS inhibition is an important correlate of 5-FU cytotoxicity. TS inhibition was highly significantly greater in malignant liver tissue than in normal liver. Among the 37 colorectal tumor biopsy specimens, 30 showed less than 85% inhibition of TS. More than 50% of the specimens with poor TS inhibition had low FdUMP levels. Inadequate cofactor (methylene tetrahydrofolate, CH_2FH_4) levels were present in only about half of the tumors.

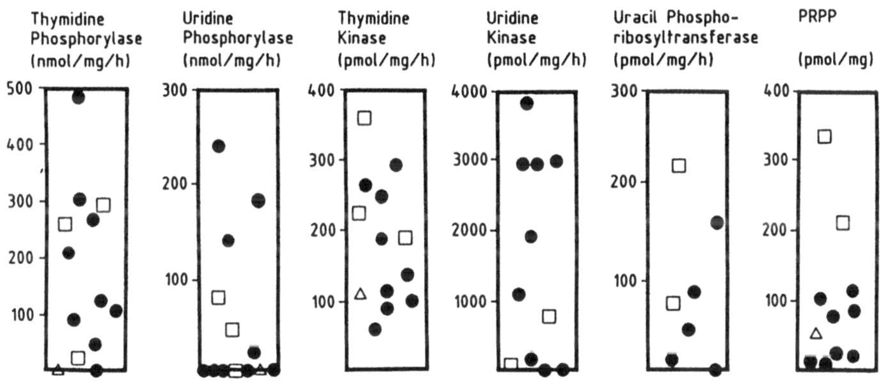

Fig. 2. Levels of 5-FU anabolic enzymes in secondary liver tumors and normal liver. Tissue specimens were obtained by biopsy from patients undergoing laparotomy. *PRPP*, phosphoribosyl pyrophosphate; • tumor; □ normal liver; △ mucosa

Table 1. Presence of mechanisms of resistance to TS inhibition

Mechanism	%
High dUMP only	20
High dUMP and low FdUMP	7
Low FdUMP only	40
Poor binding and low FdUMP	7
Poor binding only	27

Discussion

The predominant mechanism of resistance of tissues to TS inhibition in patients with gastrointestinal malignancies appeared to be low FdUMP formation. Percentage TS inhibition was significantly lower in surgical specimens of normal liver than in paired hepatic metastases. Among 30 colorectal tumors with less than 85% TS inhibition, 16 showed FdUMP levels below 75 pmol/g. We earlier postulated that a relatively high degree of inhibition of TS is required for cytotoxicity [9, 10]. Normal liver consistently showed approximately half the TS inhibition found in malignant tissues. The lower FdUMP levels in liver may be due to more rapid catabolism. A report of higher FUdR levels in liver than in tumor immediately after intra-arterial hepatic FUdR tends to support this interpretation [11].

According to our studies about half of all tumors have inadequate cofactor levels. The addition of leucovorin might help to overcome this mechanism of resistance. By increasing CH_2FH_4 it might be possible simultaneously to overcome the mechanisms of relatively low FdUMP, low folate, high dUMP, and high TS to achieve low post-5-FU free TS levels [12].

Our results demonstrate that mechanisms of resistance to TS inhibition by fluoropyrimidine therapy can be identified in the clinical setting. Such information may be useful for prospective stratification of patients. Furthermore, it seems unlikely that systemic continuous infusion of fluorinated pyrimidines can achieve the intracellular concentration of FdUMP needed for complete TS inhibition. Regional hepatic infusion, in contrast, seems more likely to succeed. However, more than one third of the tumors we studied were resistant due to deficient cofactor concentration. In the future, based on pharmacodynamic analyses of the individual tumor, some patients might be identified for whom continuous chemotherapy infusion seems rational.

References

1. Chabner BA (1981) Pharmacologic basis of cancer treatment. Saunders, Philadelphia
2. Iwatsuki S, Shaw BW jr, Starz TE (1983) Experience with 150 liver resections. Ann Surg 197:247–253
3. Collins JM (1985) Pharmacokinetics of 5-fluorouracil infusions in the rat: comparison with man and other species. Cancer Chemother Pharmacol 14:108–111
4. Wagner JG, Gyves JW, Stetson PL, Walker-Andrews SC, Wollner IS, Cochran MK, Ensminger WD (1986) Steady-state nonlinear pharmacokinetics of 5-fluorouracil during hepatic arterial and intravenous infusions in cancer patients. Cancer Res 46:1499–1506
5. Ensminger WD, Rosowsky A, Raso V et al. (1978) A clinical-pharmacological evaluation of hepatic arterial infusions of 5-fluoro-2′-deoxyuridine and 5-fluorouracil. Cancer Res 38:3784–3792
6. Kemeny N, Daly J, Oderman P et al. (1984) Hepatic artery pump infusion: toxicity and results in patients with metastatic colorectal carcinoma. J Clin Oncol 2:595–600
7. Heidelberger C, Danenberg PV, Moran RG (1983) Fluorinated pyrimidines and their nucleosides. Adv Enzymol 54:58–118
8. Houghton JA, Houghton PJ (1984) In: Fox BW, Fox M (eds) Antitumor drug resistance. Springer, Berlin Heidelberg New York, pp 515–549 (Handbook of experimental pharmacology, vol 72)

9. Spears CP, Gustavsson BG, Mitchell MS, Spicer D, Berne M, Bernstein L, Danenberg PV (1984) Thymidylate synthetase inhibition in malignant tumors and normal liver of patients given intravenous 5-fluorouracil. Cancer Res 44:4144–4150
10. Spears CP, Gustavsson BG, Berne M, Frösing R, Bernstein L, Hayes AA (1988) Mechanisms of innate resistance to thymidylate synthase inhibition after 5-fluorouracil. Cancer Res 48:5894–5900
11. Chang AE, Schneider PD, Sugarbaker PH, Simpson C, Culnane M, Steinberg SM (1987) A prospective randomized trial of regional versus systemic continuous 5-fluorodeoxyuridine chemotherapy in the treatment of colorectal liver metastases. Ann Surg 206:685–692
12. Spears CP, Gustavsson B, Carlsson G, Frösing R (1988) Fluorouracil/leucovorin pharmacodynamics: determination by serial biopsy. Proc Am Assoc Cancer Res 29:186

Central Venous Access in Children Through a Fully Implantable Drug Delivery System

L. Athlin, M. Hagberg, and Y. Wahlqvist

Surgical Clinic, University Hospital, 901 85 Umeå, Sweden

Introduction

Subcutaneously implantable delivery systems have become an alternative to the external indwelling catheter or arteriovenous fistula in patients who need safe and reliable venous access. This is especially important for patients with malignant disease who are treated with repeated infusions of anticancer agents, most of which are known to harm the peripheral veins, resulting in thrombophlebitic occlusion of the vessels used.

After first being adopted in adult patients, portals are now frequently used in children [3, 4], especially since the introduction of low-profile portals small enough to be implanted in very young individuals.

We report here on our experience of an initial series of portal systems implanted in children in our hospital.

Patients and Methods

From January 1985 to April 1988 a total of 50 portal catheters (Port-A-Cath, PAC; Pharmacia AB, Sweden) were implanted in 23 girls and 22 boys between 3 months and 18 years old (median 6 years). The diagnosis in 40 patients was a malignant disease, treated with anticancer agents, and in five patients a benign disorder, managed with specific treatment or parenteral nutrition (Table 1). The portals were also frequently used for drawing blood samples.

The catheter was inserted into the superior vena cava by cutdown to the external jugular vein in 25 cases and through the internal jugular vein in 24 cases. In one patient the right greater saphenous vein was exploited to give central venous access. The catheter was tunnelled to the chest and connected to a chamber placed in a subcutaneous pouch, usually in the anterior axillary line just above the right nipple. Low-profile portals were used in 28 treatments and adult-size portals in 22 treatments. All operations were performed under general anesthesia in the operating room. The position of the catheter tip was ascertained by fluoroscopy immediately after introduction. All systems were flushed with heparin 100 U/ml during operation

R. Jakesz/H Rainer (Eds)
Progress in Regional Cancer Therapy

Table 1. Diagnoses of the patients in the study

Diagnosis	*n*
Malignant	
ALL	18
AML	6
Cerebral tumor	5
Osteogenic sarcoma	4
Other tumor	4
Lymphoma	3
	40
Benign	
Juvenile RA	1
Hydrocephalus	2
Cystic fibrosis	1
Hemophilia	1
	5

ALL, acute lymphocytic leukemia; AML, acute myoblastic leukemia; RA, rheumatoid arthritis.

and postoperatively at least every 4 weeks. At flushing a straight Huber needle was always used. For 1 h prior to puncture the skin over the chamber was anesthesized with ointment (EMLA, Astra AB, Sweden).

Results

The median implant time (MiT) for all PAC was 9 months (range 0.5–40 months). At the end of the study period 26 patients had a still patent PAC (MiT 11 months) and 11 patients had died with working PAC in place (MiT 7 months). Six PAC were removed after completed therapy (MiT 13 months) and seven because of complications (four infections, two occlusions of system, one partial wound dehiscence; MiT, 2 months). The indication for PAC in six of the seven patients who had their portals removed early was treatment with anticancer agents.

Major complications of the implanted PAC were found in seven patients (Table 2). A local abscess was found in five patients, leading in two cases to septicemia and in four cases to removal of the PAC. One patient (no. 6 in Table 2) had a minor abscess cured by local treatment. Another (no. 5) developed septicemia following reoperation because of dislocation of the catheter tip 4 days after implantation. The infection was cured with antibiotic treatment, but the patient deteriorated and died 2 weeks later of recurrent ALL.

Positive bacterial cultures were obtained from five patients with PAC-related infections. These infections were all treated with antibiotics, but in five of six cases removal of the system was necessary for cure of the infections.

Table 2. Complications and outcome in 12/50 PACs implanted in 7/45 patients

Patient no.	Diagnosis	Age at implant	Implant	time (days)	Entry	Complication	Bacterial strain	Outcome
1	ALL	5 months	1st	45	R ext jugular	Abscess	*Staphylococcus aureus*	Removal
			2nd	27	L int jugular	Occlusion	*Staphylococcus epidermidis*	Removal
			3rd	24	R int jugular	Occlusion	—	Restored
			4th	5	R saphenous	—	—	Removal
			3rd	94	R int jugular	Wound dehiscence	—	Removal
2	Neuroblastoma	5 months	1st	205	R ext jugular	Abscess + septicemia	*Staphylococcus epidermidis*	Removal
			2nd	75	R ext jugular	—	—	Working
3	AML	15 years	1st	360	R ext jugular	(Therapy completed)	—	Removal
			2nd	14	L int jugular	Bleeding + occlusion	—	Removal
4	Juvenile RA	3 years		34	R ext jugular	Bleeding + abscess + septicemia	*Staphylococcus aureus*	Removal
5	ALL	5 years		20	R int jugular	Dislocation + septicemia	*Klebsiella*	Substitution + antibiotics
6	ALL	11 years		330	R ext jugular	Abscess	—	Local treatment
7	Sarcoma	17 years		69	R ext jugular	Abscess	*Staphylococcus aureus*	Removal

Abbreviations: see Table 1.

One patient (no. 1) received four portals during the treatment period. The first two of these were removed due to abscess and occlusion respectively. The fourth PAC was implanted due to temporary occlusion of the third, but was removed 5 days later following restoration of patency in the third. The third PAC was then patent for 3 months but was removed due to partial dehiscence of the wound over the chamber.

Two patients received two PAC systems each. One (no. 2) had his first PAC removed due to a local abscess and secondary septicemia. His second PAC was open and working at completion of the study. The other patient (no. 3) had his first PAC removed at completion of therapy, but received a second PAC 3 months later due to recurrent disease. Due to erosion of an intercostal artery and major bleeding and occlusion of the catheter, this system was removed 2 weeks after implantation. In another patient (no. 4) the PAC was removed after a chamber pouch hemorrhage followed by a local abscess and then septicemia.

Discussion

The most serious complication related to PAC in this study was septicemia, which was diagnosed in three patients. The septicemia was in two cases secondary to local abscesses, and positive bacterial cultures were obtained. However, episodes of septic fever which could not be related to the implantation or use of the PAC were not unusual. These infections were ascribed to the underlying disease and considered to be of viral etiology. Another three patients had local abscesses of the portal pouch which did not spread to the bloodstream but led to PAC removal in two cases. The total frequency of infectious episodes was 13%, which accords with results reported by others [4,10]. We could not correlate the risk of infectious complication to whether the PAC was used soon after implantation or after a delay [4]. Compared to systems using Hickman-Browiac catheters, however, the frequency of infectious complications was low with the PAC [9].

In one study [4] no correlation was found between the risk of infection and the use of perioperative antibiotics. Pegelow et al. [8] reported that infected portals were difficult to sterilize with antibiotics. Thus, if antibiotic treatment does not control the infection, early removal of the implanted system is necessary. The frequency of catheter occlusion necessitating restoration of patency with heparin or urokinase infusions has been reported to be as high as 13% [10]. In the present study occlusion was encountered in 6% of the PAC. Two portals were removed due to occlusion and one was reopened by means of heparin infusion. The difference in occlusion frequency may be explained by the use of different portals and different routines in maintenance of the systems. Moreover, when the central venous access is used for total parenteral nutrition, this seems to be associated with a high catheter occlusion rate [2].

Application of anesthetic ointment (EMLA) 1 h before puncture of the skin obviated the fear of needle punctures reported by others [2, 6].

In the Port-A-Cath system used in this study, the catheter and the chamber are separate. This gives the advantage of being able to place the catheter tip in the correct position just above the right atrium and then cut the catheter to the exact length required when connecting it to the chamber. We have not experienced accidental withdrawal of the catheter during this maneuver, or complications involving disconnection of the catheter from the chamber [1, 5, 7]. It seems important to have the catheter tip in the superior vena cava and not in the right atrium, since the latter is reported to cause tachycardia [3].

Early in the study period 22 patients received adult-size PAC. This may theoretically increase the risk of postoperative wound dehiscence, since the chamber of this model occupies a relatively large subcutaneous volume in small patients. Although the only partial wound dehiscence in the present study was observed in a 5-month-old baby with a low-profile portal, the introduction of this model offered a more attractive alternative in very young individuals, and low-profile PAC are now routinely implanted in our pediatric patients.

Minor bleedings from the wound edge were often seen in thrombocytopenic patients but could be controlled by conservative regimes. It is reasonable to assume, however, that the hemostatic surgery performed upon two patients with major bleedings contributed to the subsequent occlusion and abscess, respectively, necessitating removal of their portals.

In conclusion, this study has confirmed the positive experience reported by others. Compared to the conventional indwelling catheters, the advantages of the Port-A-Cath subcutaneously implantable delivery system are obvious: no continuous skin penetration, minimizing bacterial contamination of the bloodstream; no dressing needed when not in use; freedom of activity for the patient; no thrombophlebitis; and, with application of anesthetizing ointment, no pain at puncture.

Summary

A total of 50 portal catheters (Port-A-Cath, PAC) were implanted in 45 pediatric patients (23 girls and 22 boys) between 3 months and 18 years old (median 6 years). The diagnoses were malignancy in 40 cases and a chronic benign disorder in five. The catheter was inserted into the superior vena cava via the external jugular vein in most of the children. Low-profile portals were used in 28 patients. The median implant time (MiT) for all the PAC was 9 months range (0.5–40 months). At the end of the study period 26 patients had a still patent portal (MiT 11 months) and 11 patients had died with their PAC in place (MiT 7 months). Six PAC were removed after completion of therapy (MiT 13 months) and seven due to complications (MiT 2 months). Major complications related to PAC were found in seven patients. The most common complications were abscess (5), septicemia (3), and occlusion (3). The indication for PAC in six of the seven patients with major complications was treatment with anticancer agents. One patient received four PAC and two patients received two PAC each. Positive bacterial cultures were obtained from five patients with PAC-related infections.

The Port-A-Cath was found to be a well-tolerated system with an acceptable rate of complications, minimizing patient discomfort and psychological disturbance.

References

1. Alzen G, Mertens R, Günther R (1987) Perkutane Katheter-extraktion eines rupturierten Port-A-Cath beim Kleinkind. Klin Pädiatr 199:296–299
2. Bagnall H, Ruccione K (1987) Experience with a totally implanted venous access device in children with malignant diease. Oncol Nurs Forum 14:51–56
3. Becton DL, Kletzel M, Golladay ES, Hathaway G, Berry DH (1988) An experience with an implanted port system in 66 children with cancer 61:376–378
4. Brothers TE, Von Moll LK, Niederhuber JE, Roberts JA, Walker-Andrews S, Ensminger WD (1988) Experience with subcutaneous infusion ports in three hundred patients. Surg Gynecol Obstet 166:295–301.
5. Krul EJ, van Leeuwen EJ, Vos A, Voute PA (1986) Continuous venous access in children for long-term chemotherapy by means of an implantable system. J Pediatr Surg 21:689–690
6. Leuthardt, R, Gysler R, Morger R, Feldges A (1986) Der Port-A-Cath in der Kinderonkologie. Schweiz Rundsch Med Prax 75:582–584
7. Lokich JJ, Bothe A Jr, Benotti P, Moore C (1985) Complications and management of implanted venous access catheters. J Clin Oncol 3:710–717
8. Pegelow C, Narvaez M, Toledano S (1986) Experience with a totally implantable venous device in children. Am J Dis Child 140:69–71
9. Press OW, Ramsey PG, Larsson EB, Tefer A, Hickman RO (1984) Hickman catheter infections in patients with malignancies. Medicine (Baltimore) 63:189–200
10. Shulman R, Rahman S, Mahoney, D, Pokorny J, Bloss R (1987) A totally implanted venous access system used in pediatric patients with cancer. J Clin Oncol 5:137–140

Intraportal Chemotherapy for Colorectal Hepatic Metastases

U. Metzger and U. Laffer

Department of Surgery, University Hospital, 8091 Zürich, Switzerland

Introduction

Liver metastases are present on initial diagnosis of large bowel cancer in 25%–30% of patients [1]. After curative resection of colorectal primary tumors, the liver again is the most frequent site of relapse [2, 3]. Once liver metastases have developed the prognosis is poor, with an expected median survival time of 6–9 months [1, 4], the extent of the tumor being the most important prognostic factor [5]. A great deal of work has been done to determine the factors that influence development of liver metastases. There is evidence that tumor cells embolize into the portal venous system via the mesenteric veins and enter the liver. In 1957, Dukes [6] found evidence of venous spread in 17% of operative rectal cancer specimens. Fisher and Turnbull [7] discovered tumor cells in the mesenteric venous blood of 32% in colorectal carcinoma patients at surgery. Suggesting that manipulation of the tumor may force malignant cells into the circulation, they initiated the so-called no-touch isolation technique [8]. However, not all circulating cancer cells give rise to metastases. Several reports have shown that patients with malignant cells in the portal venous blood fare no worse than those without [9, 10].

Metachronous liver metastases may originate from microscopic deposits not visible at surgery for the primary tumor. These micrometastases are the most important target for adjuvant systemic therapy [11, 12]. Since adjuvant systemic chemotherapy has mostly failed in several prospective randomized trials [13–16], numerous studies have approached the issue of hepatic artery or portal vein infusion of fluorinated pyrimidines.

Patterns of Vascularity of Liver Tumors and Their Consequences for Different Therapeutic Approaches

In the therapeutic management of both primary and metastatic liver tumors, vascularity assumes major importance. The blood supply of these tumors constitutes a pathway for the delivery of antitumor agents. In addition, the possibility of diminishing or eliminating oxygen supply and blood flow to these tumors depends on knowledge of vascularity. The vascularity of liver tumors is more complicated

R. Jakesz/H Rainer (Eds)
Progress in Regional Cancer Therapy

than that of most other tumors because of the presence of both arterial and portal circulations. Both systems play a role in the perfusion of tumors, and arterioportal and arteriovenous shunting may further complicate the picture. Considerable work on the vascular patterns of experimental tumors has been carried out using pigmented silicone rubber (Microfil) injected into the arterial and portal circulations. The tumors were Walker carcinosarcomas implanted in the liver of rats. In these studies by Ackerman [17], tumors measuring less than 1 mm in diameter did not display any new vessel formation. Beyond this size, single, newly formed vessels began to encircle the tumors. The vessels were derived from either the arteriolar or the portal circulation in completely random fashion.

As tumors continued to grow, reaching a diameter of between 5 and 7 mm, the encircling plexus became more extensive and better developed. As this occurred, the arterial circulation became predominant, and in most specimens no portal circulation was seen. In general, portal vessels were compressed or displaced as the tumors grew. Similar results were obtained by Bassermann [32] and by Taylor et al. [18], who measured blood flow into colorectal liver metastases using ^{133}Xe clearance in patients undergoing surgery for colorectal cancer. Preoperative measurements after direct parenchymal injection showed a mean flow of 41.5 ± 22.5 ml/min/100 g which, after hepatic arterial occlusion, was reduced to a mean of 5% of the preocclusion value. Dynamic bloodflow studies using the gamma camera were performed in the postoperative period by administration of ^{131}Xe into both hepatic artery and portal vein catheters.

The initial distribution images indicated a predominantly arterial perfusion of the metastases, but after hepatic artery occlusion, portal vein perfusion to the metastases was statistically significantly increased. In the most recent study, Ridge et al. [19] demonstrated a quantitative advantage of hepatic artery infusion over portal vein infusion of colorectal hepatic metastases using nitrogen-13 amino acids and ammonia with dynamic gamma camera imaging. Data collected from the liver for 10 min after rapid bolus injection of nitrogen-13 L-glutamate, L-glutamine or ammonia were compared with ^{99m}Tc macroaggregated albumin (MAA) images produced after injection through the hepatic artery or portal vein in the same session. Tumor regions defined from the ^{99m}Tc sulfur colloid scans were compared with nearby liver areas of similar thickness. For the nitrogen-13 compounds, the area-normalized count rate at first pass maximum (Q_{max}) and the tissue extraction efficiency were computed. Results showed that more than twice as much of a nutrient substrate was delivered per volume of tumor relative to liver by the hepatic artery than by the portal vein. The delivery of substance in solution (such as nutrients or drugs) to tumor and liver tissue correlated with the distribution of colloids such as MAA after hepatic artery and portal venous injection.

From these studies, it can be concluded that the arterial route is superior to the portal for established metastatic disease, whereas the portal route might be preferable for the adjuvant setting.

Pharmacokinetics of Intraportal Chemotherapy

Almersjö et al. [20] showed the safety of intraportal 5-fluorouracil (5-FU) continuous infusion therapy. At the dose of 15 mg/kg body weight/24 h, serum concentrations were generally below 100 ng/ml, whereas the same dose given intravenously resulted in serum levels of 100–300 ng/ml.

Increasing the dose to 30 mg/kg/24 h resulted in serum concentrations below 200 ng/ml using the portal venous route, whereas intravenous systemic infusion was not feasible due to hematologic toxicities. Speyer et al. [21] measured portal circulation levels and hepatic clearance of 5-FU in humans after intraperitoneal administration. They found high levels of 5-FU in the portal vein, comparable to concentrations after direct intraportal infusion, and calculated a hepatic extraction rate of 80%–90%.

Berger et al. [22] tested systemic and local toxicity of 5-FU in Sprague-Dawley rats after systemic or locoregional infusion or bolus injection over 5 days at equimolar doses (total dose: 1220 μM/kg each). The results are listed in Tables 1 and 2. In this experimental model, continuous infusion resulted in lower systemic and

Table 1. Systemic toxicity of 5-FU after systemic or locoregional infusion or bolus injection over 5 days at equimolar doses in Sprague-Dawley rats (total doses: 1220 μM/kg each) [22]

Route	Mode	CFU-C ± SE	CFU-S ± SE	DNA-SSB ± SD
Vena cava	Infusion	43 ± 40	25 ± 24	71 ± 19
	Bolus	14 ± 5	1.3 ± 0.9	68 ± 1
Portal vein	Infusion	58 ± 26	39 ± 6	100 ± 80
	Bolus	44 ± 11	3.1 ± 0.6	137 ± 103
Proper hepatic artery	Infusion	72 ± 5.3	66 ± 13	23 ± 25
	Bolus	35 ± 15	10 ± 6.8	177 ± 9.2

CFU-C ± SE, mean colony number (in cultures) of treated bone marrow cells as a percentage of control ± standard error; CFU-S ± SE, mean colony number (in spleens) of treated bone marrow cells as a percentage of control ± standard error; DNA-SSB ± SD, single-strand breaks (radiation equivalents) in DNA of treated bone marrow cells ± standard deviation.

Table 2. Local toxicity of 5-FU after systemic or locoregional infusion or bolus injection over 5 days at equimolar doses in Sprague-Dawley rats (total doses: 1220 μM/kg each) [22]

Route	Mode	GOT ± SD	GPT ± SD	DNA-SSB ± SD
Vena cava	Infusion	108 ± 24	40 ± 9.3	43 ± 37
	Bolus	35 ± 9.9	12 ± 4.2	145 ± 37
Portal vein	Infusion	69 ± 26	32 ± 6.8	0
	Bolus	40 ± 17	14 ± 7	376 ± 277
Proper hepatic artery	Infusion	78 ± 22	46 ± 8.2	5 ± 4.9
	Bolus	71 ± 60	19 ± 9.6	270 ± 17

GOT ± SD, glutamic oxaloacetic transaminase (units/l) ± standard deviation; GPT ± SD, glutamic pyruvic transaminase (units/l) ± standard deviation; DNA-SSB ± SD, single-strand breaks (radiation equivalents) in DNA of treated liver cells ± standard deviation.

local toxicities, and in general the locoregional administration was less toxic than administration via the vena cava.

Portal Vein Infusion for Liver Metastases from Colorectal Cancer

Based on the experimental knowledge presented in the previous chapters, several investigators combined portal vein infusion with hepatic artery ligation for the treatment of established colorectal liver metastases. Laufman et al. [23] reported 19 patients with metastatic colon cancer whose bulk disease was limited to the liver, but was not amenable to surgical resection. Many of the patients had poor prognostic features: 14 had more than 30% replacement of the liver, five had poorly differentiated tumor, and five had previously failed to respond to systemic chemotherapy. All were treated with hepatic artery ligation and portal vein infusion of chemotherapy (mitomycin C and 5-FU). Two patients (10%) died within 1 month postoperatively. The remaining 17 patients all improved clinically and demonstrated a marked decrease in carcinoembryonic antigen (CEA) levels. Based on follow-up physical examination, liver function tests, computed tomographic scan and/or laparotomy, there were two complete responses, ten partial responses, four improvements, and one indeterminate result, giving an objective response rate of 63%. Median survival of all patients was 13 months after hepatic artery ligation, with four patients dying at 13, 24, 48, and 68 months respectively. Two patients died suddenly 12 and 19 days after hepatic artery ligation, and one patient experienced acute respiratory distress on the 9th postoperative day, all during or immediately after the first portal vein infusion. One death was due to pulmonary embolism, and it was suspected that thromboplastic material may be released from the liver after hepatic artery ligation and portal vein infusion [23]. In a nonrandomized comparison, Taylor [24] found mean survival of 3 months for nonresectable liver metastases for patients who had no treatment or hepatic artery ligation alone during laparotomy for the primary tumor. Patients who received intraportal 5-FU had a mean survival of 4 months, whereas the five patients who had both hepatic artery ligation and portal vein infusion survived for a mean of 10 months. Due to the small number of 24 patients included in this study, no definitive conclusions can be drawn on the value of portal vein infusion added to hepatic artery ligation for colorectal liver metastases. This subject is currently under prospective randomized investigation in EORTC trial 40794.

A randomized comparison of intra-arterial versus intraportal FUDR treatment of liver metastases has recently been published by Daly and coworkers [33]: They found four objective and three minor responses in eight intra-arterially treated patients, no response at all in 11 patients of the intraportal arm, and three objective and three minor responses in nine patients crossed over from the intraportal to the intra-arterial arm of the trial.

In the largest series of hepatic artery ligation alone, Petrelli et al. [25] found an overall median survival time of 9.5 months, with certain subgroups achieving 12.4 months' survival. Unfortunately, there is no definitive proof that any of these regional treatment modalities bears a survival advantage for liver metastases over no treatment in a strict randomized comparison.

Intraportal Infusion as an Adjuvant Modality for Colorectal Cancer

In 1957, Morales et al. [26] advocated intraportal injection of cytotoxic agents at the time of surgery for colorectal cancer in an attempt to prevent liver metastases. It is generally accepted that adjuvant therapy should be started as soon as possible after surgery, when the tumor burden is minimal [27, 28]. In addition, surgical stress, anesthetic and other drugs, hypercoagulability, blood transfusion, and impairment of immune function due to surgery possibly render the perioperative period a vulnerable phase for tumor promotion.

The renewed interest in adjuvant portal infusion is based on an early publication by Taylor et al. [29], who, in 1979, reported on a randomized study evaluating adjuvant cytotoxic liver infusion for colorectal cancer. After a mean follow-up of 26 months, 23 patients had died in the control group and seven in the infusion group. The incidence of liver metastases in the two groups (13 control, 2 infusion) was statistically significantly different. Based on these results, several cooperative groups initiated prospective randomized trials comparing intraportal infusion of various regimens to surgery alone. An overview of these studies is given in Table 3. Only randomized trials with a "no treatment" control group are included, and with the exception of Taylor's study in Liverpool, all trials are multicentric. Some do not include rectal cancer. All studies require radical en bloc resection of the primary without residual disease. Portal venous catheterization is done at laparotomy through various routes according to the protocols. The effect of heparin or fibrinolytic agents alone is tested in a three-arm trial design.

In a more recent analysis, Taylor et al. [30] reported on 127 control patients and 117 patients who received adjuvant infusion. Thirteen patients were excluded following randomization: one had cirrhosis, three were found on laparotomy to have liver metastases, and in nine there were technical problems with catheter cannulation. After a median follow-up of 4 years, 53 patients had died with recurrent disease in the control group and 25 in the infusion group.

The liver was the predominant site of recurrence: 22 patients in the control group and five in the infusion group developed hepatic metastases. Overall survival appeared to be improved in the infusion group; on closer examination, however, the only significant improvement in overall survival was among patients with Dukes' B colon tumors.

451 patients have been entered in a three-arm study at St. Mary's and surrounding hospitals in the UK. No data are yet published on this trial, but 145 of 160 control patients, 110 of 142 heparin-treated patients, and 106 of 149 patients receiving heparin + 5-FU completed the treatment according to the protocol, and liver metastases had occurred in 15.3% (control), in 8.8% (heparin alone) and in 6.5% (heparin + 5-FU) at a median follow-up of over 2 years (J.P. Fielding, personal communication).

In a Dutch study, preliminary findings at 24 months indicate a decrease in the incidence of liver metastases: 15% in the control group, 12% in the urokinase group, and 7% in the 5-FU + heparin group (J. Wereldsma, personal communication).

An interim report of our own Swiss group study SAKK 40/81 again indicates an advantage regarding disease-free survival for the patients receiving prophylactic intraportal infusion [31]. Despite the large cumulative dose of 5-FU given during

Table 3. Prospective randomized trials of adjuvant portal infusion

Study	No. of patients	Entry	Primary tumors	Treatment	Results (vs controls)
Liverpool	257	1976–1980	C + R	1 g 5-FU + heparin daily for 7 days	Survival (4 years) 70% (vs 50%) colon Dukes B 92% (vs 60%)
St. Mary's	451	1978–1983	C + R	1 g 5-FU + heparin daily for 7 days *or* 10 000 U heparin daily for 7 days	Liver metastases 6.5% vs 8.8% (vs 15.3%)
Rotterdam	303	1981–1984	C + R	1 g 5-FU + heparin daily for 7 days *or* 240 000 U urokinase over 24 h	Liver metastases (24 months) 7% vs 12% (vs 15.%)
Mayo/NCCTG	?	1980–	C	1 g 5-FU + heparin daily for 7 days	No data
NSABP	1300	1984–	C	600 mg/m^2 5-FU + heparin for 7 days	No data
EORTC 40812 + EORTC 40871	500	1983–	C	500 mg/m^2 5-FU + heparin for 7 days	No data
SAKK 40/81	533	1981–1987	C + R	500 mg/m^2 5-FU + heparin daily 7 days + 10 mg/m^2 mitomycin C on day 1	Relapses (36 months) 25.1% (vs 34.3%) Survival (36 months) 80% (vs 72%)
Australia	215	?	C	600 mg/m^2 5-FU + heparin daily for 7 days intraportal *or* same dose IV	Cancer deaths 4.5% vs 20% (vs 22%)

C, colon; R, rectum.

the immediate postoperative period, the systemic side effects were minimal and the morbidity of large-bowel surgery was only slightly increased. The overall operative mortality in all these trials is in the range of 2%–3%, considerably lower than that reported in previous multicenter trials and in the surgical literature.

Toxic deaths have been recorded in at least three trials: one in Taylor's study, due to perirectal sepsis [30], one in the St. Mary's trial in a patient over 80 years old (J.P. Fielding, personal communication), and one in the Swiss group trial, where an insulin-dependent diabetic male suffered gram-negative septicemia and leukopenia during portal infusion. For future studies, it is recommended that patients over 75 years of age, insulin-dependent diabetics, and those with any evidence of intra-abdominal sepsis at laparotomy or during the early postoperative period be excluded.

Preliminary data from four different trials at 2 years appear encouraging and tend to support the data of Taylor et al. [30]. Reduction of liver metastases, reduced overall incidence of relapse, and a tendency toward better survival for infusion patients have been consistently recorded. All these trials confirmed the feasibility of locoregional adjuvant portal chemotherapy in the period immediately following colorectal cancer surgery. Within another 2–3 years, definitive conclusions will be made on the value of adjuvant infusion.

A detailed analysis of all the studies is awaited with interest. Until these data are available, adjuvant portal infusion should continue to be restricted to well-designed protocols and is not recommended outside a clinical trial setting.

References

1. Bengmark S, Hafström L (1969) The natural history of primary and secondary malignant tumours of the liver. 1. The prognosis for patients with hepatic metastases from colonic and rectal carcinoma by laparotomy. Cancer 23:198–202
2. Cedermark BJ, Schultz SS, Bakshi S, Parthasarathy KL, Mittelman A., Evans TJ (1977) Value of liver scan in the follow-up study of patients with adenocarcinoma of the colon and rectum. Surg Gynec Obstet 144:745–748
3. Weiss L, Grundmann E, Torhost J, Hartweit F, Moberg I, Eder M, Fenoglio-Preiser CM, Napier J, Horne CHW, Lopez MJ, Shaw-Dunn RI, Sugar J, Davies JD, Day DW, Harlos JP (1986) Haematogenous metastatic patterns in colonic carcinoma: an analysis of 1541 necropsies. J Pathol 150:195–203
4. Pestana C, Reitemeier RJ, Moertel CG, Judd ES, Dockerty MB (1964) The natural history of carcinoma of the colon and rectum. Am J Surg 108:826–829
5. Wanebo H (1984) A staging system for liver metastases from colorectal cancer. Proc Am Soc Clin Oncol 3:143, C-560
6. Dukes CE (1957) Discussion on major surgery in carcinoma of the rectum, with or without colostomy, excluding the anal canal and including the rectosigmoid. Proc R Soc Med 50:1031–1052
7. Fisher ER, Turnbull RB (1955) The cytological demonstration and significance of tumor cells in the mesenteric venous blood in patients with colorectal cancer. Surg Gynecol Obstet 100:102–106
8. Turnbull RB (1970) Cancer of the colon: 5-10 years' survival rates following resection utilizing the isolation technique. Ann R Coll Surg Engl 46:243–250
9. Roberts S, Jonasson O, Long L, McGrath R, McGrew EA, Cole WH (1961) Clinical

significance of cancer cells in the circulating blood: two- to five-year survivals. Ann Surg 154:362–371
10. Sellwood RA, Kuper SW, Burn JI, Wallace EN (1965) Circulating cancer cells: the influence of surgical operations. Br J Surg 52:69–72
11. De Vita VT (1983) The relationship between tumor mass and resistance to chemotherapy. Implications for surgical adjuvant treatment of cancer. The James Ewing lecture. Cancer 51:1209–1220
12. Schabel FM (1975) Concepts for systemic treatment of micrometastases. Cancer 35:15–24
13. Metzger U, Schneider K, Largiadèr F (1982) Adjuvant therapy of colorectal cancer, an overview. Oncology 5:228–236
14. Higgins GA, Amadeo JH, McElhinney J, McCaughan JJ, Keehn RJ (1984) Efficacy of prolonged intermittent therapy with combined 5-fluorouracil and methyl-CCNU following resection for carcinoma of the large bowel. Cancer 53:1–8
15. Lawrence W, Terz JJ, Horsley S, Donaldson M, Lovett WL, Brown PW, Ruffner BW, Regelson W (1975) Chemotherapy as an adjuvant to surgery for colorectal cancer. Ann Surg 181:616–623
16. Holyoke ED, Moertel CG, O'Connell MJ and the Gastrointestinal Tumor Study Group (1984) Adjuvant therapy of colon cancer: results of a prospectively randomized trial. N Engl J Med 310:737–743
17. Ackermann NB (1974) The blood supply of experimental liver metastases. IV. Changes in vascularity with increasing tumor growth. Surgery 75:589–596
18. Taylor I, Bennett R, Sherriff S (1979) The blood supply of colorectal liver metastases. Br J Cancer 39:749–756
19. Ridge JA, Bading JR, Gelbard AS, Benua RS, Daly JM (1987) Perfusion of colorectal hepatic metastases. Cancer 59:1547–1553
20. Almersjö O, Brandberg A, Gustavsson B (1975) Concentration of biologically active 5-fluorouracil in general circulation during continuous portal infusion in man. Cancer Lett 1:113–118
21. Speyer JL, Sugarbaker PH, Collins, JM (1981) Portal levels and hepatic clearance of 5-fluorouracil after intraperitoneal administration in humans. Cancer Res 41:1916–1922
22. Berger MR, Henne TH, Aguiar JLA, Bartkowski R, Dörsam J, Geelhaar GH, Schlag P, Herfarth C, Schmähl D (1986) Experiments on the toxicity of locoregional liver chemotherapy with 5-fluoro-2'-deoxyuridine and 5-fluorouracil in an animal model. Recent Results Cancer Res 100:148–156
23. Laufman LR, Nims TA, Guy JT, Guy JF, Courter S (1984) Hepatic artery ligation and portal vein infusion for liver metastases from colon cancer. J Clin Oncol 2:1382–1389
24. Taylor I (1978) Cytotoxic perfusion for colorectal liver metastases. Br J Surg 65:109–114
25. Petrelli NJ, Bracewiecz PA, Evans JT, Ledesma EJ, Lawrence DD, Mittelman A (1984) Hepatic artery ligation for liver metastasis in colorectal carcinoma. Cancer 53:1347–1353
26. Morales F, Bell M, McDonald GD, Cole WH (1957) The prophylactic treatment of cancer at the time of operation. Ann Surg 146:588–595
27. Burchenal JH (1976) Adjuvant therapy – theory, practice, and potential. The James Ewing lecture. Cancer 37:46–57
28. Fisher B, Gunduz N, Saffer EA (1983) Influence of the interval between primary tumor removal and chemotherapy on kinetics and growth of metastases. Cancer Res 43:1488–1492
29. Taylor L, Rowling JT, West C (1979) Adjuvant cytotoxic liver perfusion for colorectal cancer. Br J Surg 66:833–837

30. Taylor I, Machin D, Mullee M, Trotter G, Cooke T, West C (1985) A randomized controlled trial of adjuvant portal vein cytotoxic perfusion in colorectal cancer. Br J Surg 72:359–363
31. Metzger U, Mermillod B, Aeberhard P, Gloor F, Bissat A, Egeli R, Laffer U et al. (1987) Intraportal chemotherapy in colorectal carcinoma as an adjuvant modality. World J Surg 11:452–458
32. Bassermann R (1986) Changes of vascular pattern of tumors and surrounding tissue during different phases of metastatic growth. Recent Results Cancer Res 100:256–267
33. Daly JM, Kemeny N, Sigurdson E, Oderman P, Thom A (1987) Regional infusion for colorectal hepatic metastases. A randomized trial comparing the hepatic artery with the portal vein. Arch Surg 122:1273–1277

Prophylactic and Adjuvant Regional Chemotherapy of the Liver in Colorectal Malignancies

H.H. Gruenagel, E. Molzahn, S. Neumann, and G.-U. Neukamp

Chirurgische Abteilung, Evangelisches Krankenhaus Düsseldorf, Kirchfeldstraße 40, 4000 Düsseldorf 1, FRG

The concept of prophylactic and adjuvant regional chemotherapy of the liver in colorectal malignancies is based on the fact that 25%–30% of the patients already have linear metastases at the time of primary resection. Of those without metastases at this time, 40%–50% develop liver metastases secondarily [2, 8]. In view of this, Taylor perfused the liver via the recanalized umbilical vein with 1 g 5-fluorouracil (5-FU) per day continuously for 7 days, starting immediately after curative resection of the tumor. He observed fewer liver metastases and better survival in the perfusion group [11].

Based on these results our management of the liver problems in colorectal malignancies is as shown in Fig. 1. If there are no hepatic metastases and the primary tumor has been completely removed we enter the patient in EORTC study 40871 (since 1987; from 1980 to 1986 we followed the Taylor protocol of prophylactic liver perfusion). If liver metastases are resectable we extirpate them and start cyclic intraportal chemotherapy. In the case of nonresectable hepatic metastases we use an arterial catheter for palliative chemotherapy.

For the prophylactic perfusion study we used the same inclusion criteria as Taylor (Table 1) [11]. In earlier reports we excluded Dukes' A cases from analysis. Later we included them after having worked out a critical check-up of each case in both the perfusion group and the control group: we excluded every patient with irregularities or complications during the postoperative days in both groups (Table 1).

During the time of our study we saw 598 patients with colorectal malignancies. Of those selected as potentially suitable, 105 were randomized to umbilical vein catheterization. In four of these patients the catheter could not be inserted for anatomical reasons. In a further 16 patients local problems (catheter blockage, leakage) hindered perfusion. In two patients the catheter could not be removed and was cut off. The remaining 11 drop-outs were due to postoperative complications (pulmonary, cardiac, and local problems). We were left with 72 patients with a completed, uncomplicated perfusion program and 67 patients in the control group. The randomization was done by means of a computerized number table. The distribution of Dukes A, B, and C tumors (Table 2) age, sex, time of entry into the

R. Jakesz/H Rainer (Eds.)
Progress in Regional Cancer Therapy

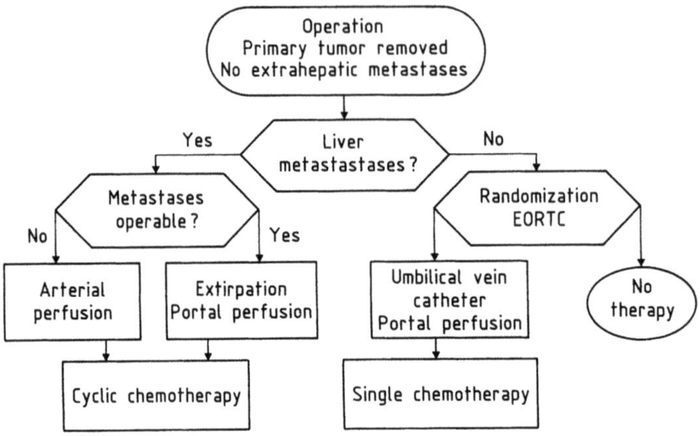

Fig. 1. Strategy for management of the liver in patients with colorectal malignancies

Table 1. Criteria for inclusion or exclusion of patients [11]

Inclusion	Exclusion
▶ Adenocarcinoma of colon or rectum	▶ Distal metastases
▶ Patient less than 70 years old	▶ Palliative operation
▶ Radical resection of tumor	▶ Pre-existing malignoma less than 5 years previously or concomitant other malignancy
▶ No liver or other metastases	▶ Leukopenia (< 4000)
▶ Normal liver parameters	▶ Thrombocytopenia (< 100 000)
▶ Dukes A, B, C	▶ Acute infection
▶ Karnofsky index above 50	▶ Postoperative radiotherapy
	▶ Patient older than 70 years

Table 2. Distribution of Dukes A, B, and C tumors in the umbilical vein perfusion study

	Perfusion	Control
Dukes A	11	8
Dukes B	40	36
Dukes C	21	23
Total	72	67

study, site, and staging are statistically equal in both groups[1]. There is also no difference in length of hospitalization between the two groups: 30.7 days in the perfused patients and 31.2 days in the controls. Like Taylor [11], we always used a rather rigid catheter (Angiographic, Plastik für die Medizin (GmbH, Köln, FRG) in

[1] We thank Prof. W. Richter of the Department of Statistics and Mathematics, Agricultural Faculty, University of Bonn, for the biostatistical analyses.

order to dilate the stenosis in the obliterated umbilical vein. We always checked the complete perfusion of the liver radiographically.

Postoperatively, the following laboratory parameters were checked every 2 days: hemoglobin, hematocrit, erythrocytes, leukocytes with differential hemogram, thrombocytes, bilirubin, serum glutamic oxaloacetic and pyruvic transaminases, alkaline phosphatase, γ-glutamyl transferase. Leukopenia (< 2000) was observed in eight patients, one of whom died. If leukopenia develops at all, it often begins at the 14th to the 16th day postoperatively, i.e., about 1 week after the end of the chemotherapy. In one patient we gave one unit of typed leukocytes on the 18th

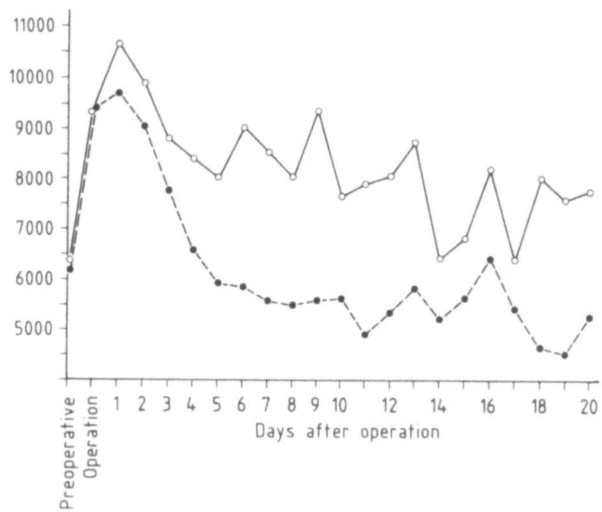

Fig. 2. Mean leukocyte counts during the first 20 days after operation in the perfusion study. •---• perfusion group; —— control group

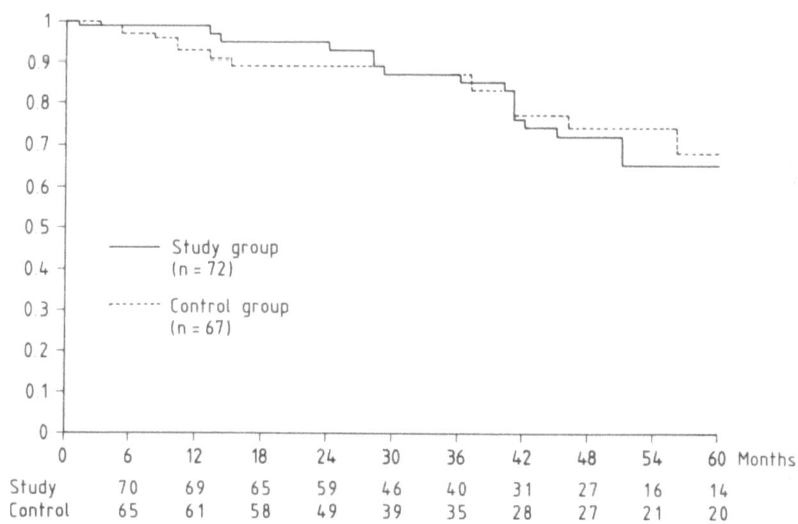

Fig. 3. Five-year survival in the perfusion study

postoperative day, and thereafter the leukocyte count rose again. The leukocyte counts of the perfused patients were very significantly lower than those of the control group patients (Fig. 2). The thrombocyte count fell below 100 000 in two cases, but thrombocytopenia was never a clinical threat. The preliminary results after 2 years showed that survival was better, though not significantly so, in the perfused group. However, after 5 years the survival rate had become worse. Regarding the number of liver metastases in our trial, the perfusion group is as bad as the control group (Table 3). If the liver metastases are resectable we always extirpate them and introduce a Port-A-Cath catheter (Pharmacia) into the umbilical vein or the portal system. In the 16 patients whose metastases were removed we administered cyclic chemotherapy with mitomycin-C (10 mg/m^2) as a bolus and 5-FU (1 g/m^2) continuously for 7 days, if possible every 6 weeks over a period of 1 year.

In this group the recurrences or the progression of the disease always occurred during the first 24 months after the operation (Fig. 4). Of the eight patients with extrahepatic progression of the disease, seven also had recurrences in the liver, hence there was no indication for surgery. One patient died of hemolytic-uremic disease.

Table 3. Liver metastases and mortality in the perfusion study (as of August 1988)

	Perfusion ($n = 72$)	Controls ($n = 67$)
Liver metastases	8	6
Postoperative death	1	0
Later death	15	15

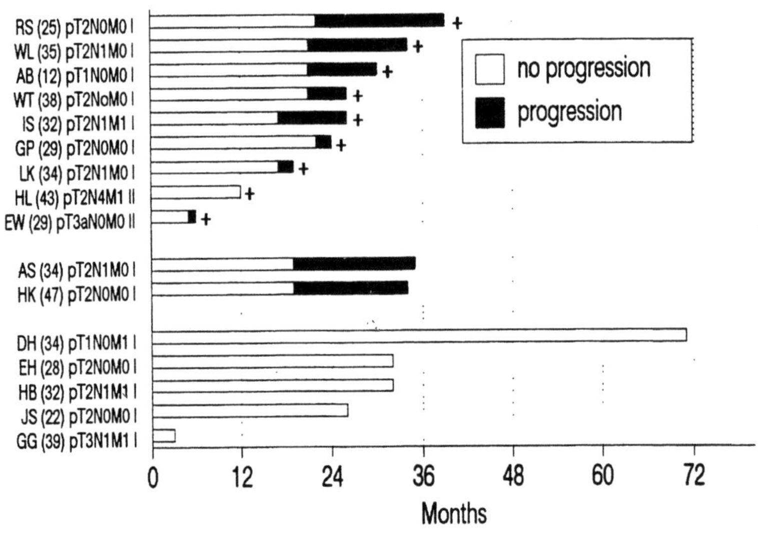

Fig. 4. Results of regional chemotherapy after metastasectomy. *RS(25)pT2NOMO I*, patient's initials/age/pTNM status/Pettavel class; +, death

On autopsy no residue of the original illness was found. Of four patients who had systemic chemotherapy, two later died and the two surviving patients were still being treated at the time of writing with the combination of 5-FU and leucovorin. Five patients are alive without signs of disease. Figure 5 shows the follow-up of one patient with no signs of recurrence or progression of the disease. In short, of 16 patients seven were still alive at the time of writing, two of them with progression of disease. There was one death due to operation, and eight more patients died between 6 months and 4 years after surgery, most of them between 13 and 36 months.

In 10% of the treatment cycles we had complications due to the chemotherapeutic agents or to the infusion system. Most of the complications involved dislocation or

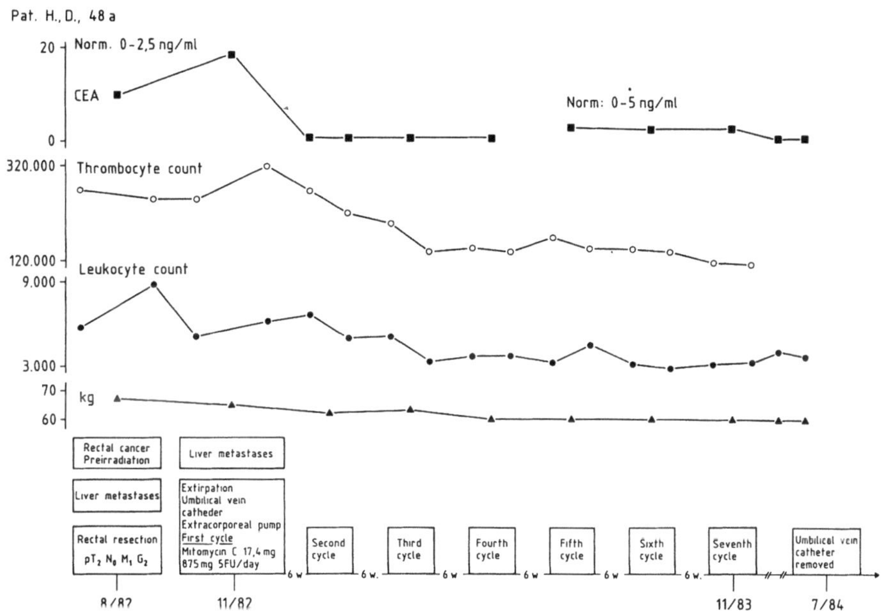

Fig. 5. Course of patient D.H., 48 years old at time of original operation. Repeated regional chemotherapy of the liver after removal of synchronous liver metastases

Table 4. Complications encountered in 113 cycles of portal liver perfusion using (Port-A-Cath) catheters after metastasectomy

	Cycles (s)	*n*
Dislocation	2, 2, 2, 2, 3, 6	6
Catheter thrombosis	3, 2	2
Subcutaneous drug infiltration	1	1
Leukopenia, thrombocytopenia	1	1
Broken needle	1	1
Total		11

thrombosis of the catheter (Table 4). Altogether, 121 patients received 218 cycles of chemotherapy (113 cycles in the 16 patients who underwent metastasectomy, one cycle each in the 105 prophylactically treated patients). The complications on the patients' side are minimal. The complications with the catheter system should decrease as surgeons' experience increases.

The chemotherapy was generally well tolerated in the two study groups. However, the number of patients was too small to allow general conclusions. Therefore in 1987 we joined the EORTC study, which should yield reliable answers in the near future.

References

1. Bengmark S, Hafström L, Jeppson B (1982) Metastatic disease in the liver from colorectal cancer: an appraisal of liver surgery. World J Surg 6:61–65
2. Denck H (1984) Ergebnisse einer intraarteriellen intermittierenden Chemotherapie mit 5-FU bei Metastasenleber sowie inoperablen Tumoren des Gastrointestinal- und Urogenitaltraktes. Onkologie 7:167–176
3. Gall FP, Scheele J, Herfarth C, Rothmund M, Funovics, J Siewert JR (1985) Therapiekonzept bei Lebermetastasen. Langenbecks Arch Chir 365:219–226
4. Ghussen F, Grundmann R, Nage K, Pichlmaier H (1985) Aktueller Stand der Therapie von Lebermetastasen kolorektaler Karzinome. Leber Magen Darm 15:76–80
5. Hohenberger P, Schlag P, Herfarth C (1986) Zur Indikationsstellung operativer Verfahren bei primären und sekundären malignen Lebertumoren (Kongreßbericht). Langenbecks Arch Chir 369:789
6. Lien MW, Ackermann NB (1970) The blood supply of experimental liver metastases. II. A microcirculatory study of the normal and tumor vessels of the liver with the use of perfused silicone rubber. Surgery 68:334–340
7. Metzger U, Schneider K, Largiadèr P (1982) Adjuvante Therapie des Kolon- und Rektumkarzinoms. Onkologie 5:228–236
8. Metzger U (1985) Efforts for the prevention of liver metastases of colorectal carcinoma. Primary and secondary liver cancer. In: Herfarth C, Hohenberger P, Schlag P (eds) Therapeutic strategies in primary and metastatic liver cancer. Springer, Berlin Heidelberg New York, pp 29–34 (Recent results in cancer research, vol 100)
9. Neuhaus P, Ringe B, Beckstein G, Pichlmayr R (1986) Ergebnisse und Bedeutung der Resektion von Lebermetastasen colorectaler Tumoren (Kongreßbericht). Langenbecks Arch Chir 369:789–790
10. Schlag P (1985) Die Chemotherapie im Rahmen der operativen Primär- und Rezidivbehandlung des colorectalen Karzinoms. Onkol Forum 3:5–8
11. Taylor J, Rowling JT (1979) Adjuvant cytotoxic liver perfusion for colorectal cancer. Br J Surg 66:833–837
12. Wolff H, Lippert H, Sterling P (1985) Die chirurgische Therapie von Lebertumoren. Klinikarzt 14:610–620

Randomized Multicenter Trial on Adjuvant Intraportal Chemotherapy for Colorectal Cancer (SAKK 40/81)

U. Laffer, U. Metzger, M. Arigoni, S. Arma, J. Barras, R. Egeli, S. Martinoli, W. Mueller, and W. Schweizer*

Chirurgische Abteilung, Kantonsspital, Universität Basel, 4031 Basel, Switzerland

Introduction

The importance and the poor prognosis of colorectal liver metastases are well known. Once liver metastases have been detected, the median survival time is in the range of 9–12 months [1–4], the extent of the tumor being the most important prognostic factor [4]. Local recurrence and liver metastases are the most common types of failure after "curative" colorectal surgery in clinical series [5].

A great deal of work has been done to prevent metachronous liver metastases of colorectal origin. With the exception of NASBP protocol C-01 [6], adjuvant systemic chemotherapy has been unsuccessful in producing significant survival benefit [7]. A strong tendency ($p = 0.0587$) toward reduction of liver metastases was seen in a recently ended Dutch multicenter study testing the no-touch isolation technique in colon cancer [8].

However, not in all cases do circulating cancer cells at the time of operation give rise to metastases. Several reports have shown that patients with malignant cells in the venous blood did not have a worse prognosis than those without [9, 10]. Metachronous liver metastases may originate from microscopic deposits not visible at the time of surgery for the primary tumor. These micrometastases are the most important target for adjuvant therapy [11]. There is strong evidence that micrometastases are more chemosensitive than established macroscopic disease [11, 12]. In experimental studies, Ackerman showed the importance of portal vascularity for lesions smaller than 1 cm in size [13, 14].

Almersjö et al. [15] showed the safety of portal venous infusion in man. They found that during continuous portal infusion of 15 mg 5-FU/kg over 24 h, systemic serum concentrations were generally below 100 μg/ml and no side effects were noted.

In 1979, Taylor et al. [16] reported a randomized study evaluating adjuvant cytotoxic liver infusion for colorectal cancer; there was significant reduction of liver metastases and prolongation of survival in the group receiving this adjuvant

*The authors wish to thank Mrs. H. Kummer and Mr. R. Fitridge MD for their help in the preparation of the manuscript, and Monica Castiglione MD and the staff of the SAKK Operations Office, Bern, for data collection.

treatment. In 1981, the Swiss Group for Clinical Cancer Research (SAKK) initiated a similar protocol to check Taylor's findings in a multicenter trial [17].

Patients and Methods

A total of 533 patients with primary adenocarcinoma of either the colon or the rectum were admitted to the SAKK trial from July 1981 to June 1987.

By preoperative randomization the patients were assigned to no adjuvant treatment or to liver infusion through the portal vein with 5-fluorouracil (5-FU) (500 mg/m^2 daily × 7, continuous infusion during the first 7 postoperative days) and mitomycin C (10 mg/m^2, 24 h postoperatively as a 2 h infusion). A portal venous catheter was placed through any side branch of the mesenteric venous system during laparotomy. All patients had normal blood counts and normal renal/liver function tests before surgery. The preoperative carcinoembryonic antigen (CEA) level was measured and liver ultrasound was performed. The trial design and treatment schema have been published [18]. Standard surgical techniques of resection were recommended, the decision on the actual procedure to be performed being left to the operating surgeon.

Postoperative blood counts and liver function tests were performed every other day until day 10, then on days 14, 28, and 42. A portal venogram was performed during the operation to ensure that the catheter was well positioned and was infusing both main portal branches equally. The operative specimens were histologically examined and described according to the Astler-Coller modification of Dukes' classification.

All patients were followed up at 3-monthly intervals for 1 year and then at 6-monthly intervals. Again, blood count, liver/renal function tests, liver scan or liver ultrasound, chest X-ray, and colonoscopy were carried out according to the protocol.

Results

The status of the study at the time of writing is given in Table 1: it is too early to obtain a valid evaluation in five patients, and 72 patients are ineligible for the adjuvant therapy, leaving a total of 456 patients (226 controls and 230 infusions) for analysis.

Table 1. Study status, August 1989

	Control	Infusion	Total
Patients entered	266	267	533
Too early	2	3	5
Analyzed	264	264	528
Ineligible	38	34	72
Evaluable	226	·230	456

Table 2. Ineligibility criteria

	Control	Infusion	Total
Liver metastases	17	14	31
Other metastases	8	7	15
Incomplete resection	0	1	1
Other histology	7	8	15
Protocol violation	6	4	10
Total	38	34	72

Table 3. Characteristics of evaluable patients

	Control	Infusion
Median age (years)	62.3	61.9
Sex		
Female	104	105
Male	122	125
Preoperative CEA (ng/ml)	8.9	9.8
Tumor location		
Right colon	47	41
Transverse colon	15	20
Left colon	85	80
Rectum	79	89

Despite preoperative ultrasound, liver or peritoneal metastases were detected at laparotomy in 46 patients (Table 2). In one patient, postoperative surgical pathology revealed incomplete resection. "Other histology" included ovarian cancer, pancreatic cancer, bladder cancer, anal cancer, non-Hodgkins lymphoma invading the bowel wall, and diverticular tumor. "Protocol violation" included mainly patients with either pre- or postoperative radiation therapy to the rectum.

The characteristics of the 456 eligible patients are similar in the two arms of the trial (Table 3, Fig. 1). Overall hospital mortality was 1.8% (5/226 control, 3/230 infusion). Cause and time (postoperative day) of death are given in Table 4. One control patient died on day 40 following reoperation for colostomy necrosis, two others died of therapy-resistant gram-negative septicaemia, both at day 15. The cytotoxic infusion was considered a contributory factor in one of these patients, a 72-year-old diabetic male. He had a persistent purulent wound secretion following right hemicolectomy. On the 11th postoperative day he developed necrotizing fasciitis of the abdominal wall with bronchopneumonia and irreversible gram-negative septicaemia. At this time he had marked leukopenia of $2200/mm^3$. Following his death, which occurred early in the study period, patients with insulin-dependent diabetes were no longer included in the trial.

The postoperative complications are shown in Table 5. Increased incidence of hemorrhage and perineal fistula was noted, especially following abdominoperineal

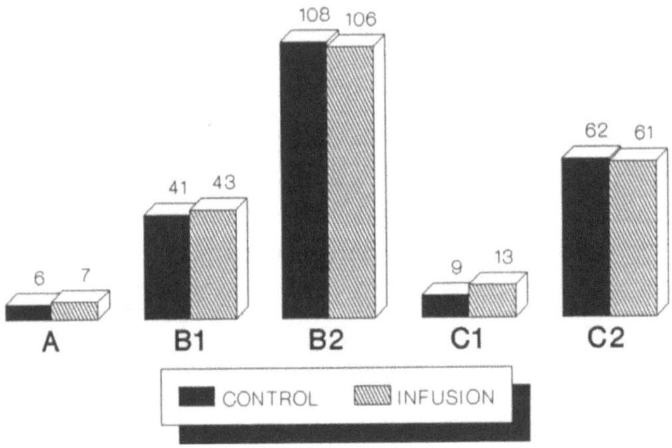

Fig. 1. Tumor stage (Astler–Coller modification of Duke's classification)

Table 4. Postoperative mortality

Cause of death	Control	Infusion
Sepsis	2 (days 15,40)	2 (days 15, 35)
Ileus	2 (days 42, 126)	—
Myocardial infarction	1 (day 1)	1 (day 6)
Total	5 (2.2%)	3 (1.3%)
	Overall: 1.8%	

Table 5. Postoperative complications

	Control	Infusion	*p*
Hemorrhage	2	11	<0.05
Perineal fistula	3	10	0.05
Wound infection	15	19	ns
Peritonitis	5	4	ns
Bowel obstruction	6	7	ns
Nausea and vomiting	0	8	<0.05
Diarrhea	4	4	ns
Cardiopulmonary	11	12	ns
Hospitalization (days, mean)	17.9	21.2	ns

resection of rectal cancer. Despite the fact that chemotherapy was given immediately following surgery, no significant negative impact was noted on rates of wound infection, peritonitis, and anastomotic dehiscence. A limited number of patients experienced mild to moderate nausea and vomiting following intraportal chemotherapy.

Six patients developed transient leukopenia (below 3000/mm^3) during infusion. The white cell count was statistically significantly lower at days 7 and 10 in the infusion group compared with the control group. The values returned to normal (with one exception) during hospitalization. There were only two cases of thrombocytopenia (56 000 and 71 000/mm^3) in the infusion group, but the mean thrombocyte count was statistically significantly lower on day 28 in the infusion group compared to the control group. These values returned to normal at the first follow-up examination. Bilirubin and other liver function tests (SGOT, SGPT, alkaline phosphatase) were not significantly influenced by the infusion treatment.

Results during follow-up are shown in Fig. 2. The overall recurrence rate after a median follow-up of 41.2 months was 32.9% (150/456). There were clearly, though not significantly, more recurrences in the control group than in the infusion group. Some 70% of all patients were still alive, while 27% had died of cancer. Overall, a significant proportion of patients ($n = 22$) died of unrelated causes, resulting in a total death rate of 29.2% (133/456), with a strong trend ($p = 0.06$) in favor of the infusion group.

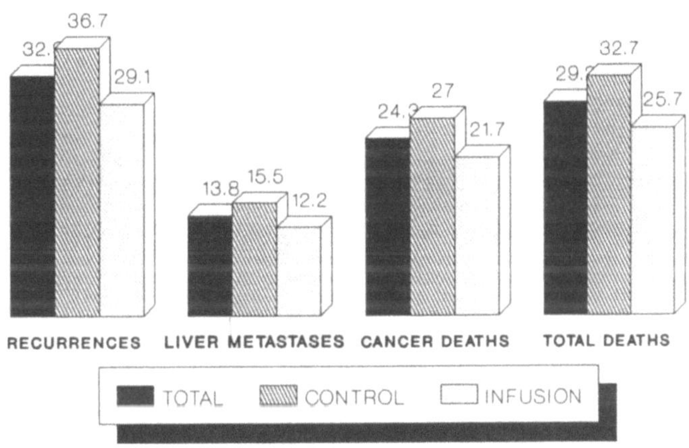

Fig. 2. Recurrence, liver metastases, and deaths (%) among all eligible patients (median follow-up 41.2 months)

Table 6. Reasons why adjuvant chemotherapy was not given

Intraoperative anesthesia problems	4
Intraoperative hemorrhage	3
Intraoperative tumor spillage	4
Catheter placement impossible	7
Refusal by surgeon	10
Incomplete resection	4
Catheter placement forgotten by surgeon	2
Other histology	1
Refusal by patient	2
Total	37

The data presented so far relate to all patients randomized. However, for the various reasons listed in Table 6, 37 patients randomized to adjuvant treatment did not receive infusion. If only those who actually underwent infusion are included in the analysis, these patients are found to have done strikingly better than control patients (Fig. 3). Such comparison is, however, not undisputed for methodological reasons, and it will be the statisticians' duty to resolve this problem. Besides, this subgroup of patients who were allocated to adjuvant treatment but did not receive complete therapy might have negative prognostic variables not known at the moment.

In contrast to Taylor's recently published data [19] we found no convincing effect of treatment on recurrences, liver metastases, and survival for patients with Dukes' B tumors. On the other hand, a clear treatment effect can be observed for patients with Dukes' C tumors (Fig. 4).

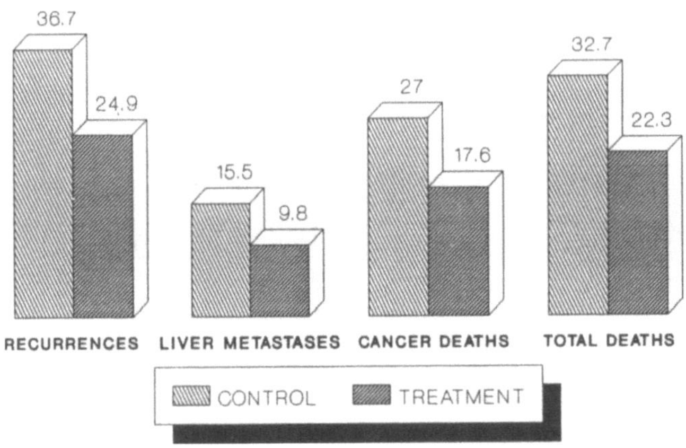

Fig. 3. Recurrences, liver metastases, and deaths (%) in the control group ($n = 226$) and in the patients who actually received adjuvant chemotherapy ($n = 193$)

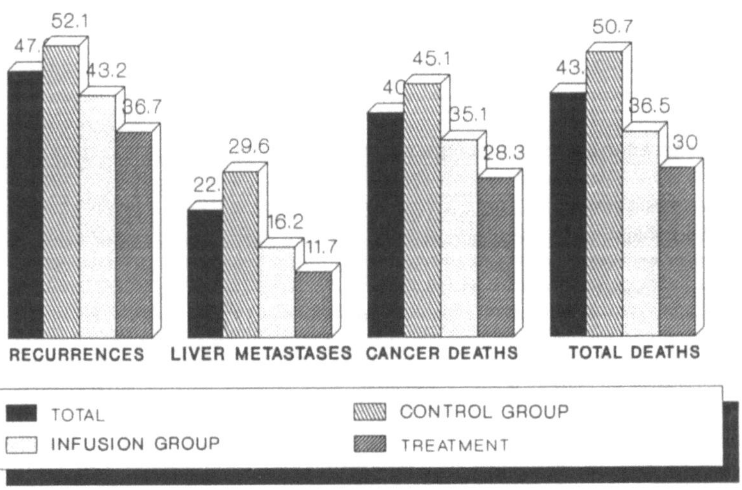

Fig. 4. Results (%) among patients with Dukes' C tumors

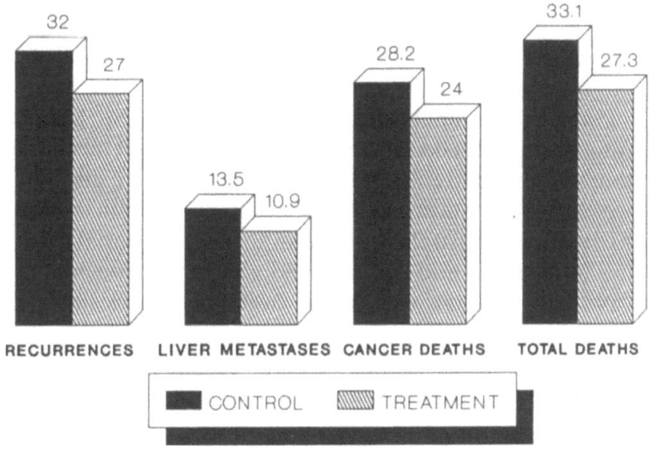

Fig. 5. Results (%) among all 533 patients entered in the study

While the treatment effect in rectal cancer patients is only slight, the infusion group seems to be doing better than the control group in patients with colon cancer.

The survival status of all 533 patients entered in the study is reported in Fig. 5. Again, a strong, but nonsignificant trend in favor of the infusion group was observed after a median follow-up of 41.2 months.

Discussion

To our knowledge, there are at least eight prospective, controlled adjuvant studies in progress using portal infusion chemotherapy following radical surgery for colorectal cancer. Only randomized trials with a "no-treatment" control group are considered here. With the exception of Taylor's study in Liverpool, all trials are multicentric. Some do not include rectal cancer. Adjuvant treatment is given immediately following surgery and consists of continuous infusion for 7 days. In two protocols the effect of anticoagulants is tested using heparin or urokinase alone in a three-arm trial design. In a similar design, the Australian group are comparing intraportal to systemic perioperative chemotherapy.

In their more recent analysis, Taylor et al. [19] reported on 127 controls and 117 patients who received adjuvant infusion. Thirteen patients were excluded following randomization, because of scirrhosis ($n = 1$), liver metastases at laparotomy ($n = 3$), or technical problems with catheterization ($n = 9$). After a median follow-up of 4 years, 53 patients had died with recurrent disease in the control group and 25 patients in the infusion group. In the control group 22 patients developed liver metastases, and in the infusion group liver deposits represented the predominant site of recurrence in five cases. The patients in the infusion group appeared to have better overall survival; however, when individual groups were analyzed, only in those with Dukes' B colon tumors was the improvement significant.

Postoperative mortality was 2.6% (five patients from each group). One patient receiving infusion died in the postoperative period, and it was felt that cytotoxicity had contributed to her death. There was evidence of perirectal sepsis at the time of surgery, and the patient died with gram-negative septicaemia and leukopenia. Following this occurrence, patients with any evidence of intra-abdominal sepsis were excluded from the study [19].

Preliminary, unpublished findings from the St. Mary's trial and the Dutch protocol indicate a decrease in the incidence of liver metastases: 15% in both control groups vs 6.5% and 8.8% in the infusion groups at a median follow-up of 24 months (personal communication). A significant reduction in the cancer death rate has been observed in an Australian study: 4.5% after intraportal treatment compared to 20% after intravenous and 22% after no adjuvant treatment.

No data are available so far from the American Cooperative Group trials. Excellent patient entry is known for the NSABP study; over 1300 patients entered within 3 years by more than 50 participating institutions. The results of the Mayo clinical trial are awaited with great interest, because this protocol has been active since 1980.

The European Organization for Research and Treatment of Cancer (EORTC) Gastrointestinal Tract Cancer Cooperative Group Study no. 40812 has been modified into a simple, large-scale, phase-III trial (EORTC 40871) with Japanese participation and minimal requirements for follow-up.

Conclusion

Perioperative intraportal chemotherapy proved to be feasible in all these trials. Preoperative randomization will lead to a relatively high proportion of ineligible patients, due to incomplete resection in some cases and to detection of occult metastases at laparotomy in others. Intraoperative randomization and operative ultrasonography of the liver is recommended for future studies [20].

Although a large cumulative dose of 5-FU was given during the immediate postoperative period, the systemic side effects were minimal and the morbidity of large bowel surgery was only slightly increased. There is a tendency toward increased postoperative hemorrhage in the patients receiving heparin, but this was not noted in all studies. However, toxic deaths have been recorded in at least three trials: one in Taylor's study, due to perirectal sepsis [19], one in the St. Mary's trial, in an over 80-year-old patient (personal communication), and in the SAKK trial. For future studies of adjuvant portal infusion, it is recommended that patients over 75 years of age, insulin-dependent diabetics, and patients with any evidence of intra-abdominal sepsis at laparotomy or during the early postoperative period be excluded.

Interestingly, the overall operative mortality in all studies cited above is in the range of 2%, considerably lower than reported by previous multicenter trials and in the surgical literature. This indicates possible advances in surgical technique and in pre-/postoperative patient management in this type of elective cancer surgery.

The preliminary findings of four different trials appear encouraging and tend to support the data of Taylor et al. [19]. Reduction of liver metastases, reduced overall incidence of relapse, and a tendency toward better survival for infusion patients have been recorded. Within another 2–3 years, definitive conclusions can be drawn concerning the usefulness of adjuvant portal infusion. Detailed analysis of all studies and meta-analysis of the different protocols is thus awaited with interest. Until these data are available, adjuvant portal infusion should continue to be restricted to well-designed protocols, and its use is not recommended outside a clinical trial setting.

Summary

A total of 533 patients from nine Swiss hospitals have been entered in a prospective randomized trial to assess the value of radical surgery plus adjuvant portal infusion of 5-fluorouracil and mitomycin C compared to radical surgery alone. After a median follow-up of 41.2 months, 150 of 456 fully evaluable patients developed tumor recurrence; the rate was 36.7% in the control arm, 29.5% in the infusion arm. Some 27% of patients in the control group and 21.7% of patients in the infusion group died of recurrent disease.

If only those patients in the infusion arm were considered who actually underwent infusion ($n = 193$), 24.9% developed recurrences (9.8% within the liver) and 17.6% died of cancer.

The study showed the feasibility of adjuvant portal infusion in a multicenter setting. After a median follow-up of 41 months, there is a clear, though not significant, reduction in overall recurrences, and analysis according to treatment strongly indicates effectiveness of adjuvant portal infusion chemotherapy. Due to the short follow-up and the low number of deaths, no conclusions regarding survival can yet be drawn.

References

1. Bengmark S, Hafström L (1969) The natural history of primary and secondary tumours of the liver. 1. The prognosis for patients with hepatic metastases from colonic and rectal carcinoma by laparotomy. Cancer 23:198–202
2. Cedermark BJ, Schultz SS, Bakshi S, Parthasarathy KL, Mittelman A, Evans TJ (1977) Value of liver scan in the follow-up study of patients with adenocarcinoma of the colon and rectum. Surg Gynecol Obstet 144:745–748
3. McDermott FT, Hughes ESR, Pihl E, Milne BJ, Price AB (1981) Comparative results of surgical management of single carcinomas of the colon and rectum: a series of 1939 patients managed by one surgeon. Br J Surg 68:850–855
4. Wanebo H (1984) A staging system for liver metastases from colorectal cancer. ASCO Proc 3:143
5. Gilbert JM, Jeffrey I, Evans M, Kark AE (1984) Sites of recurrent tumour after 'curative' colorectal surgery: implications for adjuvant therapy. Br J Surg 71:203–205
6. Wolmark N, Fisher B, Rockette H, Redmond C, Wickerham DK, Fisher ER, Jones J, Glass A, Lerner H, Lawrence W, Prager D, Wexler M, Evans J, Cruz A, Dimitrov N, Jochimesen P, other NSABP investigators (1988) Postoperative adjuvant chemotherapy or BCG for colon cancer: results from NSABP protocol C-01. Cancer Inst 80:30
7. Lise M, Gérard A, Nitti D, Zane D, Buyse M, Duez N, Arnaud JP, Metzger U (1987): Adjuvant therapy for colorectal cancer. Dis Colon Rectum 30:847–854
8. Wiggers T (1987) The no-touch isolation technique in colon cancer: report on a multicenter study with analyses of prognostic factors. CIP-DATA Koninklijke Bibliotheek, The Hague
9. Roberts S, Jonasson O, Long L, McGrath R, McGrew EE, Cole WH (1961) Clinical significance of cancer cells in the circulating blood: two- to five-year survivals. Ann Surg 154:362–371

10. Sellwood RA, Kuper SW, Burn JI, Wallace EN (1965) Circulating cancer cells: The influence of surgical operations. Br J Surg 52:69–75
11. Schabel FM (1975) Concepts for systemic treatment of micrometastases. Cancer 35:15–24
12. DeVita VT (1983) The relationship between tumor mass and resistance to chemotherapy. Implications for surgical adjuvant treatment of cancer. The James Ewing Lecture. Cancer 51:1209–1220
13. Ackerman NB (1974) The blood supply of experimental liver metastases. IV. Changes in vascularity with increasing tumor growth. Surgery 75:589–596
14. Ackerman NB (1986) Experimental studies on the role of the portal circulation in hepatic tumor vascularity. Cancer 58:1653–1657
15. Almersjö O, Brandberg A, Gustavsson B (1975) Concentration of biologically active 5-fluorouracil in general circulation during continuous portal infusion in man. Cancer Lett 1:113
16. Taylor I, Rowling JT, West C (1979) Adjuvant cytotoxic liver perfusion for colorectal cancer. Br J Surg 66:833–837
17. Metzger U, Aeberhard P, Egeli R, Harder F, Largiadèr F, Müller W, Pettavel J, Weber W, Cavalli F (1982) Adjuvante portale Leberperfusion beim kolorektalen Karzinom. Helv Chir Acta 49:175–178
18. Metzger U, Mermillod B, Aeberhard P, Gloor F, Bissat A, Egeli R, Laffer U, Martinoli S, Mueller W, Schroeder R, Weber W, Swiss Group for Clinical Cancer Research (SAKK) (1987) Intraportal chemotherapy in colorectal carcinoma as an adjuvant modality. World J Surg 11:452
19. Taylor I, Machin D, Mullee M, Trotter G, Cooke T, West C (1985) A randomized controlled trial of adjuvant portal vein cytotoxic perfusion in colorectal cancer. Br J Surg 72:359–363
20. Machi J, Isomoto H, Kurohiji T, Shirouzu K, Yamashita Y, Kakegawa T, Sigel B (1986) Detection of unrecognized liver metastases from colorectal cancers by routine use of operative ultrasonography. Dis Colon Rectum 29:405–409

Enhancement of Cytotoxic Efficacy of 5-Deoxy-5-fluorouridine in Acetoxymethyl-methylnitrosamine-Induced Colorectal Adenocarcinomas in SD Rats by Locoregional Administration into the Inferior Mesenteric Artery

E. Petru, M.R. Berger, F.T. Garzon, and D. Schmähl

Klinik für Gynäkologie und Geburtshilfe, Universität Graz, Auenbruggerplatz 14, 8036 Graz, Austria

Introduction

Colorectal cancer is one of the most frequent tumors in the western world, with rising incidence and mortality [8]. Surgery remains the only modality with curative potential, but the majority of patients with advanced neoplasms are not amenable to surgical cure. Even when resection is possible, the patients remain at high risk for recurrence and metastasis. This situation leads to the concept of combined treatment, i.e., surgery with radiotherapy, which controls the locoregional recurrence, and/or chemotherapy, which in theory controls distant micrometastasis or systemic dissemination [4]. However, most patients with advanced disease experience progression in spite of conventional chemotherapy, which is characterized by being unspecific and displaying a narrow range between marginally active and toxic doses.

Certain experimental approaches have been made, such as high-dose locoregional administration of chemotherapy to the target tissue, or high-dose systemic chemotherapy with subsequent bone marrow transplantation. Unfortunately, the benefit of these techniques has been limited. The detection of new cytotoxic agents with improved antineoplastic potency and the prediction of their clinical activity in GI tract cancer depends mainly on the preclinical system which is used to evalutate the properties of the compounds tested. The conventionally used rapidly proliferating rodent tumors have failed to identify new agents. The former NCI system, which was based on transplanted mouse models, was recently supplemented by tumors of human origin inoculated into nude mice. Once again, this system failed to predict or select compounds active against tumors of the GI tract.

Acetoxymethyl-methylnitrosamine (AMMN)-induced autochthonous colorectal cancer in SD rats appears to be a more reliable model than transplanted tumors for the prediction of the efficacy of new compounds [2,5]. The tumors are well-differentiated adenocarcinomas with a relatively long volume-doubling time (18.5 days, 95% confidence limits 15.7–22.5 days) [2]. Furthermore, the chemoresistance of this tumor increases the model's similarity to the human situation [6]; their growth within the colorectum can be diagnosed endoscopically. 5-fluorouracil is one of the classical agents used in chemotherapy of colorectal cancer [5]. Its prodrug 5-deoxy-5-fluorouridine (5′dFUR) has shown a better therapeutic index in several

R. Jakesz/H Rainer (Eds)
Progress in Regional Cancer Therapy

murine systems. Moreover, 5′dFUR has shown a 26% response rate in a phase II clinical study on advanced colorectal adenocarcinoma (cited in [6]).

Locoregional chemotherapy increases the drug concentration in the infused area and, at the same time, reduces the availability of the drug and its metabolites in the systemic circulation [1]. Consequently, locoregional treatment is expected to lower the overall toxicity. A limited number of clinical studies have been carried out in which patients with advanced colon cancer have been treated intra-arterially. This treatment modality has shown substantial benefits in patients with advanced pelvic neoplasms and uncontrollable pain not amenable to any surgical maneuver [7]. The purpose of the present experiment was to investigate the efficacy of 5′dFUR against colon cancer using the access to the inferior vena cava (systemic treatment) as compared to the antitumor effect of locoregional chemotherapy following cannulation of the arterial access to the large intestine via the inferior mesenteric artery.

Material and Methods

Male Sprague-Dawley rats (Charles River Breeding, Sulzfeld, FRG) were purchased at a weight of 140–160 g and kept thereafter under conventional conditions. Colorectal carcinomas were induced using 0.2% solutions of AMMN in physiological saline: 2 mg/kg was administered intrarectally at weekly intervals for 10 weeks by means of a rectal tube, the tip of which reached the colonic flexure when fully inserted. At the beginning of the 5th week after completion of the 10-week induction period, the animals were anesthesized using chloral hydrate (3 kg/kg↔IP, diluted in physiological saline). This was followed by an endoscopic examination of the colon using a pediatric bronchoscope (Olympus BF, Type4C2, Olympus Optical Co., Tokyo); animals showing evidence of tumors were randomly allocated to experimental groups. Cannulas with a length of 40 cm (PP 10, Portex, Hythe, England) were used. The musculature of the left abdominal wall was transfixed and a needle (2 × 240 mm) was pushed under the subcutaneous tissue up to the midscapular area, where the skin was transfixed. Through a needle the distal part of the polyethylene catheter was positioned in the peritoneal cavity. The proximal part of the catheter was protected by a steel spiral (2.5 × 180 mm) equipped with a 20-mm-diameter metal swivel attached to the superior end which was used for hanging the spiral from the cage covering. The spiral was fixed in place with two stitches of 3–0 nylon to the midscapular skin. Cannulation of the inferior vena cava was performed through the iliolumbar vein (Fig. 1). After isolation and distal ligation of the iliolumbar vein through a transverse incision, the catheter was inserted into the inferior vena cava and pushed cephalad. The catheter was fixed in place with 6–0 silk.

The descending colon was retracted to the right side, and with the aid of an operating microscope (10-fold magnification) the left iliolumbar artery and inferior mesenteric arteries were dissected (Fig. 1). The aorta was laid open as far as the renal arteries to facilitate clamping. The iliolumbar artery was ligated distally, and the aorta was clamped temporarily. The distal end of the polyethylene catheter was narrowed, and through a transverse incision of the iliolumbar artery the catheter was inserted up to the inferior mesenteric artery via the aorta and fixed in place there.

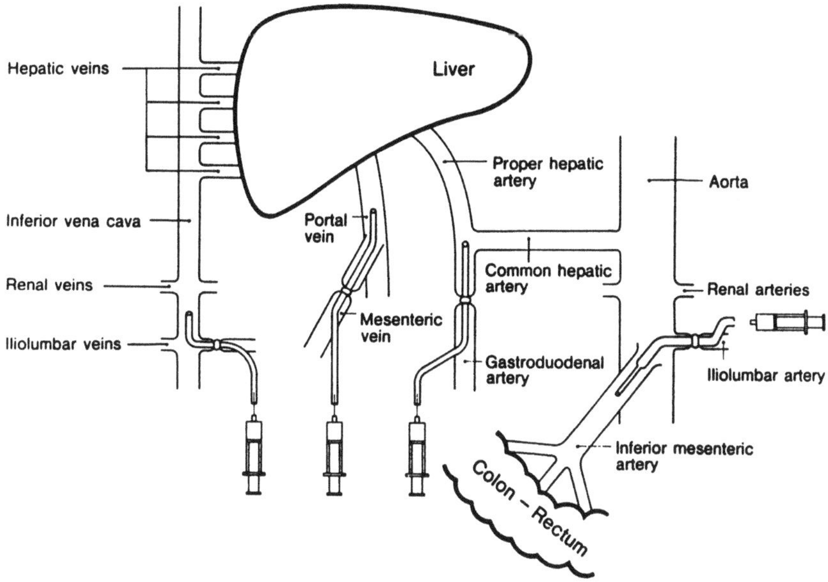

Fig. 1. Cannulation routes for drug administration

A quantity of 300 mg/kg 5'dFUR (Grenzach-Wylen, FRG) was administered twice a week over a 2-h period using an infusion pump (Perfusor V, Braun, Melsungen, FRG) connected to respective catheters Heparin solution was given daily. Animals were sacrificed after the treatment period; they were dissected and the last 20 cm of the gut was removed, opened and weighed. The volume of each tumor was estimated by measuring three diameters according to the formula axbxc/2. For statistical analysis a multiple rank sum test according to Dunn was applied [3].

Results

The antitumor activity of systemic 5'dFUR versus intra-arterial 5'dFUR is shown in Table 1 and Fig. 2. The difference in median tumor volumes between control animals and rats receiving intra-arterial chemotherapy, was significant ($p < 0.05$), whereas that between controls and animals treated systemically was not.

Discussion

Since 5'dFUR is one of the new fluoropyrimidines in clinical use with response rates around 30% (cited in [6]), we compared the efficacy of this compound given systemically via the inferior vena cava and intra-arterially via the inferior mesenteric artery in AMMN-induced colorectal rat adenocarcinoma.

In the present experiment, the antitumor effect of 5'dFUR was only slightly greater after locoregional than after systemic administration (Table 1, Fig. 2).

Table 1. Systemic versus locoregional chemotherapy with 5'dFUR in AMMN-induced colorectal adenocarcinoma starting at week 15 following endoscopic diagnosis of tumors

Group	No. of animals	Median tumor volume in mm^3 (95% confidence limits)	Median tumor volume relative to controls	Median no. of tumors per rat (95% (confidence limits)
Control	15	192 (97–232)	100	6 (3–4)
Inferior vena cava	15	115 (61–177)	56	5 (3–6)
Inferior mesenteric artery	15	95 (83–156)	49	5 (3–6)

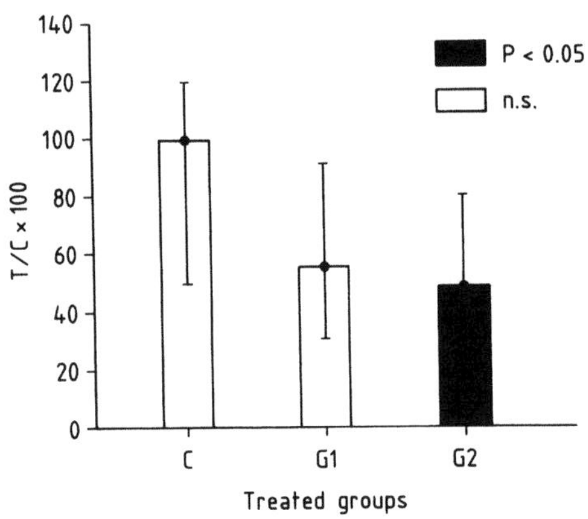

Fig. 2. Relative median tumor volumes. *C*, controls; *G1*, systemic treatment via the inferior vena cava; *G2*, locoregional treatment via the inferior mesenteric artery

However, this experimental model seems particularly well suited for future studies on the pharmacokinetics of new antineoplastic agents [1, 5].

In recent experiments, a new metal compound, budotitane, has shown outstanding antineoplastic activity in this tumor model [5]. Moreover, this titanium derivative was remarkably nontoxic, thus making it suitable for prolonged therapy. Furthermore, water-soluble, heterocyclic coordinated complexes such as imidazole-bis-tetrachloro-ruthenium have produced encouraging results in primary screening models and also in this tumor model [5, 6]. These results have prompted the initiation of phase I and II clinical studies. It is hoped that these new compounds will be able to improve the poor results of chemotherapy in slowly growing tumors such as colorectal cancer.

Summary

Fluoropyrimidines are currently used for the adjuvant or palliative treatment of colorectal cancer. The efficacy of 5'deoxy-5-fluorouridine (5'dFUR) in acetoxymethyl-methylnitrosamine (AMMN)-induced colorectal adenocarcinoma in rats, when administered systemically or locoregionally, was investigated. Rats received a dose of 2 mg/kg AMMN each week for 10 weeks. Five weeks after the end of this induction period, endoscopic diagnosis of tumors was performed. One group served as controls, another received systemic treatment via the inferior vena cava, and a third received locoregional therapy via the inferior mesenteric artery. A dose of 300 mg/kg 5'dFUR was administered twice weekly by an infusion pump. After 5 weeks of therapy, 5'dFUR via systemic and locoregional administration resulted in inhibition of median tumor volume by 44% and 51%, respectively, compared to controls. The difference in median tumor volumes between controls and animals treated locoregionally proved to be significant ($p < 0.05$). 5'dFUR increased the antineoplastic effect in AMMN-induced autochthonous colorectal adenocarcinoma when it was administered intra-arterially.

References

1. Aguiar JL, Bartkowski R, Berger MR, Petru E, Schlag P, Schmähl D, (1987) Feasible model for locoregional and systemic longterm administration of drugs and concomitant blood sampling in Sprague Dawley rats. J Cancer Res Clin Oncol 113:27–30
2. Berger MR, Bischoff H, Fritschi E, Henne T, Herrmann M, Pool BL, Satzinger G, Schmähl D, Weiershausen U (1985) Synthesis, toxicity, and therapeutic efficacy of 4-amino-*N*-(2'-aminophenyl)-benzamide: a new compound preferentially active in slowly growing tumors. Cancer Treat Rep 69:1415–1424
3. Dunn OI (1964) Multiple comparisons using rank sums. Technometrics 6:241–252
4. Fischerman K, Briand P, Olsen J, Nilsen OV (1974) Intra-arterial combined cancer chemotherapy in technically inoperable carcinoma of the anus and rectum. Acta Chir Scand 140:416–421
5. Garzon FT, Berger MR, Bischoff H, Schmähl D (1988) New drug development in gastrointestinal-tract cancer. Recent Results Cancer Res 110:286–296
6. Garzon FT, Berger MR, Keppler B, Schmähl D (1987) Comparative antitumor activity of ruthenium derivatives with 5'deoxy-5-fluorouridine in chemically induced colorectal tumors in SD rats. Cancer Chemother Pharmacol 19:347–349
7. Heim S, Eberwein S, Georgi M (1983) Palliative therapy of pelvic tumors by intra-arterial infusion of cytotoxic drugs. Recent Results Cancer Res 86:37–40
8. Silverg E, Lubera J (1986) Cancer statistics 1986. CA 36:9–25

Second Hepatic Resections in Patients with Liver Metastases from Colorectal Carcinoma

K.D. Griffith, A.E. Chang, and P.H. Sugarbaker

National Cancer Institute, Bethesda, MD 20892, USA

Introduction

Over the past 20 years, data have been presented indicating surgical resection as the primary treatment for isolated hepatic metastases from colorectal carcinoma. In most series reporting long-term follow-up (i.e., >5 years), a salvage rate of approximately 25% is reported for completely resectable lesions numbering less than four [1–16]. As this therapy has gained acceptance, the question of appropriate follow-up and repeat resections for recurrent metastatic cancer of the liver has become relevant. We present our own experience with hepatic re-resection as well as an overview of those few anecdotal case reports to be found in the literature.

Patients and Results

Between 1970 and 1987, 106 patients had undergone a resection of colorectal liver metastases at the US National Cancer Institute (84 patients) or Emory University School of Medicine (22 patients). Among these patients, nine underwent a second hepatic resection of recurrent liver metastases (seven at NCI, two at Emory). Median follow-up for these patients was 21 months (range 9–67 months) from the time of their second liver resection. The data on these nine patients are summarized in Table 1. Their median age at follow-up was 57 years (range 44-70 years). There were six males and three females. At the first operation all but one of the patients had wedge resections of their hepatic metastases. Wedge resections were classified as operations which entailed the removal of less than a major lobe. Seven patients had solitary metastases, two (patients 3 and 5) had bilobar metastases. Six of the nine patients had their hepatic resections performed at the time of their primary tumor excisions. The remaining three patients had resection of metachronous liver tumors which were all diagnosed by elevations in carcinoembryonic antigen (CEA) levels.

The median disease-free interval from the time of the first hepatic resection to the diagnosis of the hepatic recurrence was 21 months (range 1–39 months). Recurrent disease was initially diagnosed by elevations in CEA levels in six patients and by computed tomography (CT) scans in the other three patients. Preoperative

R. Jakesz/H Rainer (Eds.)
Progress in Regional Cancer Therapy

Table 1. Summary of data on nine patients who had second hepatic resections for colorectal metastases at the National Cancer Institute or Emory University School of Medicine

		Primary tumor[a]	First hepatic resection			Second hepatic resection				
Patient	Age/sex	Location/stage	DFI[b]	No. of Nodules	Operation	DFI[c]	No. of nodules	Operation	Adj.[d]	Follow-up
1	56/M	Sigmoid/B2	18	1	R wedge	3	5	R lobectomy	+	NED, 67 mo
2	63/M	Sigmoid/C2	0	1	R wedge	33	4	R lobectomy	+	NED, 50 mo
3	57/M	Rectal/C2	0	3	R wedge (2) L wedge (1)	37	1	L lobectomy	+	NED, 25 mo[e]
4	67/F	Right colon/B2	0	1	L wedge	25	1	R trisegmentectomy	+	Died 4th day after operation
5	62/F	Sigmoid/B2	0	2	R + L wedge	39	1	R lobectomy	+	NED, 31 mo
6	70/M	Rectal/C2	0	1	L wedge	19	1	R wedge	+	AWD, 16 mo
7	44/M	Rectal/C2	0	1	R wedge	1	1	R lobectomy	–	NED, 21 mo[e]
8	59/M	Sigmoid/C2[f] Rectum/C2	18	1	L wedge	8	1	R wedge	–	NED, 9 mo
9	53/F	Sigmoid/B2	34	1	R lobectomy	21	1	L wedge	–	NED, 19 mo

R, right; L, left; NED, no evidence of disease; AWD, alive with disease.
[a] site and locoregional stage of primary tumor utilizing Astler and Coller classification system.
[b] Disease-free interval in months from time of resection of primary tumor to diagnosis of hepatic metastasis (synchronous = 0).
[c] Disease-free interval in months from time of first hepatic resection to diagnosis of second hepatic metastasis.
[d] Adjuvant therapy: + represents administration of adjuvant intraperitoneal 5-FU.
[e] Resection of solitary pulmonary metastasis 11 and 18 months after second hepatic resection in patients 3 and 7, respectively.
[f] Patient initially had sigmoid lesion resected and was found to have a metachronous rectal tumor.

evaluation to exclude extrahepatic metastases included barium studies of the large bowel, CT scan of the chest and abdomen, and a bone scan. Intraoperative abdominal exploration involved careful palpation and biopsies of hepatic lymph nodes when clinically suspect. Seven patients had solitary nodules, while the two remaining patients had four and five tumor nodules respectively. Second hepatic resections includes six lobectomies, one trisegmentectomy, and two wedge resections. The one post-operative death involved patient 4, who had the trisegmentectomy: the cause of death was a myocardial infarction sustained on the 4th postoperative day. Six patients had adjuvant intraperitoneal 5-fluorouracil (5-FU) therapy via a Tenckhoff catheter as previously described [4]. The median survival in all patients was 21 months, with two patients remaining free of disease for over 4 years.

Three patients have suffered recurrences after the second hepatic resection. Patients 3 and 7 developed solitary pulmonary nodules 11 and 18 months, respectively, after the second hepatic procedure. They underwent pulmonary metastasectomy and have been free of disease for 14 and 3 months, Patient 6 was found to have respectively unresectable disease in the liver 12 months after the second hepatic resection and remains alive with disease.

Discussion

It is estimated that approximately 10% of all patients who develop hepatic metastases from colorectal cancer may benefit by liver resection [17]. The Registry of Hepatic Metastases reported a collected series of 859 patients who had undergone resection of colorectal liver metastases and had a 5-year survival rate of 33% [12]. In a follow-up study reported by the Registry, the site of recurrence in those patients who had complete resection of liver metastases was examined [18]. The liver was the most common site, with 28% of patients having recurrences confined to the liver and 11% having recurrences in the liver plus other sites. Recurrent tumor confined to the liver most likely develops from tumor deposits present but undetected at the initial liver resection. This possibility is supported by the observation that patients who had positive pathologic margins or bilobar metastases at the time of liver resection were at increased risk for developing hepatic recurrences [18]. The increasing use of intraoperative ultrasound may improve the ability of the surgeon to detect smaller lesions not identified by CT scanning or manual palpation, as well as aid in achieving adequate surgical margins [19].

Data from the literature and our experience suggest that approximately one-third of isolated liver recurrences are technically resectable. In the past, the major deterrent to aggressive metastasectomy of the liver has been the potential operative morbidity. However, advances in hepatic parenchymal dissection and in the diagnostic evaluation of the colorectal cancer patient have helped to improve the feasibility of hepatic metastasectomies. Careful monitoring of CEA levels can lead to the earlier detection of recurrent liver disease which may be more amenable to surgical resection [20]. Likewise, newer diagnostic scanning techniques have improved the sensitivity and resolution of diagnosing smaller hepatic nodules. The Cavitron ultrasonic surgical aspirator has been shown to provide a more controlled dissection of the hepatic parenchyma with improved identification of vasculobiliary

Table 2. Summary of cases of second hepatic resection for metastases of colorectal cancer reported in the literature

Author	No. of patients	First procedure	Second procedure	Follow-up[a]
Nordlinger et al. [11]	6	Wedge resection	R trisegmentectomy	Died, 25 mo
		Wedge resection	R trisegmentectomy	AWD, 23 mo
		Wedge resection	R trisegmentectomy	NED, 17 mo
		Wedge resection	R lobectomy	NED, 42 mo
		Wedge resection	R lobectomy	AWD, 41 mo
		Wedge resection	Wedge resection	NED, 40 mo
Butler et al. [6]	2	Wedge resection	Lobectomy	NED, 6 mo
		Wedge resection	Lobectomy	NED, 17 mo
Tomas-de la Vega et al. [9]		Not reported	Not reported	AWD (2), NED (2): mean 22 mo
Fortner [23]	3	Lobectomy	Wedge resection	AWD, 39 mo[b]
		Lobectomy	Wedge resection	Alive, 5 + mo[c]
		Lobectomy	Wedge resection	Died, 16 mo

R, right; L, left: NED, no evidence of disease; AWD, alive with disease.
[a] Follow-up status in months from second hepatic resection.
[b] Recurrent disease documented 7 months after second liver resection in lung and pelvis: had four subsequent operations for localized recurrent disease.
[c] Had second recurrence inliver and underwent third liver resection: alive 5 months later.

structures, which can decrease operative blood loss [21]. Increased blood loss and transfusion requirements have been reported to increase postoperative complications and decrease disease-free and overall survival after liver resections [4, 22].

We have presented the largest reported series of patients who have undergone second liver resections for colorectal metastases. Four previous reports have commented on a total of 15 patients who have had repeat liver resections for metastases [6, 9, 11, 23]. These reports are summarized in Table 2. Seven of these 15 patients remained alive and disease-free at the time of follow-up from 6 to 42 months after their second hepatic resection. Among the nine patients reviewed in our series, two have remained disease-free for more than 4 years, longer than any patient in previous reports. Combining the data on all the patients with individual follow-up information from our series and others, the median survival after second liver resection was 22 months ($n = 20$).

Of note in our series was that six of the nine patients received adjuvant intraperitoneal 5-FU; however, the role of adjuvant chemotherapy in patients surgically rendered free of metastatic disease in the liver has yet to be established. An effective adjuvant treatment after liver metastasectomies is an important area for future investigation. The data presented here and a review of the literature suggest that aggressive repeat resection of recurrent colorectal metastases confined to the liver may be beneficial in selected patients.

Summary

One hundred six patients were identified who had undergone complete resection of isolated hepatic metastases from colorectal carcinoma primaries. Nine of these patients subsequently underwent repeat liver resection for isolated hepatic recurrences. There was one postoperative death related to the second hepatectomy, and one patient has developed an unresectable second liver recurrence. The remaining seven patients remain alive and free of detectable malignancy with a median follow-up period of 21 months. Two of these survivors has undergone resection of a subsequent pulmonary metastasis to re-establish their disease-free status. The remaining five of nine patients remain free from recurrent disease at 9, 19, 31, 50, and 67 months after their second hepatic resection. These results compare very favorably with the reported survival in patients with unresected hepatic metastases and demonstrate that prolonged survival can follow repeat hepatic resection in selected patients.

References

1. Fortner JG, Silva JS, Golbey RB, Cox EB, MacLean BJ (1984) Multi-variate analysis of a personal series of 247 consecutive patients with liver metastases from colorectal cancer. Ann Surg 199:306–316
2. Petrelli NJ, Nambisan RN, Herrera LM, Mittelman A (1985) Hepatic resection for isolated metastases from colorectal carcinoma. Am J Surg 149:205–209
3. Adson MA, van Heerde JA, Adson MH, Wagner JS, Ilstrup DM (1984) Resection of hepatic metastases from colorectal cancer. Arch Surg. 199:647

4. August DA, Sugarbaker PH, Ottow RT, Gianola FJ, Schneider PD (1985) Hepatic resection of colorectal metastases: influence of clinical factors and adjuvant intraperitoneal 5-FU via Tenckhoff catheter. Ann Surg 201:210–218
5. Cady B, McDermott WV (1985) Major hepatic resection for metachronous metastases from colon cancer. Ann Surg 201:204–209
6. Butler J, Attiyeh FF, Daly JM (1986) Hepatic resection for metastases of the colon and rectum. Surg Gynecol Obstet 162:109–113
7. Gennari L, Doci R, Bignami P, Bozzetti F (1986) Surgical treatment of hepatic metastases from colorectal cancer. Ann Surg 203:49–54
8. Coppa GF, Eng K, Ranson JCH, Gonge TH, Localio SA (1985) Hepatic resection for metastatic colon and rectal cancer: an evaluation of preoperative and postoperative factors. Ann Surg 202:203–208
9. Tomas-de la Vega JE, Donahue EJ, Doolas A et al. (1984) A ten year experience with hepatic resection. Surg Gynecol Obstet 159:223–228
10. Iwatsuki S, Shaw BW, Starzl TE (1983) Experience with 150 liver resections. Ann Surg 197:247–253
11. Nordlinger B, Parc R, Delva E, Quilichini MA, Hannou L, Huguet C (1987) Hepatic resection for colorectal liver metastases. Ann Surg 205:256–263
12. Hughes KS, Simon R, Songhorabodi S, Adson MA et al. (1988) Resection of the liver for colorectal carcinoma metastases: a multi-institutional study of indications for resection. Surgery 103:278–288
13. Hughes KS, Rosenstein RB, Songhorabodi S et al. (1988) Resection of the liver for colorectal carcinoma metastases. Dis Colon Rectum 31:1–4
14. Liotta LA (1987) Overview of the biology of cancer invasion and metastases. In: Rosenberg SA (ed) Surgical treatment of metastatic cancer. Lippincott, Philadelphia, pp 1–36
15. Kern KA, Pass HI, Roth JA (1987) Surgical treatment of pulmonary metastases. In: Rosenberg SA (ed) Surgical treatment of metastatic cancer. Lippincott, Philadelphia, pp 69–100
16. August DA, Ottow RT, Sugarbaker PH (1984) Clinical perspectives on human colon cancer metastases. Cancer Metastasis Rev 3:303–324
17. Hughes KS, Simon R, Songhorabodi S et al. (1986) Resection of the liver for colorectal carcinoma metastases: a multi-institutional study of patterns of recurrence. Surgery 100:278–284
18. Machi K, Isomoto H, Yamashita Y et al. (1987) Intraoperative ultrasonography in screening for liver metastases from colorectal cancer: comparative accuracy with traditional procedures. Surgery 101:678–684
19. Rizzoni WE, Pass HI, Wesley MN et al. (1986) Resection of recurrent pulmonary metastases in patients with soft-tissue sarcomas. Arch Surg 121:1248–1252
20. Wanebo HJ, Stearns M, Schwartz MK (1978) Use of CEA as an indicator of early recurrence and as a guide to a selected second-look procedure in patients with colorectal cancer. Ann Surg 188:481–492
21. Ottow RT, Barbieri SA, Sugarbaker PH, Wesley RA (1985) Liver transection: a controlled study of four different techniques in pigs. Surgery 97:596–601
22. Stephenson KR, Steinberg SM, Hughes KS et al (1988) Perioperative blood transfusions are associated with decreased time to recurrence and decreased survival after resection of colorectal liver metastases. Ann Surg 208:679–687
23. Fortner JG (1988) Recurrence of colorectal cancer after hepatic resection. Am J Surg 155:378–382

Six Years of Experience with Local Chemotherapy of the Liver

C. Hottenrott, M. Lorenz, R.P. Baum, M. Kirkowa-Reimann, T. Herrhausen, and R. Inglis*

Department of Surgery, Johann Wolfgang Goethe-University, Theodor-Stern-Kai 7, 6000 Frankfurt/Main, FRG

Introduction

Since the first description of regional chemotherapy of the liver, many reports [1–4] have demonstrated more theoretical advantage than clinical benefits. Not toxic but catheter complications seemed to limit the potential of the new method [5]. Totally implantable drug pumps and ports (Infusaid, Shiley Infusaid, Inc., Norword, Mass., USA) in the late reduced the risk of technical problems. Using continuous intra-arterial floxuridine (FUDR) with an extraction of more than 90% in the liver [6], response rates of 30%–88% were reported [7, 8]. A methodological standard for the first time allowed reliable clinical studies[9–12]. Local treatment seemed superior to conventional systemic chemotherapy, although prolongation of survival was only demonstrated using historical control groups. Our own investigations in this field have tremendously increased the number of patients undergoing hepatic surgery in our institution. Since 1982 we have treated 516 patients with hepatic only malignancies, of whom 128 have undergone liver resection or transplantation.

Material and Methods

Of 162 patients receiving palliative treatment for liver metastases from colorectal cancer 112 underwent local chemotherapy of the liver via implantable pumps (Infusaid; Medtronic, USA) or ports (Infusaid; Fresenius, Oberursel, FRG; Pharmacia, Lund, Sweden) and external pumps (Siemens, Erlangen, FRG; Pharmacia; Travenol, Baxter, USA). Standard therapy was continuous intrahepatic arterial FUDR (0.2 mg/kg/day for 14 days every 4 weeks) via an implanted pump (Infusaid) in 52 patients (group I).

Group I was compared with 30 patients receiving FUDR for only 5 days (1 mg/kg/day every 4 weeks (group II). This treatment modality had shown less toxicity. Ambulatory use of external pumps with ports was possible.

*We thank Peter Kempkes for the assistance in computerized analysis of data and preparation for publication.

R. Jakesz/H Rainer (Eds)
Progress in Regional Cancer Therapy

Table 1. Local chemotherapy of "liver-only" metastases of colorectal cancer at the University of Frankfurt, 1982-1988: characteristics of patient groups

	Total		Group I		Group II		Group III		Group IV	
n	112		52		30		26		4	
Number male	70	62%	36	69%	18	60%	12	46%	4	100%
Extent of Primary										
T1	3	3%	2	4%	0	0%	1	4%	0	0%
T2	21	19%	6	12%	7	23%	5	19%	3	75%
T3	62	55%	36	68%	13	43%	12	46%	1	25%
T4	10	9%	3	6%	4	13%	3	12%	0	0%
TX	16	14%	5	10%	6	21%	5	19%	0	0%
Synchroneous	43	38%	20	38%	11	37%	10	38%	2	50%
Tumor volume (Frankfurt class.)										
I	36	32%	21	40%	10	33%	4	15%	1	25%
II	72	64%	30	58%	18	60%	21	81%	3	75%
III	4	4%	1	2%	2	7%	1	4%	0	0%
CEA > 20 ng/ml	76	68%	35	67%	18	60%	21	81%	2	50%
AP > 195 U/dl	54	48%	27	52%	11	37%	14	54%	2	50%
LDH > 215 U/al	43	38%	17	33%	13	43%	11	42%	2	50%
Loss of weight	29	26%	14	27%	2	7%	12	46%	1	25%

CEA, carcinoembryonic antigen; Ap, alkaline phosphatase; LDH, lactate dehydrogenase.

Table 2. Frankfurt classification of liver metastases [13–15]

Stage I	< 25% Tumor volume (intraoperative staging)
Stage II	25%–75% Tumor volume
Stage III	> 75% Tumor volume
F	Disturbance of liver function: Bilirubin or AP > twice normal value
S	Symptomatic patient (weight reduction, liver enlargement, pain in upper abdomen)
E	Extrahepatic disease

In a randomized phase III trial, 26 group I patients were compared to 26 patients receiving additional systemic treatment (group III).

Four patients with continuous intraportal FUDR treatment only because of arterial abnormalities not allowing complete arterial perfusion (group IV) were not evaluable due to the smallness of the group.

In all patients extrahepatic disease was excluded by chest X-ray, ultrasound, computed tomography, and immunoscintiscan. Arterial supply was regularly studied by preoperative angiography (aortography, celiacography, and mesenterico-graphy), and catheter implantation (up to three per patient) was performed by the Watkins technique, avoiding arterial ligation. Incomplete perfusion and malperfusion were excluded (intra operative fluorescein and postoperative scintiscan). Patients with primary malfunction of the pump or change of therapy because of severe early side effects were excluded as well.

All patients were classified according to the Frankfurt classification (Table 2), and sex, age, location, and extent of the primary and chronicity and side of liver metastases were registered. All patients had histological improvement of liver metastases, and the gallbladder was removed if possible. The pump, always primed with heparin (5000 units/50 ml), was located in a separate pocket in the right lower abdominal wall. Regular treatment of the patients and regular follow-up was guaranteed by two full-time oncologists registering all data prospectively in a dBase III program. The following results were calculated, comparisons being done by chi square test and log rank test (software: Test, IDV, Munich, FRG).

Results

Table 3 shows that patients with continuous FUDR infusion for 14 days have a better outcome than those with a higher dosage infused over only 5 days per month. Although response and median survival time are increased in group. I (Fig. 1), the only statistically significant difference is in median time to extrahepatic progression [16]. The rationale for the group II protocol was severe local toxicity (biliary sclerosis), and indeed the incidence of this complication was 27% in group I but only 4% in group II [16–18].

Table 3. Liver-only colorectal metastases: results of infusing FUDR via a totally implantable pump (Infusaid) for 14 days (Group I) or 5 days (group 2) per cycle

	Total		Group I		Group II	
n	82		52		30	
Response (WHO)						
Complete	2	3%	2	4%	0	0%
Partial	31	38%	25	48%	6	20%
Stable disease	24	29%	12	23%	12	40%
Progression	25	30%	13	25%	12	40%
Death	56	68%	44	84%	12	40%
Progression, liver	56	68%	41	78%	15	50%
Progression, extrahepatic	47	57%	30	58%	17	56%
Lung	30	37%	20	38%	10	33%
Median time to liver progression (months)	8		8		8	
Median time to extrahepatic progression (months)	10		12		6	
Median survival (months)	14		16		10	

*P = 0.01.

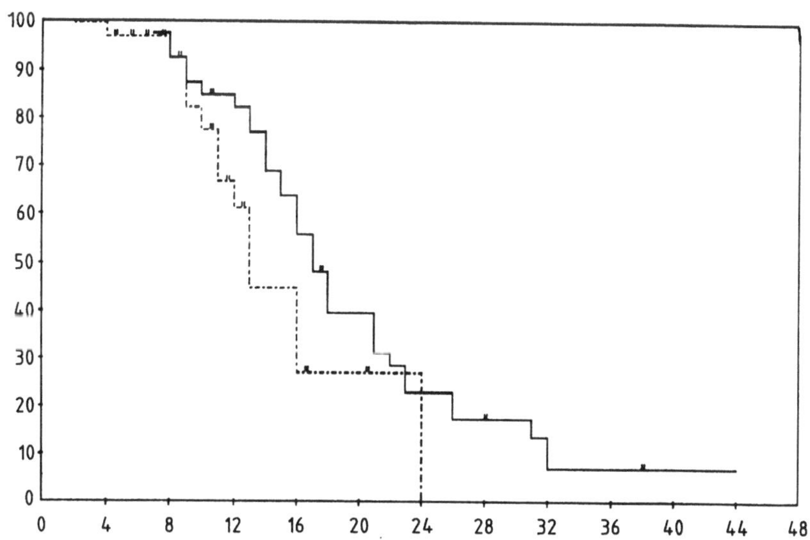

Fig. 1. Kaplan–Meier survival curves from patients with colorectal liver metastases: group I ($n = 52$, *continuous line*) vs group II ($n = 30$, *broken line*). No significant difference

As found in other series [19], the majority of all patients died from extrahepatic progression such as lung metastases, which could be found retrospectively in 7% of cases at the time of pump implantation but which had not been diagnosed earlier. The reason why more patients suffer extrahepatic relapse under local chemotherapy than after liver resection is unknown. Different extent of disease, selection of patients, and a change in immune function could be an explanation.

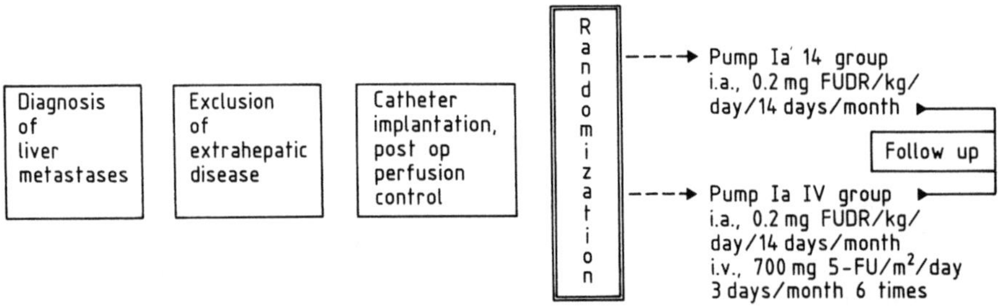

Fig. 2. Stratification of patients with colorectal liver metastases for a randomized multicenter trial. Patient with stage III tumors (> 75% tumor replacement) were excluded, as were those with malperfusion. Intra-arterial treatment was identical in both groups. The *pump IA IV* group (group I) received an additional six cycles of 5-FU

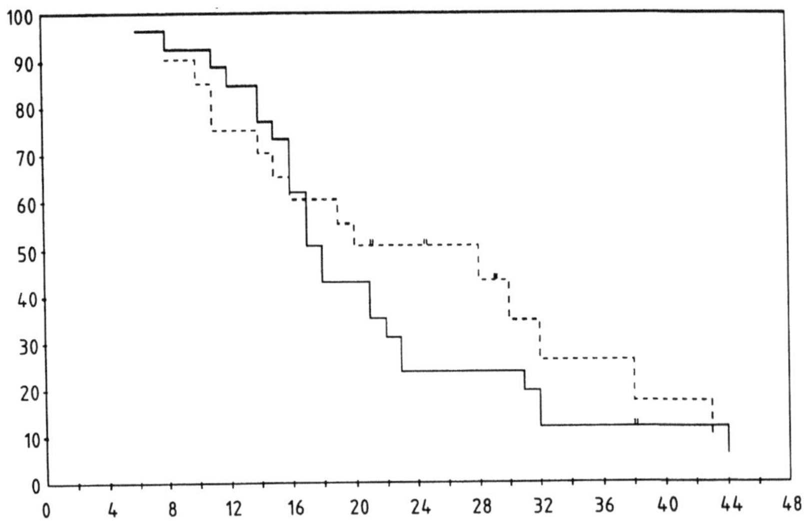

Fig. 3. Kaplan–Meier survival curves according to regional IA treatment (group I, *continuous line*) or combined IA + IV treatment (group III, *broken line*) in patients with liver-only metastases from colorectal cancer (censored observations, $n = 7$)

To test whether systemic treatment additional to the standard local therapy could prevent extrahepatic disease 52 patients were randomized as shown in Fig. 2. Patient accrual was limited to 2 years. The final data after the death of most patients are presented.

Important details demonstrating the comparability of these two groups are shown in Table 4. There was, however, a difference in tumor volume according to the Frankfurt classification favoring patients without additional systemic therapy.

The survival curves of both groups are shown in Fig. 3. Although the response rate in patients with additional systemic treatment (65%) is higher than in patiehts without (50%), there is no significant difference in survival, and again most patients (57%) die from extrahepatic disease.

Table 4. Randomized multicenter trial comparing local chemotherapy (group I) with local chemotherapy plus systemic treatment (group III): patient characteristics

	Group I		Group III		Total		
Randomized	26		26		52		
Evaluable	26		20		46		
Median age (years)	57		61		58		NS
Location of primary tumor							
Colon							
Ascending	1	(4%)	3	(15%)	4	(9%)	NS
Transverse	2	(8%)	0		2	(4%)	
Descending	2	(8%)	3	(15%)	5	(11%)	
Sigmoid	6	(23%)	7	(35%)	13	(28%)	
Rectum	15	(58%)	7	(35%)	22	(48%)	NS
Synchronous	5	(38%)	10	(50%)	22	(43%)	NS
Tumor volume							
Stage I < 25%	12	(46%)	3	(15%)	15	(33%)	P = 0.0314
Stage II 25%–75%	14	(54%)	17	(85%)	31	(67%)	
Extent of infiltration							
Solitary	3	(12%)	2	(10%)	5	(11%)	NS
Multiple	18	(66%)	13	(65%)	31	(66%)	
Diffuse	5	(19%)	5	(25%)	10	(22%)	
Anatomy of hepatic supply							
Normal	17	(65%)	17	(85%)	34	(74%)	NS
Abnormal	9	(35%)	3	(15%)	12	(26%)	
Dual catheter pump	3	(12%)	2	(10%)	5	(11%)	
CEA (Range 4–2760 ng/ml)							
> 10 ng	21	(81%)	17	(85%)	38	(83%)	NS
> 100 ng	15	(58%)	13	(65%)	26	(57%)	
AP (Range 89–944 U/dl)							
195 U/dl	15	(58%)	12	(60%)	27	(59%)	NS
> 400 U/dl	3	(12%)	6	(30%)	9	(20%)	

NS, not significant.
Participating centers: Chirurgische Universitätsklinik Mainz, Heinz-Kalk-Klinik Bad Kissingen, Chirurgische Universitätsklinik Ulm, Chirurgische Universitätsklinik München-Großhadern Städtisches Krankenhaus Kaiserslautern, Chirurgische Universitätsklinik Tübingen, Chirurgische Universitätsklinik Lübeck, Städtisches Krankenhaus Koblenz.

Table 5. Results of intra-arterial pump chemotherapy (continuous FUDR) of liver-only colorectal metastases in 542 patients; review of literature upto 1986 [16]

	Mean	Range
Response	59%	15%–88%
Time to progression	10	8–13
Survival time	14	10–18
Biliary sclerosis	9.4%	5%–33%
Extrahepatic recurrence	45%	23%–70%

Table 6. Results of intra-arterial chemotherapy of liver-only metastases of colorectal cancer compiled from 14 centers in German-speaking countries

	Chemo-embolization[a]	Continuous FUDR via pump	5-FU via port[a]	Chemo-perfusion of isolated liver	Total
n	58	115	126	16	647
Technical complications (%)	16	10	13	12	23
Toxic complications (%)	5	24	3	0	8.6
Response (%)	72	54	25	69	42
Months to progression	9.8	8.1	10.4	4.5	8.2
Survival (months)	17.2	16.6	13	11.5	12.9

[a] Various methods.
Participating centers: CU Bonn, Marienhospital Düsseldorf, CU Frankfurt, CU Gießen, CU Hannover, CU Heidelberg, CU Köln-Lindenthal, CU Mainz, CU München-Innenstadt, CU München-Großhadern, 1. CU Ulm, CU Wien, CJ Zürich.

The overall median survival time after pump implantation in this prospective control study is 17 months. When all publications in the USA up to 1986 were compiled, the mean of the median survival times of a total of 542 patients was found to be only 14 months (Table 5). This corresponds with the results of 14 specialized centers in German-speaking countries, where median survival time was 12.9 months in 647 patients treated using different modalities in different institutions (Table 6). Identical requests for data were made blindly from hospitals having major experience in this field with substantial numbers of patients.

These data make early reports on local chemotherapy of the liver [7,8] seem too optimistic from today's point of view. Treatment under controlled conditions, however, betters the results, as is shown in our own experience but also in a study randomizing patients to local and systemic treatment (median survival time 17 and 12 months respectively) [20]. Despite a significant advantage of the intra-arterial therapy in this trial, these important findings have to be confirmed in further studies, and local chemotherapy of liver-only metastases from colorectal cancer cannot yet be seen as obligate standard therapy.

The only convincing concept in the treatment of such metastases at the moment is resection of solitary or lobe-restricted tumors [21–23]. Whether adjuvant local chemotherapy of the resected liver is beneficial is unknown [24, 25].

In our own series it was possible to compare patients with curative resection (> 1 cm tumor-free margin), palliative resection, and no resection (Table 7). All of them had either adjuvant, or palliative local chemotherapy comprising continuous infusion of FUDR via a pump. There was a marked difference in survival (Table 7, Fig. 4); however, the groups were not comparable regarding the extent (tumor volume) and severity (alkaline phosphatase, carcinoembryonic antigen) of the disease.

Table 7. Influence of hepatic resection on the outcome of local chemotherapy of liver-only metastases

	Curative resection[a]		Palliative resection[a]		No resection[b]	
n	26		5		112	
Tumor volume						
I	21	81%	3	60%	36	32%
II	5	19%	2	40%	72	64%
III	0	0%	0	0%	4	4%
AP > 195 U/dl	8	31%	1	20%	54	48%
CEA > 20 ng/ml	11	42%	1	20%	76	68%
Solitary	16	62%	1	20%	9	8%
Bilateral	6	23%	4	80%	86	77%
Median time to live progression (months)	37		5		11	
Median time to extrahepatic progression (months)	30		18		10	
Death	7	35%	0	0%	76	68%
Survival after 24 months (%)	67		—		23	

[a]Adjuvant intra-arterial FUDR (0.2 mg/kg/day for 14 days every 4 weeks).
[b]Total results from Table 1.

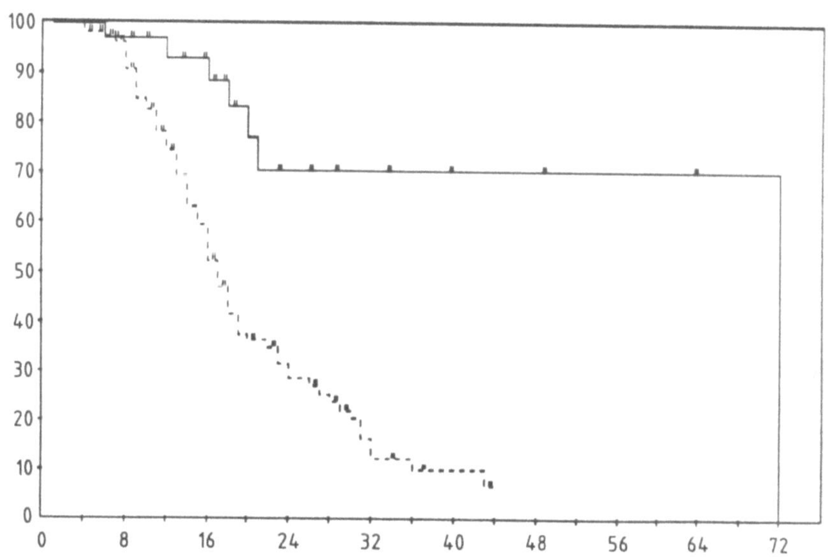

Fig. 4. Kaplan–Meier survival curves of patients with colorectal liver metastases and local chemotherapy: resection ($n = 31$, *continuous line*) vs no resection ($n = 112$, *broken-line*) (see Table 7)

Table 8. Influence of primary extrahepatic disease at the time of pump implantation on the outcome of local chemotherapy of the liver

	Hepatic and extrahepatic disease			Liver-only metastases	
n	19			112	
Tumor volume					
I	5	26%	36		32%
II	9	47%	72		64%
III	5	26%	4		4%
AP > 195 v/dl	9	47%	54		48%
CEA > 20 nm/ml	10	53%	76		68%
Solitary	4	21%	9		8%
Bilateral	14	74%	86		77%
Liver progression	5	26%	79		70%
Extrahepatic progression	4	21%	67		60%
Death	9	35%	76		68%
Median survival (months)	10	*		15	
Median time to extrahepatic progression (months)	4	**		11	
Median time to liver progression	5			10	

* $p = 0.02$.
** $p = 0.002$.

However, as few patients in the resection groups have died as yet, an even more pronounced prolongation of life following resection can be expected in a final analysis.

As demonstrated before, most patients die from extrahepatic disease, and the follow-up of our patients demonstrates that it is not possible with modern diagnostic means, including immunoscintiscan, to state with certainty that metastases are restricted to the liver. To evaluate the influence of primary extrahepatic disease on the outcome of local chemotherapy of the liver, 19 patients with minor extrahepatic disease which had been resected at the time of catheter implantation were compared with "hepatic only" patients (Table 8).

As would be expected, there is a significant reduction in median time to further extrahepatic progression, and consequently in survival (Fig. 5), with known extrahepatic disease, and the prognosis for these patients do not differ generally from that for patients with untreated liver metastases.

Table 9. Technical complications of local chemotherapy of the liver: comparison of port and pump patients

	Port	Pump
Number of patients	77	87
Observation time (patient months)	722	1295
Catheter occlusion	9%	4.6%
Septum damage	9%	0%
Catheter dislocation	8%	4.6%
Thrombosis of hepatic artery	10%	3.4%
Pump or pouch infection	6%	4.6%
Skin perforation	5%	3.4%
Pump dislocation	0%	2.3%
Pump malfunction	0%	2.3%
Overall	46%	23%

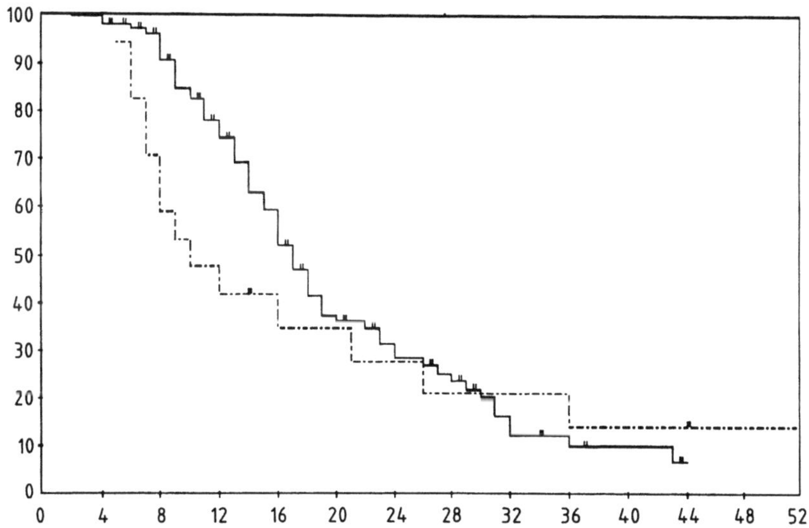

Fig. 5. Kaplan–Meier survival curves of patients with colorectal liver metastases: comparison between patients with disease restricted to the liver ($n = 112$, *continuous line*) and those with coexisting extrahepatic metastases ($n = 19$, *broken line*)

Finally, regarding [26] complications of the method, in our patients it is obvious that technical complications are twice as frequent with ports as with pumps, although the observation time is longer for the pumps (Table 9). Both groups had continuous FUDR treatment. A possible explanation is the reduced number of punctures and the continuous heparin clearance of the catheter in pump patients.

Although there were increased technical problems with earlier ports, we are now satisfied with Port-A-Cath (Pharmacia); the rate of treatment interruptions with ports, however, is still higher than with implanted pumps. This fact and the increased effectiveness with longer continuous infusion of FUDR favor totally implanted pumps. Our own calculation of treatment costs, including hospital stays because of port and pump complications and taking account of the higher initial price of pumps, shows a clear advantage for pumps.

Conclusions

In the palliative treatment of metastases of colorectal cancer restricted to the liver, intra-arterial administration of FUDR seems to be more effective than intravenous treatment. The average value for median survival time is 17 months. Most patients die with extrahepatic recurrence, which cannot be prevented by additional systemic 5-FU.

There is currently no alternative local chemotherapy superior to continuous FUDR. Administration of FUDR in a higher daily dose over a shorter period reduces local toxicity but is also less effective. The resection of liver metastases prolongs survival. Primary extrahepatic disease contraindicates intra-arterial infusion therapy. Due to the unsatisfactory overall results, further treatment modalities should be investigated only under controlled conditions.

References

1. Sullivan RD, Norcross JW, Watkins E (1964) Chemotherapy of metastatic liver cancer by prolonged hepatic-artery infusion. N Engl J Med 270:321–327
2. Oberfield RA, McCaffrey JA, Polio JP, Clouse ME, Hamilton T (1979) Prolonged and continuous percutaneous intraarterial hepatic infusion chemotherapy in advanced metastatic liver adenocarcinoma from colorectal primary. Cancer 44:414–423
3. Patt YZ, Mavligit GM, Chuang VP, Wallace S, Johnston S, Benjamin RS, Valdivieso M, Hersh EM (1980) Percutaneous hepatic arterial infusion (HAI) of mitomycin C and floxuridine (FUDR)—an effective treatment for metastatic colorectal carcinoma in the liver. Cancer 46:261–265
4. Reed ML, Vaitkevicius VK, Al-Sarraf M, Vaughn CB, Singhakowinta A, Sexon-Porte M, Izbicki R, Baker L, Straatsma GW (1981) The practicality of chronic hepatic artery infusion therapy of primary and metastatic hepatic malignancies. Cancer 47:402–409
5. Watkins E, Khazei AM, Nahra KS (1970) Surgical basis for arterial infusion chemotherapy of disseminated carcinoma of the liver. Surg Gynec Obstet 130:581–605
6. Ensminger WD, Roskowsky A, Raso V et al. (1978) A clinical-pharmacological evaluation of hepatic arterial infusions of 5-fluoro-2-deoxyuridine and 5-fluorouracil. Cancer Res 38:3784–3792
7. Balch CM, Urist MM, Soong SJ, McGregor M (1983) A prospective phase II clinical trial of continuous FUDR + regional chemotherapy for colorectal metastases to the liver using a totally implantable drug infusion pump. Ann Surg 198:567
8. Niederhuber JE, Ensminger W, Gyves J, Thrall J, Walker S, Cozzi E (1984) Regional chemotherapy of colorectal cancer metastatic to the liver. Cancer 53:1336–1343
9. Cohen AM, Schaeffer N, Higgins J (1986) Treatment of metastatic colorectal cancer with hepatic artery combination chemotherapy. Cancer 57:1115–1117
10. Johnson LP, Rikvin SE (1985) The implanted pump in metastatic colorectal cancer of the liver: risk versus benefit. Am J Surg 149:595–598

11. Shepard KV, Levin B, Karl RC, Faintuch J, DuBrow RA, Hagle M, Cooper RM, Beschorner J, Stablein D (1985) Therapy for metastatic colorectal cancer with hepatic artery infusion chemotherapy using a subcutaneous implanted pump. J Clin Oncol 3:161–169
12. Schwarz SI, Jones LS, McLune CS (1985) Assessment of treatment of intrahepatic malignancies using chemotherapy via an implantable pump. Ann Surg 201:560–567
13. Pettavel J, Morgenthaler F (1978) Protracted arterial chemotherapy of liver tumors – an experience of 107 cases over a 12 year period. Prog Clin Cancer 7:217–233
14. Gennari L, Poci R, Bozze HF Veronesi U (1982) Proposal for a clinical classification of liver metastases. Tumori 68:443–449
15. Lahr CJ, Soong SJ, Cloud G, Smith JW, Urist MM, Balch CM (1983) A multifactorial analysis of prognostic factors in patients with liver metastases from colorectal carcinoma. J Clin Oncol 1:720
16. Hottenrott C, Lorenz M (1987) Stellenwert der regionalen Chemotherapie der Leber. Z Gastroenterol 25:364–373
17. Hohn DC, Rayner AA, Economon JS, Ignoffo RJ, Lewis BJ, Stagg RJ (1986) Toxicities and complications of implanted pump hepatic arterial and intravenous floxuridine infusion. Cancer 57:465–470
18. Herrmann G, Lorenz M, Kirkowa-Reimann M, Hottenrott C, Hübner K (1987) Morphological changes after intraarterial chemotherapy of the liver. Hepato-gastroenterology 34:5–9
19. Balch CM, Christ MM (1984) Intraarterielle Chemotherapie mit einer implantierbaren Infusionspumpe bei Lebermetastasen colorectaler Tumoren und Hepatomen. Chirurg 55:485–493
20. Kemeny N, Daly J, Reichmann B, Geller N, Botet J, Odermann P (1987) Intrahepatic or systemic infusion of fluorodeoxyuridine in patients with liver metastases from colorectal carcinoma. Ann Intern Med 107:459–465
21. Hegemann G, Mühe E (1976) Extirpation von Metastasen. Langenbecks Arch Chir 342:261–268
22. Adson MA, von Herden JA (1980) Major hepatic resection for metastatic colorectal cancer. Ann Surg 191:576–583
23. Iwatsuki S, Shaw B, Storzl T (1983) Experience with 150 liver resections. Ann Surg 197:247–253
24. Kemeny MM, Goldberg D, Beatty JD et al. (1986) Results of a prospective randomized trial of continuous regional chemotherapy and hepatic resection as treatment of hepatic metastases from colorectal primaries. Cancer 57:492–498
25. Hodgson WJB, Friedland M, Ahmed T, Mittelmann A, Berman H, Katz S, Morgan J, Byrne D (1986) Treatment of colorectal hepatic metastases by intrahepatic chemotherapy alone or as an adjuvant to complete or partial removal of metastatic disease. Ann Surg 210:420–425
26. Jaffe BM, Donegan WL, Watson F, Spratt J (1968) Factors influencing survival in patients with untreated hepatic metastases. Surg Gynecol Obstet 127:I–II
27. Lorenz M, Hottenrott C, Seufert RM, Kirkowa-Reimann M, Encke A (1986) Dauerhafter intravenöser oder intrarterieller Zugang mit einer subkutan liegenden implantierbaren Infusionskammer. Dtsch Med Wochenschr 111:772–779

Regional Therapy of Hepatic Metastases: Prognostic Factors*

J.A. Stephenson, A.L. Wiley, Jr., G.W. Wirtanen, and G. Ramirez

Department of Human Oncology and Radiology, University of Wisconsin School of Medicine, 600 Highland Avenue, Madison, WI 53792, USA

Introduction

The liver is a common first site of metastatic involvement of colorectal adenocarcinoma. Progressive hepatic destruction and eventual failure to control metastatic disease are responsible for 25%–33% of the 20000 deaths each year in the United States from this tumor [6, 12]. Clinical trials utilizing systemic 5-fluorouracil (5-FU) for colorectal metastases began at the University of Wisconsin shortly after the discovery of this drug in 1957 [11]. Response rates of up to 20% were observed following systemic administration; however, systemic 5-FU administration was limited by toxicity, including mucositis, diarrhea, and myelosuppression. In addition, progressive hepatic disease continued to be a major cause of clinical failure [1, 4].

A program of intra-arterial continuous infusion of 5-FU was initiated in 1964 with the goal of reducing systemic toxicity while maximizing the drug concentration delivered to the liver [3]. Utilization of percutaneous transbrachial catheterization techniques allowed for selective catheterization of the common or proper hepatic artery [14]. Patients remained ambulatory by means of a portable pump (Cormed, Medina, New York, USA) and infusion lasted for as long as several months (typically 21 days). 5-FU doses of 15–30 mg/kg/day were routinely administered, with the most common side effects being abdominal cramping and nausea (20%), diarrhea (20%), stomatitis (10%), and low-grade myelosuppression (20%). Acute side effects generally resolved with a break of several days. Thromboembolic events, drug toxicity, and septic episodes occurred in less than 5% of patients treated with 3-week infusion courses. Intrahepatic 5-FU therapy was reported in 293 patients with measurable disease. The tumors of 75% of these patients had progressed on systemic 5-FU. Intrahepatic infusions produced a 55% response rate by objective clinical and radiographic measurements. This was 2–3 times the response rate observed with most systemic administration schemes [2].

Due to the magnitude of the problem, multiple investigators have analyzed the natural history and treatment of colorectal hepatic metastases with surgery,

*This work was supported in part by the National Cancer Institute through USPHS grant 5-P02-CA-06295RAD.

R. Jakesz/H. Rainer (Eds.)
Progress in Regional Cancer Therapy

chemotherapy, radiotherapy, and combinations of these modalities [5, 8]. No one method of therapy has clearly emerged as the treatment of choice for hepatic metastases. One reason for this may be the general heterogeneity of the patient population entered into therapeutic clinical trials.

Methods

We report the results of a prospective randomized trial in which 38 patients with hepatic metastases from colorectal adenocarcinoma underwent percutaneous transbrachial catheterization of the common or proper hepatic artery. Patients received a 21-day continuous intra-arterial 5-FU infusion (20 mg/kg/day × 4 days, 15 mg/kg/day × 17 days). After a 14-day break, 19 patients went on to receive external hepatic irradiation (25.5 Gy divided into 17 fractions) by anteroposterior and posteroanterior photon fields with megavoltage linear accelerators. All patients received weekly systemic maintenance 5-FU (600 mg/m^2).

Results

Patients who had hepatic infusion and irradiation had a median survival of 6 months, compared with 8 months for patients treated by infusion alone ($p = 0.106$). A response was defined as a reduction of over 50% in the sum of the products of the perpendicular diameters of measurable lesions on liver/spleen scintigraphy, arteriography, or computerized tomography for at least 3 months. Patients treated by infusion and irradiation had a 37% response rate compared with 50% for infusion alone.

Toxicity was higher for those patients who were randomized to receive hepatic infusion and irradiation: 42% developed diarrhea, 26% abdominal pain or cramping. Those patients treated with infusion alone had a 17% incidence of diarrhea and abdominal cramping. Several patients in each group were found to have guaiac-positive stools or stomatitis. Three patients had gastrointestinal bleeding – one bleeding esophageal varices, two hematemesis. In all three cases the complication resolved within several days of stopping aterial drug infusion. One death was attributed to small bowel toxicity several days after completion of arterial infusion. There were no infections of catheterization site during infusion.

Patient Heterogeneity

Patients were prospectively categorized according to a number of prognostic criteria. The sex ratio was nearly 1:1 for those patients who received infusion and irradiation, and survival was roughly equal in males and females in this group. Only two female patients were randomized to infusion alone. These two women had a mean survival of 32 months compared with 9 months for female patients treated with infusion and irradiation. In spite of these small numbers, female patients who received infusion alone were found to have significantly improved survival ($p = 0.0441$).

Table 1. Percent hepatic replacement with tumor (PHR) and median survival

PHR	Number of patients CT + RT n(%)	CT n(%)	Total n(%)	Median survival (months) CT + RT	CT
75%–100%	9 (47)	14 (78)	23/33 (70)	6	8
50%–74%	2 (11)	1 (6)	3/33 (9)	7	1
25%–49%	6 (32)	0 (0)	6/33 (18)	10	—
0%–24%	1 (5)	0 (0)	1/33 (3)	6	—
Unknown	1 (5)	3 (17)	—	0	6

CT + RT, infusin and irradiation; CT, infusion alone.

A performance status of less than 0 on the ECOG scale was observed in 43% of patients. No difference in median survival was observed in patients with poor performance status ($p = 0.315$). Sixty-eight percent of patients had progressive tumor growth during previous systemic therapy (generally 5-FU). No differences in survival were observed in these patients ($p = 0.909$). Elevated liver function tests were observed in 65% of patients. The addition of hepatic irradiation did not influence these patients' survival ($p = 0.129$). The median age of all patients was 60 years. No survival differences were observed between younger and older patients ($p = 0.237$).

A number of investigators recommend staging hepatic metastases by percent hepatic replacement by tumor (PHR). There is evidence that patients with minimal tumor burden survive longer than those with a large tumor burden. Pattavel has proposed the Lausanne classification, which has three stages (0%–25%, 25%–75%, and 75%–100%) and takes into account liver function tests and symptomatology [13]. Gennari has proposed a more complicated system which has three stages (0%–25%, 25%–50%, and 50%–100%) and is modified by a number of factors, including the number of metastases, synchronicity, infiltration, liver function, and cirrhosis [10]. Since PHR is the major component of these staging systems, patients with stage III (75%–100%) disease and measurable hepatomegaly were specifically selected for the current series in an effort to eliminate bias which might be introduced if too many patients had a low tumor burden. Table 1 demonstrates that 70% of patients had 75%–100% PHR. The only appreciable subset with less tumor burden comprised six patients treated with infusion plus irradiation: their duration of survival was marginally longer (10 months), but the difference was not statistically significant ($p = 0.156$).

Histologic Grading

Pathologic review of surgical and biopsy specimens was performed so that histologic tumor grade could be analyzed. Dukes and Bussey, in their 1958 article analyzed the survival of 2097 surgically treated patients by tumor grade. Patients with well-differentiated (grade I) tumors displayed 77.3% corrected 5-year survival,

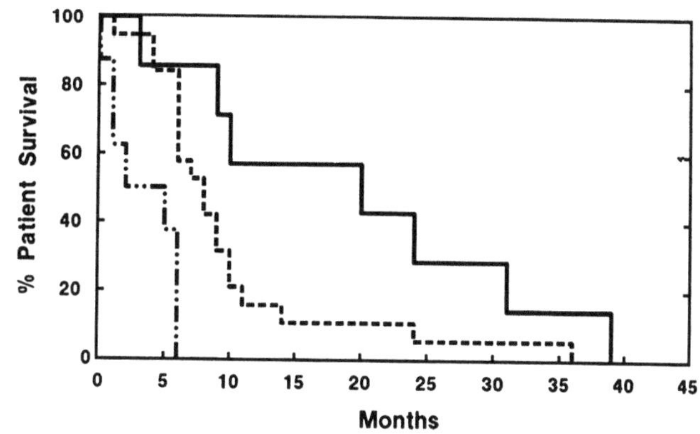

Fig. 1. Survival according to tumor grade. ——grade I; - - - grade II; -··- grade III. $p = 0.0001$, log rank test

compared with 60.6% for moderately well differentiated (grade II) tumors and 28.9% for poorly differentiated (grade III) tumors [9]. In this current series, regardless of therapy, patients with grade I tumors had a median survival of 20 months, against 8 months for grade II and 5 months for grade III (Fig. 1). Grade I histology was highly predictive of a favorable response to regional therapy ($p = 0.0001$).

Tumor Vascularity

Hepatic metastases derive their major blood supply from the hepatic artery [7]. We analyzed the angiograms of 540 patients with hepatic metastases from a variety of primary tumors and expressed the findings on a scale of 0–4 +, where 0 represented no vascularity documented, 1 + was neovascularity minimally greater than normal hepatic vascularity, 4 + was extreme hypervascularity with dense arrangement of vessels and intense tumor stain, and 2 + and 3 + were intermediate between 1 + and 4 +.

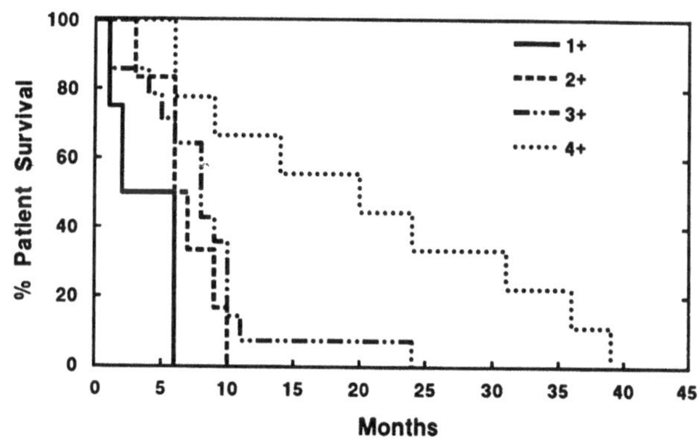

Fig. 2. Survival according to tumor vascularity. $p = 0.0009$; log rank test

In this current series of 38 patients, four had 1+ vascularity and median survival of 6 months, six had 2+ vascularity and median survival of 7 months, 14 had 3+ vascularity and median survival of 8 months, and nine had 4+ vascularity and median survival of 20 months (Fig. 2). Tumor vascularity of 4+ on angiography was highly predictive of a favorable response to regional therapy ($p = 0.0009$).

Patients with both grade I histology and 4+ vascularity exhibited median survival of 27.5 months ($p = 0.0019$). Both grade ($p = 0.034$) and vascularity ($p = 0.036$) were significant in the presence of each other. The addition of irradiation did not affect the significance of either vascularity ($p = 0.0449$) or grade ($p = 0.0312$).

Conclusion

Death from hepatic metastases continues to be a major clinical problem. Numerous studies have been undertaken of various treatment modalities to maximize palliation and survival. Patients with hepatic metastases of colorectal primary tumors represent a heterogeneous group. Unfortunately, conclusions have frequently been based on small patient numbers with little attention paid to identifying subgroups of patients who might benefit from more aggressive regional therapy. Staging the percent hepatic replacement by tumor has been proposed by some investigators as a way of rendering treatment results comparable. It appears from this current study that tumor vascularity and histologic grade are important prognostic variables which deserve consideration when regional therapeutic modalities are being investigated. Our 25 years' experience with percutaneous catheterization of the common or proper hepatic artery and prolonged continuous infusion of 5-FU suggests that this technique can be safely performed, that toxicity is less than with systemic administration, and that this therapy is capable of providing consistently high response rates in patients who have progressive disease, whether previously treated with systemic chemotherapy or not.

References

1. Ansfield FJ, Klotz J, Nealon T, Ramirez G, Minton J, Hill G, Wilson W, Davis H, Cornell G (1977) A phase III study comparing the clinical utility of four regimens of 5-fluorouracil. Cancer 39:34–40
2. Ansfield FJ, Ramirez G, Davis HL, Wirtanen GW, Johnson RO, Bryan GT, Manalo FB, Borden EC, Davis TE, Esmaili M (1975) Further clinical studies with intrahepatic arterial infusion with 5-fluorouracil. Cancer 36:2413–2417
3. Ansfield FJ, Ramirez G, Skibba J, Bryan GT, Davis HL Jr, Wirtanen GW (1971) Intrahepatic arterial infusion with 5-fluorouracil. Cancer 28:1147–1151
4. Ansfield FJ, Schroeder JM, Curreri AR (1962) Five years' clinical experience with 5-fluorouracil. JAMA 181:295–299
5. Barone RM, Byfield JE, Goldfarb PB, Frankel S, Ginn C, Greer S (1982) Intra-arterial chemotherapy using an implantable infusion pump and liver irradiation for the treatment of hepatic metastases. Cancer 50:850–862
6. Bergmark S, Hofstrom L (1969) Natural history of primary and secondary malignant tumors of the liver. Cancer 23:198–204

7. Breedis C, Young G (1949) Blood supply of neoplasms of the liver. Fed Proc 8:351–354
8. Byfield JE, Frankel SS, Sharp TR, Hornbeck CL, Callipari FB (1985) Phase I and pharmacologic trial of 72-hour infused 5-fluorouracil and hyperfractionated cyclical radiation. Int J Radiat Oncol Biol Phys 11(4):791–800
9. Dukes CE, Bussey HJR (1958) The spread of rectal cancer and its effect on prognosis. Br J Cancer 12:309–320
10. Gennari L, Doci R, Bozzetti F, Veronesi U (1982) Proposal for a clinical classification of liver metastases. Tumori 58:443–449
11. Heidelberger C (1957) Fluorinated pyrimidines, a new class of tumor inhibitory compound. Nature 179:663
12. Jaffe B, Donegan W, Watson F (1968) Factors influencing survival in patients with untreated hepatic metastases. Surg Gynecol Obstet 127:1–11
13. Pettavel J, Leyveras S, Douglas P (1984) The necessity for staging liver metastases and standardizing treatment response criteria. The case of secondaries of colorectal origin. In: Van de Velde CJH, Sugarbaker PH (eds) Liver metastasis. Basic aspects, detection and management. Nijhoff, Boston, pp 154–168
14. Wirtanen GW (1973) Percutaneous transbrachial artery infusion chatheter techniques. Am J Roentgenol 117:696–700

Regional Therapy with 5-Fluorouracil: Dependence of Systemic Concentrations on the Infusion Rate

A. Schalhorn, G. Peyerl, W. Heinlein, and W. Wilmanns

Medizinische Klinik III, Klinikum Großhadern, Ludwig Maximilian-Universität, Marchioninistraße 15, 8000 München 70, FRG

Introduction

Hepatic artery infusion (HAI) with floxuridine (FUDR) has resulted in CT-confirmed remission rates between 30% and 50% in patients with liver metastases from colorectal cancer [5]. In spite of very optimistic reports, especially that by Balch and Urist [1], long-term results are less impressive. There is a relatively high risk of local toxicity due to chemical hepatitis and/or sclerosing cholangitis [3]. A high proportion of the patients will eventually develop extrahepatic metastases, and no statistically significant survival advantage for patients treated by HAI with FUDR has yet been demonstrated [4, 6].

Taking into account the high costs of regional FUDR therapy, its hepatic toxicity and its unsatisfactory long-term results, new efforts are being undertaken to make effective use of 5-fluorouracil (5-FU), with or without folinic acid, in the regional chemotherapy of colorectal liver metastases. The rationale is the very low hepatic toxicity of 5-FU and the easy administration using simple low-priced port systems connected with the arterial catheter. To gain better insight into the mechanisms of HAI with 5-FU, we measured systemic (venous) 5-FU blood levels during and after regional chemotherapy.

We wanted to anwser the following questions: Can any 5-FU be detected in the systemic circulation? And if so, what is the influence of the infusion rate on the systemic concentration?

Patients and Methods

Twenty-six patients with isolated but inoperable liver metastases from colorectal cancer were treated with regional 5-FU. 5-FU doses of 750–2000 mg were infused via the hepatic artery over a period of 60–240 min with infusion rates ranging from approximately 5 to 20 mg 5-FU/min. At different time intervals during and in some cases after HAI, venous blood was taken to determine the 5-FU levels by means of a simple HPLC method [7, 8]. After deproteinization, 20-μl aliquots were injected onto a 5-μm Shandon ODS Hypersil column (250 mm × 4.5 mm). Elution was

R. Jakesz/H. Rainer (Eds.)
Progress in Regional Cancer Therapy

performed with 10 mM phosphate buffer pH 3.93. With UV detection at 266 nm, the lower detection limit is in the range of 3–5 μM 5-FU [7].

Results

In all 26 patients, with infusion rates between 5 and 33 mg/min, 5-FU could be demonstrated in the systemic circulation. Depending on the infusion rate, steady-state systemic 5-FU levels ranged from 2.4 to 144 μM. With 5-FU infusion rates up to 10 mg/min, maximum systemic 5-FU levels were $< 26\ \mu M$, and with flow rates > 15 mg/min they were always above 50 μM. The dependence of steady-state systemic 5-FU levels on the arterial infusion rate is well demonstrated in single patients: One patient received a constant 5-FU dose of 1000 mg over different periods. If this dose was infused rapidly over 30 min, the systemic serum 5-FU increased to 100 μM. With lower infusion rates the steady-state 5-FU levels remained lower. If the 5-FU infusion time was 60 min, for example, the systemic 5-FU reached a maximum of 10 μM, and with a further extension of the infusion time up to 90 min, the systemic 5-FU levels peaked at only 4 μM.

Figure 1 shows the systemic 5-FU levels of a patient treated with increasing 5-FU doses via HAI. When 1000 mg 5-FU was infused over 90 min, a flow rate of 11 mg/min, systemic 5-FU levels of 25 μM were measured. Flow rates of 17 mg/min (1500 mg/90 min) and 22 mg/min (2000 mg/90 min) resulted in serum 5-FU levels of 76 and 144 μM respectively. Thus, in spite of the regional application, HAI with 5-FU can result in high, possibly toxic systemic 5-FU concentration (see below)

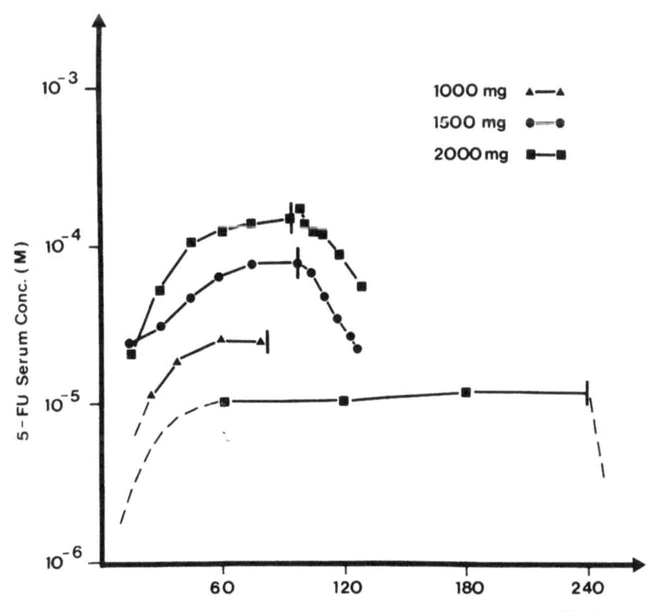

Fig. 1. Course of serum 5-FU in a male patient with HAI of different 5-FU doses over different periods

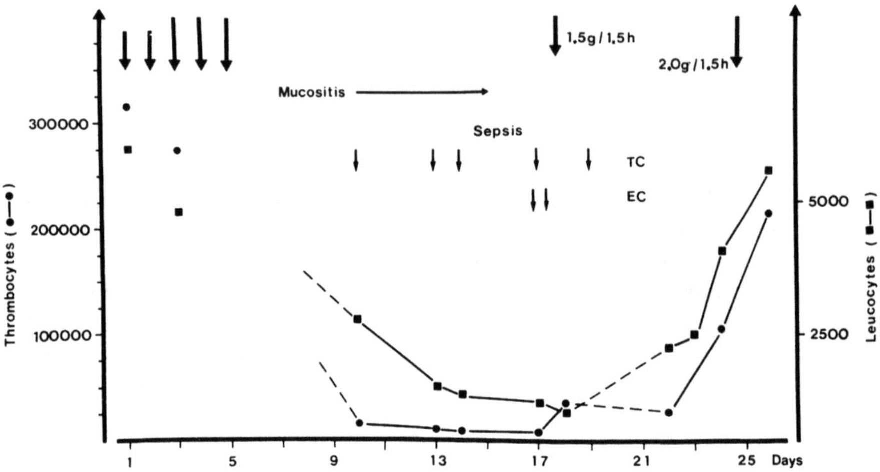

Fig. 2. Clinical course of a patient treated with a 5-day course of high 5-FU doses (1500 and 2000 mg) at high infusion rates (17 and 22 mg/min respectively). *TC*, thrombocyte concentrate; *EC*, erythrocyte concentrate

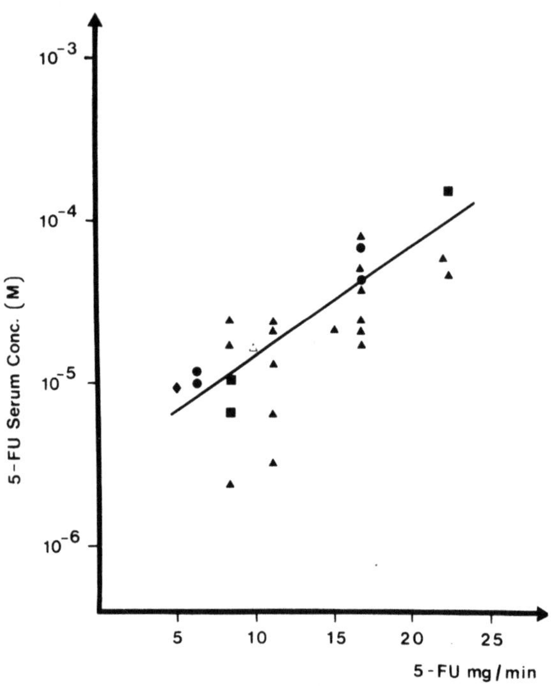

Fig. 3. Steady-state systemic levels of 5-FU depending on the 5-FU HAI rate. Total 5-FU dose: ◆ 750 mg; ▲ 1000 mg; △ 1250 mg; ● 1500 mg; ■ 2000 mg

when high doses are infused over short periods. When the flow rate was reduced to 8 mg/min and the infusion of 2000 mg 5-FU thus extended to 4 h, only low systemic 5-FU levels, in the range of 10 μM, were detected.

The influence of high 5-FU doses and high flow rates is illustrated in Fig. 2. With a 5-day course of 1500 or 2000 mg 5-FU administered intra-arterially over 90 min, the high systemic 5-FU levels mentioned above were detected. Some days post treatment the patient experienced severe toxicity. Leukocyte and thrombocyte counts rapidly dropped below 1000/μl and 25000/μl respectively. In addition to severe mucositis, the clinical course was complicated by an *E. coli* sepsis. With intensive supportive care the critical phase could be overcome, and starting from day 21 all pathologic findings normalized rapidly.

During the next treatment course the total 5-FU dose remained unaltered, but the flow rate was diminished considerably to 8 mg/min. With an infusion time of 4 h for 2000 mg 5-FU, steady-state systemic 5-FU levels now peaked at only 10 μM. Therefore, this treatment course with a high total 5-FU dose of 10 g caused no toxic side effects.

The pharmacokinetic results were similar for all other patients and treatment courses investigated so far. Due to different 5-FU doses and infusion times, the 5-FU flow rates ranged from 5 to 33 mg/min. As demonstrated in Fig. 3, steady-state systemic 5-FU levels differed considerably, but increased with increasing arterial 5-FU flow rates. Roughly a fourfold increase of 5-FU infusion rate from 5 to 20 mg/min caused a tenfold increase in the mean systemic 5-FU level from approximately 7 to 70 μM.

Discussion and Conclusion

The results presented here demonstrate that hepatic 5-FU clearance is always incomplete. In all cases of 5-FU HAI with flow rates > 5 mg/min, steady-state systemic 5-FU levels were $> 2\,\mu M$. As we did not measure the 5-FU concentrations in the hepatic artery and the hepatic veins, we cannot say exactly how much 5-FU is cleared in the liver. According to Ensminger and Gyves [2] the hepatic extraction of FUDR is high, between 69 and 99%, explaining the near absence of systemic toxicity during FUDR therapy. These authors state a lower hepatic extraction rate for 5-FU, only 19%–51% of the total dose infused intra-arterially. Our data presented here indirectly confirm the results of Ensminger and Gyves: due to the low hepatic 5-FU extraction, the mean 5-FU serum concentration increased from 7 to 70 μM when the 5-FU infusion rate was raised from 5 mg/min to 20 mg/min.

The rather high systemic 5-FU concentrations achieved during HAI are of considerable clinical importance. First, in contrast to regional FUDR therapy, high doses of 5-FU (> 1500 mg) at high flow rates (> 15 mg/min) can cause severe systemic toxicity, at least in some individuals. Second, even during regional 5-FU therapy systemic 5-FU levels can be achieved which might be effective against extrahepatic metastases from colorectal carcinoma. Further studies are necessary to define more clearly the role of 5-FU dosage and flow rate and the possible influences of liver size and metastatic involvement. We believe, however, that regular monitoring of 5-FU serum levels during HAI provides the possibility of preventing undesired systemic toxicity in individual patients. In addition, appropriate doses and infusion rates of 5-FU can be selected which result in high regional concentrations and effective but tolerable concentrations in the systemic circulation.

Summary

During hepatic artery infusion (HAI) with 5-fluorouracil (5-FU) we studied the course of systemic serum 5-FU concentrations. 5-FU dosages ranging from 750 to 2000 mg were infused over 30–240 min, representing an infusion rate of 5–33 mg/min. In spite of the regional application, systemic 5-FU levels ranged from 2.4 to 144 μM. With 5-FU infusion rates up to 10 mg/min, maximum systemic 5-FU levels were $< 26\ \mu M$, and with flow rates > 15 mg/min they were always above 50 μM. Though steady-state serum 5-FU levels differed considerably, a clear dependence on the infusion rate could be demonstrated: a fourfold increase of the 5-FU infusion rate from 5 to 20 mg/min resulted in a tenfold increase of steady-state systemic 5-FU levels from 7 to approximately 70 μM. These findings reveal incomplete hepatic 5-FU clearance. As we demonstrated in an individual patient, higher 5-FU doses (> 1500 mg) at high infusion rates (> 15 mg/min) result in high systemic 5-FU levels and bear the risk of severe systemic toxicity. The pharmacokinetic conditions prevailing during HAI provide the possibility of selecting dosages of 5-FU which result in high regional concentrations and effective but tolerable concentrations in the systemic circulation.

References

1. Balch CM, Urist MM (1984) Intraarterielle Chemotherapie mit einer implantierbaren Infusionspumpe bei Lebermetastasen colorectaler Tumoren und Hepatomen. Chirung 55: 485–493
2. Ensminger WD, Gyves J (1983) Clinical pharmacology of hepatic arterial chemotherapy. Semin Oncol 10:1876–1882
3. Hohn D, Rayner AA, Economou JS, Ignoffo RJ, Lewis BJ, Stagg RJ (1986) Toxicities and complications of implanted pump hepatic arterial and intravenous floxuridine infusion. Cancer 57:465–470
4. Hohn D, Stagg R, Friedman M, Ignoffo R, Rayner A, Hannigan J, Lewis B (1987) The NCOG randomized trial of intravenous versus hepatic arterial FUDR for colorectal cancer metastatic to the liver. ASCO Proc 6(333):85
5. Kemeny N, Daly J, Oderman P, Shike M, Chun H, Petroni G, Geller N (1984) Hepatic artery pump infusion: toxicity and results in patients with metastatic colorectal carcinoma. J Clin Oncol 2:595–600
6. Kemeny N, Daly J, Reichman B, Geller N, Botet J, Oderman P (1987) Intrahepatic or systemic infusion of fluorodeoxyuridine in patients with liver metastases from colorectal carcinoma. Ann Intern Med 107:459–465
7. Peyerl G (1986) Pharmakokinetik von 5-Fluorouracil bei der isolierten Leberperfusion und sein chromatographischer Nachweis im Serum. Dissertation, München
8. Schalhorn A, Peyerl G, Denecke H (1988) Pharmacokinetics of 5-fluorouracil during isolated liver perfusion. Reg Cancer Treat 1:21–27

Combined Regional and Systemic Chemotherapy in Hepatic Metastases of Colorectal Carcinoma: Continuous IA Vs Simultaneous IA/IV FUDR Infusion

F. Safi, R. Roscher, R. Bittner, K.H. Link, and H.G. Beger

Abteilung für Allgemeine Chirurgie, Universität Ulm, Steinhövelstraße 9, 7900 Ulm, FRG

Introduction

The recent literature shows that response rates of liver metastases to regional intra-arterial perfusion of fluorodeoxyuridine (FUDR) can vary between 43% and 80%. On the basis of these rates, median survival time is said to range between 17 and 26 months [1,3]. Rates from 42% to 75% are reported for the occurrence of extrahepatic metastases after the beginning of regional chemotherapy. It is the formation of metastases that causes the death of most patients, even those responding to regional chemotherapy [1,3].

The role of continuous hepatic artery infusion of the liver and of adjuvant systemic therapy is a related area of investigation. This study addresses both issues in a randomized prospective fashion in an attempt to establish the efficacy of both regional and systemic FUDR therapy of isolated hepatic metastases from colorectal cancer. The aim of adjuvant systemic therapy is to delay or prevent the occurrence of extrahepatic metastases during the course of regional chemotherapy. This report also reviews the response and survival of patients with colorectal carcinoma involving the liver in our pilot and randomized study.

Patients and Methods of Treatment

All patients with histologically confirmed adenocarcinoma of the colon and rectum who had measurable hepatic metastases were eligible for the study.

The first 20 patients, who received a hepatic artery infusion of FUDR, were entered in a phase 1 (pilot) study. An additional 50 patients were stratified by primary tumor stage (TNM classification) and the proportion of the liver involved ($< 50\%$ vs $> 50\%$) and were then randomly assigned before surgery to receive either intrahepatic or intrahepatic and systemic therapy. The IA group ($n = 25$) were treated only intra-arterially. In the IA/IV group ($n = 25$), IA/IV dual-catheter Infusaid pumps (Shiley Infusaid, Inc., Norwood, Mass., USA) were implanted. The characteristics of the patients are shown in Table 1. The patients in the two randomized groups were comparable with respect to the stage of primary tumor ($p < 0.2$), metastatic spread in the liver ($p < 0.8$), age, and sex (both $p < 0.7$). The

R. Jakesz/H. Rainer (Eds.)
Progress in Regional Cancer Therapy

Table 1. Regional chemotherapy in liver metastases of colorectal carcinoma: patient characteristics

	Total	Pilot study	*Randomized study* IA	IA/IV
	$n = 70$	$n = 20$	$n = 25$	$n = 25$
Age (years)[a]	36–77	36–77	46–70	36–77
Average	57	57	57	57
Sex[a]				
Female	$n = 28$	$n = 10$	$n = 10$	$n = 8$
Male	$n = 42$	$n = 10$	$n = 15$	$n = 17$
Primary tumor stage[b]				
T1–3 N0	31 (44%)	6	10	15
T1–3 N1	33 (48%)	13	11	9
T1–3 N2	6 (8%)	1	4	1
Volume of metastases[c]				
< 50% of liver volume	49 (70%)	12	19	18
> 50% of liver volume	21 (30%)	8	6	7

[a] $p < 0.7$.
[b] $p < 0.2$.
[c] $p < 0.8$.

serum concentrations of carcinoembryonic antigen (CEA) and liver enzymes (median values) were also similar in the two groups.

All patients had abdominal laparotomy to position the catheter and the Infusaid pumps. Extrahepatic intra-abdominal tumor spread was found in three patients of the IA/IV group, and in another patient of this group lung metastases were overlooked preoperatively. The placement of the catheter in the hepatic artery was performed according to the technique of Balch and Urist [1]. The arterial catheter was also implanted in the common hepatic artery in those patients in whom an IA/IV pump had been placed. The venous catheter was inserted into the testicular or the ovarian vein and positioned at the junction of the inferior vena cava.

The FUDR therapy was initiated on the 8th to the 14th day after pump implantation. FUDR was the basic chemotherapeutic agent (0.2 mg/kg/day) administered in 2-week cycles alternating with double-distilled water. This was the dosage administered to all patients who had IA pumps. Patients with IA/IV pumps were given FUDR at a dose of 0.3 mg/kg/day, during the course of which 0.21 mg/kg was perfused intra-arterially (regionally) and 0.09 mg/kg intravenously (systemically). Thus, the regional dose was the same in both the IA and IA/IV groups.

Monitoring the Regional Chemotherapy

The following parameters were investigated preoperatively and at 2-week intervals postoperatively: blood count, liver parameters (γ-glutamyl transferase, γ-GT; glutamic pyruvic transaminase, GPT; alkaline phosphatase, AP; lactate dehydrogenase, LDH; bilirubin), and CEA. Arterial computer tomographic angiography (angio-CT) of the liver, sonography of the abdomen, and chest X-ray were performed preoperatively and every 3 months during treatment.

We refer to "chemical hepatitis" when a twofold increase of two liver parameters above the normal values (glutamic oxaloacetic transaminase, GOT; GPT; APH; γ-GT) is present. Biliary sclerosis indicates bilirubinemia and strictures of the biliary tract; intrahepatic tumor progression and metastases in the liver hilum must be excluded.

Statistics

Patient survival time from the time of pump implantation was calculated in accordance with the Kaplan-Meier method. The test of Mantel and Haenzel was used for comparison of survival rates. For categorical variables, the chi-square test and Fisher's exact test were used [4].

Results

FUDR Toxicity

Gastroduodenitis or duodenal ulcers occurred in 18% of the patients. In 47%, a twofold elevation of the liver parameters was observed (chemical hepatitis). In an additional 16 patients (23%), a sclerosing cholangitis could be detected by means of endoscopic retrograde cholangiopancreatography or percutaneous transhepatic cholangiography after elevation of serum bilirubin. Sclerosing cholangitis was reversible in only seven patients after discontinuation of the FUDR therapy. Seven patients (two in the IA group and five in the IA/IV group) complained of diarrhea that was severe enough for them to be hospitalized for hydration. Stomatitis was seen in four patients (one in the IA and three in the IA/IV group). Myelosuppression, alopecia, and emesis did not occur with either treatment. Gastrointestinal tract and liver toxicities were not significantly different between the IA and the IA/IV treated patients ($p > 0.1$).

Response

With regard to the development of intrahepatic metastases, the control angio-CT scans showed a complete response in 20 patients, i.e., there were no detectable metastases. The median duration of the complete response was 15 months (range 6–39 months). Another 20 patients showed a reduction in metastatic volume by more than 25%. The median duration of this partial response was 14 months (range 6–27 months). In 12 other cases no change in metastatic size was seen on CT scan. Progression of metastases in spite of FUDR therapy was observed in 18 patients.

Some 88% of the patients ($n = 62$) had a CEA level of over 4 ng/ml before the beginning of chemotherapy. Regression of more than 60% (compared to the starting values) was seen in 24% of the patients and normalization in 30% of the entire group. In accordance with the identical intra-arterial dose, the metastases in the two randomized groups responded equally to regional chemotherapy. Remission of the metastases (partial or total) was evident in 56% ($n = 14$) of the patients in the IA group and in 64% ($n = 16$) of those in the IA/IV group. A decrease of the serum CEA level exceeding 60% or normalization of the serum levels during the course of treatment could be found in 14 patients of the IA group (56%) and in 18 patients of the IA/IV group (72%).

Extrahepatic Spread of Metastases During Therapy

The median observation time for the patients in our pilot study was 19 months (range 3–47 months). In this period of time, 15 patients developed extrahepatic metastases (75%). During treatment, 72% ($n = 17$) of the IA and 29% ($n = 6/21$) of the IA/IV group developed extrahepatic metastases in the lung, peritoneum, and bone. This spreading of the carcinoma was found at a median duration of observation of 16 months. The difference between the two groups was significant at that point in time ($p < 0.01$).

Survival

The 1-year survival rate of the entire population ($n = 70$) was 80%, the 2-year rate 45%, and the 3-year rate 20%. The median survival time was 20 months (Fig. 1). No difference in survival rate was found between the IA and the IA/IV treated patients ($p < 0.7$).

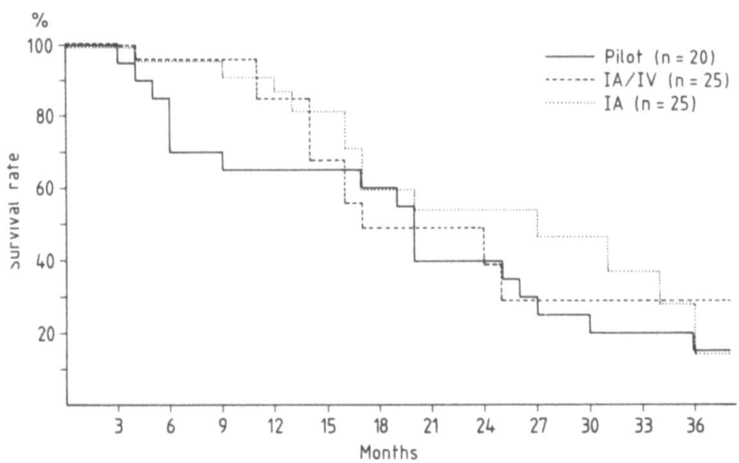

Fig. 1. Survival in the pilot study and in the two arms of the randomized study

Discussion

The efficacy of hepatic artery infusion of FUDR using an implantable pump for the treatment of hepatic metastases from primary colorectal carcinoma has yet to be proven in a prospective, randomized study. The value of this type of therapy has been controversial, mainly because of the development of extrahepatic metastases responsible for the patient's death [1, 3, 5].

The IA and IA/IV arms were well matched regarding important prognostic factors (metastatic spread in the liver), as well as by other prognostic variables such as initial liver function tests and CEA serum levels. The IA and IA/IV groups responded similarly to chemotherapy (56% vs 64% as assessed by CT and 56% vs 72% by tumor marker criteria). This observation is not surprising, since, prior to the onset of therapy, the metastatic spread in the two groups had been identical and the FUDR intra-arterial dose amounted to 0.2 mg/kg/day in the IA resp. IA/IV treated patients. The adjuvant IV therapy appeared to prevent extrahepatic spread of metastases, which tends to occur during regional therapy. Extrahepatic tumor progression occurred in 75% of the patients in the pilot study, 72% of those in the randomized IA group, and only 29% (6/21) of those in the randomized IA/IV group. This difference is statistically significant ($p < 0.01$). The literature reports high rates of extrahepatic metastasis after the onset of regional chemotherapy. Balch and Urist state an incidence of 42% [1], Niederhuber et al. 73% [3], Rothmund et al. 77% [4], and Kemeny et al. 56% [2].

Using the pump catheter system and treatment with FUDR, Balch and Urist [1] achieved a median survival time of 26 months, and Niederhuber et al. [3] reported 25 months from the diagnosis of metastases and 18 months from the beginning of the therapy. The response rate in their studies was above 80%. In all of our patients ($n = 70$) the response rate was 57% and 54% by CT and tumor marker criteria respectively. The median survival time of these patients is 20 months from pump implantation.

We found no improvement of short-term survival in the two randomized groups during the 36-month observation period. Later, 30% of the IA/IV patients were found to survive beyond 36 months.

References

1. Balch CM, Urist MM (1984) Intraarterielle Chemotherapie mit einer implantierbaren Infusionspumpe bei Lebermetastasen colorektaler Tumoren und Hepatomen. Chirung 55:485–493
2. Kemeny N, Daly J, Reichmann B, Geller N, Botet J, Oderman P (1987) Intrahepatic or systemic infusion of fluorodeoxuridine in patients with liver metastases from colorectal carcinoma. Ann Intern Med 107:459–465
3. Niederhuber JE, Ensminger W, Gyves J, Thrall J, Walker S, Cozzi E (1984) Regional chemotherapy of colorectal cancer metastatic to the liver. Cancer 53:1336–1343
4. Ramm B, Hofmann G (1982) Biomathematik. Enke, Stuttgart
5. Rothmund M, Brückner R, Keller E, Quint B, Knuth A, Schicketanz KH (1986) Regionale Chemotherapie bei Lebermetastasen kolorektaler Karzinome mit implantierbaren Druckpumpen. Dtsch Med Wochenschr 17:652–658

Intra-arterial Chemotherapy of Liver Metastases

F. Sturba, R. Bencivenga, A. Paccapelo, L. Zepponi, M. Bonsignori, F. Mingolla, A. Cavicchi, F. Feliciotti, and S. Occhipinti

Oncology Department, Regional Hospital Torrette, 60020 Ancona, Italy

Introduction

The liver is the first and most frequent site of metastasis of gastroenteric cancer; in 10% of cases such pathology is already present at the time of diagnosis of the primary neoplasm. Metachronous metastases occur within 5 years in 20% of patients. The average survival in the case of untreated liver metastases from large bowel cancer is 6–8 months; 30%–35% of such patients are alive after 6 months and only 15%–18% at 1 year [1, 5]. The therapy of liver metastases is based on surgical resection, systemic chemotherapy, and radiotherapy, but response rates are not good. Surgery is indicated only when the liver presents a single metastasis or multiple metastases confined to one lobe; this is the case in 20%–25% of patients, and no more than 5%–10% cases are actually operable. Chemotherapy is indicated in all other patients, and because systemic treatment is ineffective many groups throughout the world have been using locoregional intra-arterial therapy [6, 9].

Material and Methods

Since March 1980 we have been conducting a series of studies of locoregional intra-arterial chemotherapy of liver metastases from large bowel cancer. At first the proper hepatic artery was catheterized percutaneously via the femoral artery (Seldinger's technique) [10]. Since January 1986 we have been conducting a study, utilizing totally implantable systems, to evaluate the effect of hepatic artery infusion (HAI) in patients with liver metastases from already resected large bowel cancer. The therapeutic protocol stipulates the insertion through a laparotomy, of a totally implantable apparatus delivering drug directly into the proper hepatic artery rather than via the gastroduodenal artery. The device can be implanted at the time of the operation on the primary neoplasm, or later in the case of metachronous metastasis. The totally implantable system has two different parts:

1. A subcutaneous drug reservoir with a silicon membrane (volume 0.4 ml), normally placed in the presternal subcutaneous region
2. A Silastic catheter, connected with the reservoir and the proper hepatic artery (or portal vein)

R. Jakesz/H Rainer (Eds)
Progress in Regional Cancer Therapy

The therapeutic program can start 15–20 days after the insertion of the implantable system. The portal vein is used if the arterial route is not feasible. It is important to heparinize the system weekly.

Therapy Scheme

For infusion of the liver we use mitomycin C 10 mg/m^2 over 24 h followed by 5-fluorouracil 15 mg/kg/day continuously up to a total dose of 4000 mg. The interval between cycles is 4 weeks, and we generally administer at least six cycles. So for the study includes 16 patients (11 evaluable for response): eight males and eight females with an average age of 59 years (range 47–74 years). In 11 patients the access was via the hepatic artery, in the remaining five cases via the portal vein. The average proportion of the liver involved by the metastases was 36% (range 10%–70%).

Results

For evaluating the results we used the following parameters: *Objective response*: Two of the 11 evaluable patients exhibited partial responses (average duration 5 months), and in the other nine cases progression of the disease was halted for an average of 4 months. We observed no progressions within 3 months of therapy.
Performance status: The performance status was good for all patients, showing excellent tolerance of the therapy. Their quality of life was good, normally right up to the time of death. *Survival*: Nine of the 11 evaluable patients were alive after 6 months and six after 12 months; this latter result is better than that in untreated controls (55% vs 15%–18%). The average survival of our treated patients from the time of diagnosis of hepatic metastases, was 13.36 months at the time of writing; four were still alive with an average survival of 14.75 months.
Toxicity: 6 patients had no side effects at all. Two others presented moderate leukopenia. Six patients displayed local toxicity, and in one of these cases we stopped the treatment because of severe gastralgia during the second cycle. Finally, two patients showed combined systemic and local toxicity. One of them had very severe acute hepatic necrosis followed by severe pancreatitis, and we stopped the treatment during the second cycle.
Local reaction to implant: Nine patients showed moderate erythema and seroma near the site of access to the implantable system, but we were able to resolve this pathology easily without stopping the therapy. Fracture of the catheter during the second cycle of therapy in one case and the detachment of the catheter from the reservoir in two other cases (during the first two cycles) determined interruption of the therapy (drop-out patients).

Finally, in one case we observed occlusion of the subcutaneous reservoir but after surgical exchange the new reservoir functioned well.

Conclusions

Our good results (in agreement with reports in the literature) and the excellent quality of life of patients with totally implantable systems encourage continuation of the trial. Another very interesting fact is that with the implantable systems we no longer observed the side effect we encountered frequently with the percutaneous catheter used in our earlier trial:

- Detachment of the catheter from the artery
- Bleeding often severe, at the site of percutaneous access to the catheter
- Infections.

References

1. Wallace S, Chuang VP (1982) Transcatheter management of the cancer patient. In: De Vita V (ed) Cancer principles and practise of oncology. Lippincott Philadelphia, pp 1862–1877
2. Gennari L, Doli R, Orefice S et al. (1982) Trattamento infusionale locoregionale dei tumori primitivi e metastatici del fegato. Meeting multidisciplinare su: "Tecniche speciali di somministrazione di farmaci antiblastici", Verona, 15 Oct 1982
3. Lokich J et al. (1981) Concomitant hepatic radiation and intraarterial fluorinated pyrimidine therapy. Cancer 48:2569–2574
4. Friedman M et al. (1979) Combined modality therapy of hepatic metastasis. Cancer 44:906–913
5. Ramming KP, Sporks FC, Eilber FR et al. (1979) Il trattamento delle metastasi epatiche. Aggiorn Oncol Clin V (4): 323–341
6. Oberfield RA (1979) Prolonged and continuous percutaneous intraarterial hepatic infusion chemotherapy in advanced metastatic liver adenocarcinoma from colorectal primary. Cancer 44:414–423
7. Ansfield FJ, Ramirez G, Davis HL et al. (1971) Further clinical studies with intrahepatic arterial infusion with 5-FU. Cancer 36:2413–2417
8. Ansfield FJ, Ramirez G et al. (1971) Intrahepatic arterial infusion with 5FU. Cancer 28:1147–1151
9. Cady B, Oberfield RA (1974) Regional infusion chemotherapy of hepatic metastases from carcinoma of the colon. Am J Surg 127:220–227
10. Sturba F, Bonsignori M, Rossi G et al. (1984) Chemioterapia infusionale intraepatica per via percutanea delle metastasi epatiche da neoplasie del tratto gastro-enterico. Paper presented at congress "Terapie d'avanguardia in oncologia", Ancona, 28–29 Sept 1984

Current Standards and Limits in Treatment of Hepatic Metastases

R. Bittner, F. Safi, K.H. Link, and H.G. Beger

Abteilung für Allgemeine Chirurgie, Universität Ulm, Steinhövelstraße 9, 7900 Ulm, FRG

Introduction

Hepatic metastases represent a common site of dissemination for a number of primary malignancies, partly because of the dual blood supply, the large blood flow, and the receptive environment of the hepatic parenchyma. Primary gastrointestinal neoplasms are particularly prone to develop hepatic metastases. Most of what we have learned concerns the treatment of metastases of colorectal cancers, because these primary lesions are very common, usually can be removed widely along with regional lymphatic spread, and thus often give rise to resectable hepatic metastases that appear to be the only residual sites of growth.

Experience with surgical treatment of hepatic metastases from primary lesions other than colorectal cancer is too limited for determinant analysis. Moreover, in the cases of dissemination of these tumors – especially those of the stomach or pancreas – to the liver, there are usually locoregional recurrences or additional extrahepatic tumor sites. For these reasons we will confine ourselves to hepatic metastases of colorectal carcinomas.

Clinical Importance and Natural History

Today, in the Federal Republic of Germany, colorectal neoplasms are the second most frequent cancers in men and are nearly as frequent as breast cancer in women. Whereas in 1952 only about 10000 patients died of colorectal cancer, by 1979 this number had more than doubled. Hepatic metastases are evident in 25%–30% of patients at the time of operation. Some 40%–70% of patients with progressive disease have liver involvement. After curative resection of the primary tumor, the liver is the most frequent site of relapse (40%–50% of patients).

In evaluating the effect of different treatment regimens, it is most important to know the true natural history of entirely untreated liver metastases, the standard against which the effectiveness of any treatment should be measured. But what is known about the natural course of disease? Here the problems begin. Untreated controls cannot be used in prospective studies when the value of some kind of

R. Jakesz/H Rainer (Eds.)
Progress in Regional Cancer Therapy

treatment has been established. There is therefore a need to study the natural history retrospectively, but many difficulties are associated with studies of this kind.

In the past, most tumors were comparatively advanced at the time of discovery; today, however, modern diagnostic tests permit early detection of hepatic metastases. For this reason alone, patients in more recent studies should survive longer from diagnosis than those in earlier series. Second, it is difficult in retrospective studies to get information on important prognostic factors such as the percentage of liver replaced by tumor, the performance status of the patient, liver function, and the presence or absence of intra-abdominal extrahepatic disease. Third, inadequate methods for estimating survivals are used in some investigations. One thing, however, remains clear: the presence of hepatic metastases confers an extremely poor prognosis – and the most important determinant of survival is the extent of liver involvement by the tumor. According to Wood et al. [1], patients with widespread metastases involving both lobes of the liver have a 1-year survival rate of only 5.7%. Patients with several metastases confined to one segment or lobe of the liver have a rate of 27%, while in those with solitary metastases the figure is as high as 60%.

Rationale for Surgical Treatment

The most important single point is that the liver is the sole site of initial tumor recurrence in up to 30% of patients with metastatic disease. Furthermore, today the risks involved in hepatic resection for metastatic tumors are relatively low. Two reasons for the considerable improvement in operative results over the past 20 years can be mentioned: First, improved understanding of the anatomical organization of the liver, especially of the distribution of the portal pedicles and hepatic veins, allows not only safe major resections such as right or left hemihepatectomy, but also the extirpation of single segments without the removal of large amounts of normal parenchyma [2]. Second, surgical techniques have improved. Above all, bleeding can be controlled more effectively. Complete hemostasis is now possible without large, traumatizing sutures; in this way necrosis and infection are avoided. As a result of this progress, one question is becoming more and more important: "As more surgeons are now able to remove large portions of the liver with little risk, it is time to ask not how such surgery can be done safely but when it should be done – or when it is worthwhile" [3].

Summarizing the results shown in Table 1, surgical resection of all hepatic metastases can yield a 5-year survival rate of about 25% among resectable patients. Analyzing a number of factors that might predict failure or success of therapy, Adson [3] found three statistically significant determinants of prognosis which might guide the choice of treatment: (a) the sex of the patient, (2) the locoregional stage of the primary lesion, and (3) the presence or absence of extrahepatic metastases. In addition, several authors [4, 7, 9–11] have found survival to be limited after resection of more than three hepatic metastases, and some now consider such multiplicity to be an absolute contraindication for resection with curative intent.

In summary, surgical therapy can bring about long-term survival in some cases, but the proportion of patients with hepatic metastases who will benefit from hepatic

Table 1. Results of resection for hepatic metastases of colorectal cancer

Reference	No. of patients	Operative deaths	Survival rate (%)		
			3 years	5 years	10 years
Foster [4]	259	13 (5.0%)	44	22	—
Logan et al. [5]	19	1 (5.0%)	—	21	—
Adson et al. [3]	141	2 (1.4%)	—	25	—
Kortz et al. [6]	16	1 (6.0%)	54	—	—
Fortner et al. [7]	65	5 (8.0%)	57	—	—
Butler et al. [8]	62	6 (10.0%)	50	34	21

resection is small – about 5%–10%. The greatest enhancement of survival is achieved in the case of female patients with Dukes A or B primary tumors and no extrahepatic metastases whose hepatic disease is limited to a single lobe. The great majority of patients are candidates for other treatment regimens, for example systemic chemotherapy.

Systemic Chemotherapy of Liver Metastases

The interpretation of the results of systemic chemotherapy is difficult, because of inconsistent definitions of tumor "response" and difficulties in determining tumor size reproducibly. 5-Fluorouracil (5-FU) is the standard chemotherapeutic agent. Various dosage schedules for 5-FU have been proposed in the effort to maximize clinical response and reduce toxicity. Patients receiving continuous infusion or bolus 5-FU therapy have shown overall response rates of 15%–25% [12]. The results of systemic treatment with other chemotherapeutic agents – fluorodeoxyuridine (FUDR), CCNU, mitomycin C – alone or in combinations, have not been significantly better than those of 5-FU alone.

In summary, however, regardless of the response rates observed with systemic treatment, prolongation of survival by comparison with untreated patients has not been demonstrated with confidence. Disappointment with the results of systemic chemotherapy has led researchers to evaluate such other modes of treatment as direct chemotherapy of the liver.

Rationale for Regional Chemotherapy

The rationale for regional chemotherapy of the liver is that the hepatic artery is the major source of blood supply to hepatic metastases. The advantages of this kind of therapy are as follows:

1. It delivers higher concentrations of drug directly to the liver tumor avoiding the dilutional effect that otherwise occurs with systemic intravenous injection.
2. Many antimetabolites are more effective as antineoplastic agents when administered by chronic infusion than by pulse injection.

3. There is significant hepatic extraction of many drugs when they are injected directly into the hepatic circulation; this is particularly true of FUDR. This further increases the concentration of the drug at the site of the liver neoplasm.
4. Continuous infusion results in lower peak serum concentrations, thus decreasing toxicity such as marrow depression.

Numerous researchers have found measurable tumor response rates of 50%–70%. Unfortunately, using the Seldinger technique of external catheter placement, complications, notably hepatic artery thrombosis and catheter displacement, have been observed in up to 80% of the patients. To eliminate these complications and to avoid patients having to stay in the hospital, a totally implantable infusion pump has been introduced [13].

This implantable pump delivery system offers several potential advantages: reduction in catheter-related sepsis, ease of drug administration, and greater patient acceptance without bulky external devices.

Recent studies have reported response rates of between 30% and 90% (Table 2). This wide range can be explained by differences in response criteria, which vary among researchers, and by the heterogeneity of the patients treated with hepatic arterial infusion. The median duration of survival has been approximately 16 months.

Despite the reductions in technical, infectious, and mechanical complications with the use of an implantable pump, substantial complications of chronic hepatic arterial infusions continue to occur (Table 3). In our experience the most serious complication is sclerosing cholangitis, which occurs in up to 20% of patients. We have found that all patients treated with continuous regional chemotherapy show a gradual increase in alkaline phosphatase. In a significant number of patients, therapy has to be discontinued because of intra- and extrahepatic bile duct strictures. Continued jaundice requiring extrahepatic duct drainage has been noted

Table 2. Results of clinical trials of continuous regional chemotherapy (nonrandomized)

Author(s)		Reference(s)	No. of patients	Response rates	Median survival (months)
Ensminger/Niederhuber	1981/1984	[14, 15]	93	91%[b]/79%[c]	19
Barone	1982	[16]	18	56%[c]	12
Cohen	1983	[17]	50	54%[c]	12
Balch	1983/1986	[18, 19]	110	83%[a]	18
Daly	1984	[20]	40	41%[c]	?
Shepard	1985	[21]	62	33%[c]	17
Kemeny, N.	1986	[22]	42	69%[b]	15
Patt	1986	[23]	29	52%[c]	12
Hottenrott	1987	[24]	52	75%[a]	16
Present Authors	1987		64	54%[b]	18

[a] CEA↓ > 33%.
[b] CEA↓ 50%.
[c] 50% reduction in volume on X-ray.

Table 3. Hepatic and systemic toxicity encountered in continuous regional therapy of hepatic metastases ($n = 64$, Ulm)

Complication	n	%
Diarrhea	3	4.0
Ulcer	4	6.0
Stomatitis	8	12.0
Gastritis	10	15.6
Biliary sclerosis	15	23.0
Chemical hepatitis	37	57.0

by some authors in up to 10% of patients. Thus the improvement in tumor response achieved by higher arterial drug concentrations has been offset by the increase in treatment-related complications.

In view of the fact that up to now no definite proof of the benefit of regional hepatic chemotherapy has been afforded, we close this rather pessimistic assessment of the current situation with a quotation from our colleagues at the Mayo Clinic [25]. They point out the three main problems in the treatment of hepatic metastases:

To try to show what might be good or bad to do is not easy because our view of cancer is so clouded. Fulfillment of our obligations is precluded by three aspects of our ignorance:

1. Our blindness to a tumor's real stage,
2. Our limited knowledge of the natural history of disease, and
3. Lack of really good clinical determinants of prognosis derived from treated patients.

References

1. Wood CB, Gillis CR, Blumgart LH (1976) A retrospective study of the natural history of patients with liver metastases from colorectal cancer. Clin Oncol 2:285–288
2. Bismuth H (1982) Surgical anatomy and anatomical surgery of the liver. World J Surg 6:3–9
3. Adson MA (1987) Resection of liver metastases—when is it worthwhile? World J Surg 11:511–520
4. Foster JH (1978) Survival after liver resection for secondary tumors. Am J Surg 135:389–394
5. Logan SE, Meier SJ, Ramming KP, Morton DL, Longmire WP Jr (1982) Hepatic resection of metastases colorectal carcinoma: a ten year experience. Arch Surg 117:25–28
6. Kortz WJ, Meyers WC, Hanks JB et al. (1984) Hepatic resection for metastatic cancer. Ann Surg 199:182–186
7. Fortner JG, Silva JS, Golbey RB, Cox EB, Maclean BJ (1984) Multivariate analysis of a personal series of 247 consecutive patients with liver metastases from colorectal cancer. Ann Surg 199:306–316

8. Butler J, Attiyeh FF, Daly JM (1986) Hepatic resection for metastases of the colon and rectum. Surg Gynecol Obstet 162:109–113
9. Cady B, Oberfield RA (1974) Regional infusion chemotherapy of hepatic metastases from carcinoma of the colon. Am J Surg 127:220–227
10. Ekberg H (1986) Colorectal liver cancer, resection and regional chemotherapy. Thesis. Bulletin no. 61, Department of Surgery, Lund University, Lund, Sweden pp 1–62
11. Iwatsuki S, Byers W, Starzl TE (1983) Experience with 150 liver resections. Ann Surg 197:247–253
12. Kemeny N (1983) The systemic chemotherapy of hepatic metastases. Semin Oncol 10:148–158
13. Balch CM, Urist MM (1983) Vollständig implantierbare Infusions-pumpe. Eine neue Behandlungsmöglichkeit für ausgewählte Patienten mit Lebertumoren. Dtsch med Wochenschr 26:1008–1013
14. Ensminger W, Niederhuber J, Dakhil S, Thrall J, Wheeler R (1981) Totally implanted drug delivery system for hepatic arterial chemotherapy. Cancer Treat Rep 65:393–400
15. Niederhuber JE, Ensminger W, Gyves J, Thrall J, Walker S, Cozzi E (1984) Regional chemotherapy of colorectal cancer metastatic to the liver. Cancer 53:1336–1343
16. Barone RM, Byfield JE, Goldfarb PB, Frankel S, Ginn S, Greer S (1982) Intraarterial chemotherapy using an implantable infusion pump and liver irradiation for the treatment of hepatic metastases. Cancer 50:850–862
17. Cohen AM, Kaufman SD, Wood WC, Greenfield AJ (1983) Regional hepatic chemotherapy using an implantable drug infusion pump. Am J Surg 145:529–533
18. Balch CM, Urist MM, Soong SJ, McGregor M (1983) A prospective phase II clinical trial of continuous FUDR regional chemotherapy for colorectal metastases to the liver using a totally implantable drug infusion pump. Ann Surg 198:567–573
19. Balch CM, Urist MM (1986) Intraarterial chemotherapy for colorectal liver metastases and hepatomas using a totally implantable drug infusion pump. In: Recent Results Cancer Res 100:234–247
20. Daly JM, Kemeny N, Oderman P, Botet J (1984) Long-term hepatic arterial infusion chemotherapy: anatomic considerations, operative technique and treatment morbidity. Arch Surg 119:936–941
21. Shepard KV, Levin B, Karl RC, Faintuch J, DuBrow RA, Hagle M et al. (1985) Therapy for metastatic colorectal cancer with hepatic artery infusion chemotherapy using subcutaneous implanted pump. J Clin Oncol 3:161–169
22. Kemeny N, Reichman B, Oderman P, Daly J, Geller N (1986) Update of randomized study of intrahepatic (H) vs systemic (S) infusion of fluorodeoxyuridine (FUDR) in patients with liver metastases from colorectal carcinoma (CRC). Proc Am Soc Clin Oncol 5:47
23. Patt YZ, Boddie AW, Charnsangavej C, Ajani JA, Wallace S, Soski M et al. (1986) Hepatic arterial infusion with fluoxuridine and cisplatin: overriding importance of antitumor effect versus degree of tumor burden as determinants of survival among patients with colorectal cancer. J Clin Oncol 4:1356–1364
24. Hottenrott C, Lorenz M (1987) Stellenwert der regionalen Chemotherapie der Leber. Z Gastroenterol 25:364–373
25. Wagner JS, Adson MA, van Heerden JA, Adson MH, Ilstrup DM (1984) The natural history of hepatic metastases from celorectal cancer. A comparison with resective treatment. Ann Surg 199:502–508

Degradable Starch Microspheres in Intra-arterial Tumor Treatment: An Overview

L. Håkansson and H. Starkhammar

Department of Oncology, University Hospital of Linköping, 581 85 Linköping, Sweden

Introduction

Tumor drug concentration may be of major importance for the cytotoxic effect of cytostatic drugs [10]. Therefore, intra-arterial (IA) administration has been used in an attempt to improve upon the often poor results of systemic chemotherapy. Hepatic artery infusion of colorectal liver metastases mainly with 5-fluorouracil (5-FU) or floxuridine (FUDR), has significantly increased the remission rate [e.g. 12, 21].

The total body clearance of a drug and the blood flow of the infused artery have a major influence on regional drug delivery [6].

To improve treatment efficacy, reduced flow during IA chemotherapy of liver tumors has been obtained by ligation of the artery, by exteriorized tourniquets around the artery, by inflating balloon-tipped catheters, or by injection of particles of various materials. The effect of permanent arterial ligation alone is of short duration, mainly due to the rapid appearance of collateral arteries [1]. Infusion of FUDR into the ligated artery resulted in about 50% objective tumor regression in several studies but was associated with a high frequency of liver abscesses [1]. The liver function tests were usually only minimally affected. However, total embolization with nondegradable material (e.g., Ivalon) causes a deterioration in the liver function [3].

Degradable starch microspheres (DSM; Spherex, Pharmacia, Sweden) might further improve the efficacy and safety of regional chemotherapy because a temporary vascular blockade of distal arteries can be induced under controlled conditions.

Degradable Starch Microspheres

Characteristics

Degradable starch microspheres have a mean diameter of 45 μm and induce vascular occlusion at the arteriolar level. They are degraded by serum alpha-amylase and have an in vitro half-life of about 20–30 min at 37°C in human serum.

R. Jakesz/H Rainer (Eds.)
Progress in Regional Cancer Therapy

Due to a high degree of cross-linkage at the periphery, the microspheres maintain their size and shape during degradation until they finally collapse and blood flow is restored [14].

DSM efficiently reduce the arterial blood flow, as has been demonstrated in several in vivo studies of different animal species and humans using various methods, e.g., the electromagnetic flow probe technique [14, 23] angiography [7], and xenon wash-out [9]. Vital microscopy of the exteriorized hamster cheek pouch demonstrated the microsphere passage within the vascular tree [24].

Simultaneous injection of various substances and cytostatic drugs with DSM gave a high regional concentration in normal tissues and tumors [15, 17]. In agreement with these results, a reduced systemic concentration has been demonstrated for several cytostatic drugs (e.g., carmustine, doxorubicin, mitomycin C) when given IA together with DSM [7, 11, 22].

Optimal Use

The great individual variation in size and vascularity of liver tumors and the occurrence of A-V shunts, explains the observed variation in the effects of DSM in tumor patients when standard doses were given [7, 11]. In patients with minimal metastatic disease, total vascular occlusion could be achieved with the injection of about 300 mg DSM, whereas in large, highly vascularized tumors more than 3000 mg was needed [19].

As the objective must be to treat all the tumor and avoid back-flow of microspheres along with the cytostatic drug to unintended areas, the dose of DSM obviously has to be individualized.

Monitoring of Treatment

A method for the monitoring of DSM treatment should give the following data during treatment sessions: (1) the effect of DSM on vascular occlusion, (2) the effect of DSM on the degree of retention of the coinjected labeled marker/drug, and (3) the degree of arteriovenous (A-V) shunting. A simple method (Spherex monitoring system, SMS) for monitoring the dose of DSM was developed. It is based upon changes in the kinetics of the passage of a labeled marker, $^{99}Tc^{m}$-methylene diphosphonate ($^{99}Tc^{m}$-MDP) through the target organ when coinjected with the microspheres. Details of this procedure have been described [19].

Percutaneously or surgically inserted catheters were placed in the proper hepatic artery distal to the gastroduodenal artery. The passage of $^{99}Tc^{m}$-MDP through the liver was continuously registered by a sodium iodide scintillation detector placed over the clavicular area because the count rates after injection of $^{99}Tc^{m}$-MDP rapidly achieved a plateau and also because radioactivity lodged in the top of the ipsilateral lung could be registered. This enabled determination of A-V shunting as passage of $^{99}Tc\text{-}^{m}$-labeled macroaggregated albumin ($^{99}Tc^{m}$-MAA) through the target organ to the lungs. The $^{99}Tc^{m}$-MAA passage was expressed in arbitrary units. The detector was connected via a single-channel analyzer to a counter and a computer.

Registration of Data

A typical recording of a treatment session is shown in Fig. 1. In the cumulative curve, the increase in systemic concentration after each injection (marked by a vertical line) is demonstrated. The substracted curves are more detailed and show only the registration from the most recent injection together with the reference curve. These curves showed that two kinetic parameters—the passing fraction (PF) and the rate at which the marker passed through the target organ (marker flow rate, MFR)— were influenced by the microspheres.

In order to calibrate the system, $^{99}Tc^{m}$-MDP was given alone, without DSM or cytostatic drug, in two reference injections and the average increase in the count rates was recorded and taken to represent 100% passage of the marker. The cytostatic drug, mixed with DSM and 20–40 MBq of ^{99}Tc-^{m}-MDP was given in repeated injections after the reference injections. The content of each syringe was vigorously mixed before injection and injected manually over a period of 20 s. The intervals between the injections were generally 2–3 min. The increase in count rates after each injection of DSM was expressed in percent (PF) of the mean of the two reference values (Fig. 1).

The MFR was calculated as the maximum count rate increase per 10 s, in percent of the total increase after the injection. MFR was expressed in arbitrary units (Fig. 1). The reduction of MFR of the first or second DSM injection compared to the mean of the reference injections was called marker flow rate reduction (MFRR)

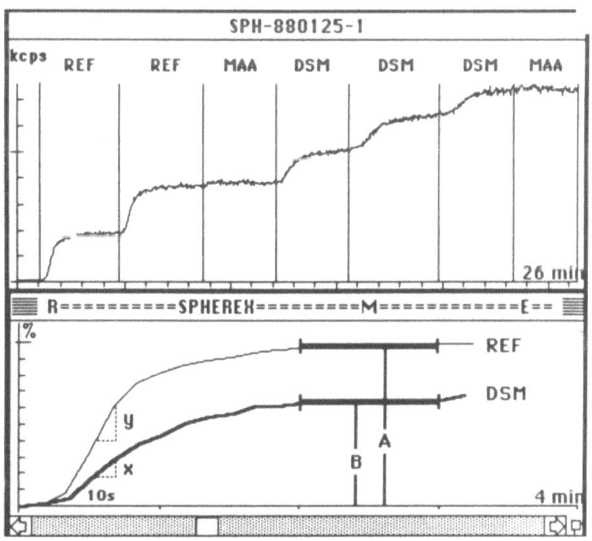

Fig. 1. A typical recording of a treatment session. The cumulative curve (*upper panel*) shows increase in systemic concentration after each injection (*vertical lines*). The subtracted curve (*lower part*) shows a DSM injection and calculation of the kinetic parameters. $PF = B/A \times 100$; MFR for reference $(REF) = y\,(\max)/A \times 100$; MFR for DSM injection $= x\,(\max)/B \times 100$; $MFRR = (MFR_{REF} - MFR_{DSM\,1,2})/MFR_{REF} \times 100$. *MAA*, macroaggregated albumin

and was expressed in percent of the MFR of the references. All injections used for the calculation of MFRR were given over a period of 20 s.

The effect of DSM on the passage of the labeled marker was analyzed in 50 patients, each given 300 mg of DSM over 20 s in their first DSM injection during the first treatment session. PF was 70% or less in 12 patients, between 71% and 80% in 19 patients, and 81% or more in another 19 patients.

Results

Correlation Between SMS Parameters and Angiographic Findings

Twenty-three patients were studied with liver angiography before and immediately after Spherex treatment. The lowest PF registered and the highest MFRR of the first or second DSM injection were used in this study. The degree of vascular blockade achieved by the microspheres (after administration of the total dose of DSM) was classified as flow not reduced (no visible effect on the passage of the contrast medium) or flow reduced (prolonged passage time, backflow, or complete cessation of the arterial blood flow). As demonstrated in Table 1, in 6/12 patients with a PF of more than 65% there was no reduction of blood flow, whereas all 11 patients with PF below 65% had reduced flow. MFRR identified five of the six patients who, despite a PF of above 65%, had flow reduction angiographically.

Importance of the Portal Flow for the Passage of an Intra-arterially Injected Labeled Marker Through the Liver

Surprisingly, the PF value was never reduced to below 30%–40%, even if complete or nearly complete cessation of the blood flow was demonstrated angiographically. This apparent paradox was studied further in a pig liver model. The portal flow turned out to be of great importance for the passage of low-molecular-weight substances injected into the hepatic artery. In one series of experiments a reference

Table 1. Correlation between SMS parameters and angiographic findings

Kinetic parameters of the labeled marker	Angiographic findings: Flow not reduced (*n*)	Angiographic findings: Flow reduced (*n*)
PF > 65% all patients	6	6
MFRR < 25	3	1
> 25	3	5
PF < 65% all patients	0	11
MFRR < 25	0	1
> 25	0	10

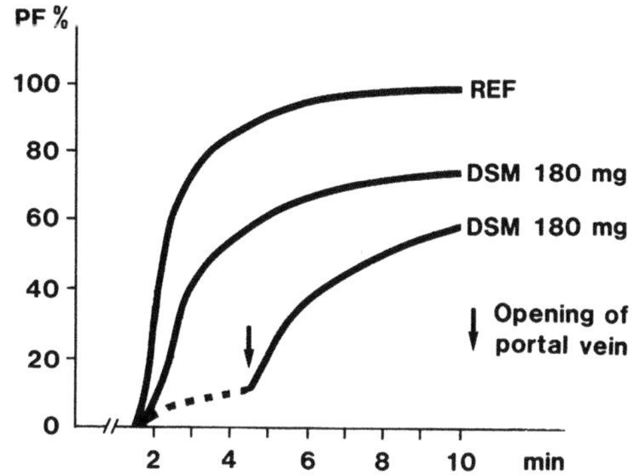

Fig. 2. Effect of DSM and the portal blood flow on the passage of a labeled marker injected into the hepatic artery

dose of $^{99}Tc^{m}$-MDP was injected as described above. The portal vein was then clamped and a second injection of the marker was given. The passage into the systemic circulation was reduced to about 70% as long as the portal vein was clamped, but when this vessel was reopened the remaining amount of the marker entered the systemic circulation.

When 180 mg of DSM mixed with $^{99}Tc^{m}$-MDP was injected with the portal flow intact and the arterial perfusion maintained, about 75% of the marker passed the liver in 120 s (Fig. 2). However, when the portal flow was stopped and these experiments repeated, 180 mg of DSM reduced the passage of $^{99}Tc^{m}$-MDP to about 20% [20]. This might explain why the passage of $^{99}Tc^{m}$-MDP coinjected with DSM could not be reduced below 30%–40% in tumor patients even if the arterial flow was almost completely blocked.

Tumor Selective Uptake

As the portal flow drained a considerable fraction of an intra-arterially injected, labeled marker substance even when the arterial flow was completely blocked by DSM [20], it can be assumed that cytostatic drugs lodged distal to the microspheres in normal liver tissue will be washed out. Thus, cytostatic drugs will be retained by the microspheres in liver tumor tissue but not in normal liver tissue. Tumor-selective, increased uptake of doxorubicin in VX-2 liver tumors in the rabbit and of FUDR in human liver tumors was achieved when these drugs were given together with DSM [17]. Similarly, DSM increased the tumor concentration of $^{99}Tc^{m}$-DTPA by a mean of 1.71-fold, whereas the hepatic exposure was increased by 1.46-fold [16]. These experiments have now been extended, using the SMS, for $^{99}Tc^{m}$-MDP and doxorubicin in a rat liver tumor model (Cooke and Chang, next chapter).

Retention in Vascular and Tissue Compartments

The increased retention of low-molecular-weight substances induced by coinjection of starch microspheres can be due either to trapping in blocked vessels or to increased first-passage extraction. To analyze which mechanism prevails, the effect of the microspheres on the retention of $^{99}Tc^{m}$-MDP was compared with $^{99}Tc^{m}$-labelled erythrocytes. About 100% of the $^{99}Tc^{m}$-labelled erythrocytes passed through the liver in eight of 10 patients when coinjected with DSM, even when the passage of $^{99}Tc^{m}$-MDP was reduced. However, the passage of the erythrocytes was significantly delayed by DSM.

Therefore, it can be concluded that as long as there is not a complete cessation of blood flow the substances retained by coinjection with DSM are not lodged within the vessel compartment to any large extent but actually diffuse out into the tissues [18].

Occurrence and Importance of A-V Shunt Circulation

Arteriovenous shunting through liver tumors, when measured as the passage of intra-arterially injected $^{99}Tc^{m}$-MAA to the lungs, has been reported by Kaplan et al. [13]. As discussed by Bledin et al. [2], $^{99}Tc^{m}$-MAA should not pass through a normal liver.

Arteriovenous shunt circulation reduces the effect of DSM. If the passage of MAA before DSM injection was more than 20 arbitrary units, PF of the first DSM injection of the first treatment session was less than 80% in only 4/13 patients, compared to 35/41 patients in whom MAA passage was less than 20%. Arteriovenous shunt circulation before and after DSM treatment was analyzed in 34 patients. The passage of macroaggregates before administration of DSM was more than 20 arbitrary units in nine of the 34 patients. After DSM treatment, however, the passage of $^{99}Tc^{m}$-MAA increased markedly (more than 10 arbitrary

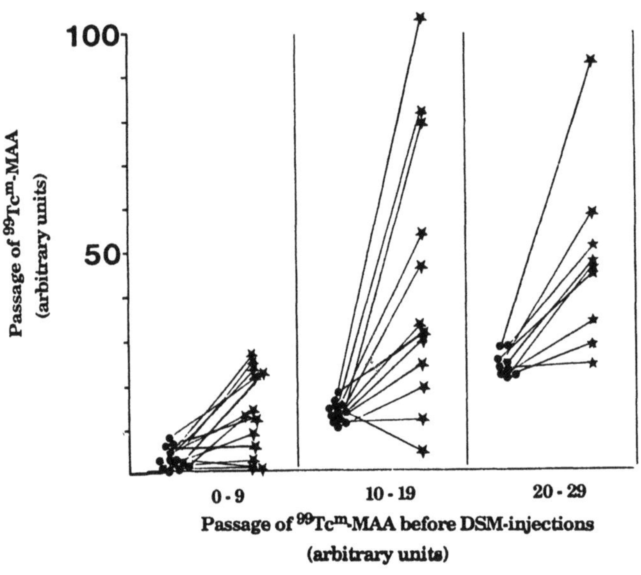

Fig. 3. Passage of $^{99}Tc^{m}$-MAA before (●) and after (★) injection of DSM. The passage before DSM injection is divided into three groups

units) in another 21 patients irrespective of the pretreatment passage (Fig. 3). An increased passage of $^{99}Tc^{m}$-MAA after DSM injections was also reported by Zeissman et al. [25] and Gyves et al. [11].

Distribution and Diversion of Flow

A positive correlation between the hypervascularity of liver tumors and the efficacy of cytostatic drugs has been described (e.g. [81]). The effect of DSM on the arterial blood flow to liver metastases and normal liver tissue was studied in four patients using a CT scanner with a dynamic program [4]. Density plots were obtained after an injection of contrast medium. After DSM injection the calculated area under the curve was reduced by a mean of 82% in 10 parenchymal areas and by 94% in a single hypervascular colorectal metastasis. However, in six of eight hypovascular colorectal metastases the area under the curve was dramatically increased [4]. After ligation of aberrant hepatic vessels, perfusion scanning with $^{99}Tc^{m}$-MAA showed reduced perfusion of the areas supplied by the ligated artery. After infusion of DSM a nearly normal perfusion of the ischemic lobe was achieved in all four patients [5].

Conclusions

Degradable starch microspheres as a tool to induce vascular occlusion have several advantages:

1. An increased regional concentration can be achieved.
2. The blood flow is only temporarily reduced during drug injection and then restored which allows repeated treatment sessions.
3. Peripheral vascular occlusion avoids the development of collateral circulation.
4. Blood flow can be diverted to hypovascular areas of the tumor.
5. A tumor-selective increased drug uptake has been demonstrated for liver tumors.

The Spherex monitoring system is a simple nuclear medicine procedure which provides information on vascular occlusion, the degree of retention of the coinjected marker, and the degree of A-V shunting continuously throughout the treatment session. It thereby considerably increases the safety of microsphere administration by reducing the risk of backflow of the microspheres along with the cytotoxic drugs to unintended areas, and it also provides an early warning so that administration of microspheres through A-V shunts to the lungs can be avoided.

References

1. Bengmark S, Peterson-Dahl E, Fredlund PE (1979) Hepatic dearterialization and infusion treatment of liver tumours. In: Peterson HI (ed) Tumor blood circulation: angiogenesis, vascular morphology and blood flow of experimental and human tumors. CRC Boca Raton, pp 203–216
2. Bledin AG, Kim EE, Harle TS, Haynie TP, Chuang VP (1984) Technetium-99m-labeled macroaggregated albumin arteriography for detection of abnormally positioned arterial catheters during infusion chemotherapy. Cancer 53:858–862

3. Chuang VP, Tsai C-C, Soo C-S, Wright K, Wallace S, Charnsangavej C (1982) Experimental canine hepatic artery embolization with polyvinyl alcohol foam particles. Radiology 145:21–25
4. Civalleri D, Rollandi G, Simoni G, Mallarini G, Repetto M, Bonalumi U (1985) Redistribution of arterial blood flow in metastases-bearing livers after infusion of degradable starch microspheres. Acta Chir Scand 151:613–617
5. Civalleri D, Scopinaro G, Simoni G, Claudiani F, Repetto M, DeCian F, Bonalumi U (1986) Starch microspheres induced arterial flow redistribution after occlusion of replaced hepatic arteries in patients with liver metastases. Cancer 58:2151–2155
6. Collins JM (1986) Pharmacologic rationale for hepatic arterial therapy. Recent Results Cancer Res 100:140–147
7. Dakhil S, Ensminger W, Cho K, Niederhuber J, Doan K, Wheeler R (1982) Improved regional selectivity of hepatic arterial BCNU with degradable microspheres. Cancer 50:631–635
8. Daly JM, Butler J, Kemeny N, Yeh SDJ, Ridge JA, Botet J, Bading JR, De Cosse JJ, Benua RS (1985) Predicting tumor response in patients with colorectal hepatic metastases. Ann Surg 202:384–393
9. Egeli RA, Ritschard J (1985) Transient ischemia of the liver by biodegradable starch microspheres. In: Proceedings of International Congress on Regional Chemotherapy, Geissen, abstracts, p 64
10. Frei E, Canellos GP (1980) Dose: critical factor in cancer chemotherapy. Am J Med 69:585–594
11. Gyves JW, Ensminger WD, VanHarken D, Niederhuber J, Stetson P, Walker S (1983) Improved regional selectivity of hepatic arterial mitomycin by starch microspheres. Clin Pharmacol Ther 34:259–265
12. Huberman MS (1983) Comparison of systemic chemotherapy with hepatic arterial infusion in metastatic colorectal carcinoma. Semin Oncol 10:238–248
13. Kaplan WD, Come SE, Takvorian RW, Laffin SM, Gelman RS, Weiss GR, Garnick MB (1984) Pulmonary uptake of technetium 99 m macroaggregated albumin: a predictor of gastrointestinal toxicity during hepatic artery perfusion. J Clin Oncol 2:1266–1269
14. Lindberg B, Lote K, Teder H (1984) Biodegradable starch microspheres – a new medical tool. In: Davis SS, Illum L, McVie JG, Tomlinson E (eds) Microspheres and drug therapy. Elsevier, Amsterdam, pp 153–188
15. Lörelius LE, Benedetto AR, Blumhardt R, Gaskill HV, Lancaster JL, Stridbeck H (1984) Enhanced drug retention in VX2 tumors by use of degradable starch microspheres. Invest Radiol 19:212–215
16. Pfeifle CE, Howell SB, Ashburn WL, Barone RM, Bookstein JJ (1986) Pharmacologic studies of intra-hepatic artery chemotherapy with degradable starch microspheres. Cancer Drug Deliv 3:1–14
17. Sigurdson ER, Ridge JA, Daly JM (1986) Intra-arterial infusion of doxorubicin with degradable starch microspheres; improvement of hepatic tumor drug uptake. Arch Surg 121:1277–1281
18. Starkhammar H, Håkansson L (1987) Effect of starch microspheres on the passage of labeled erythrocytes and a low molecular weight marker through the liver. Acta Oncol 26:361–365
19. Starkhammar H, Håkansson L, Morales O, Svedberg J (1987) Effect of microspheres in intra-arterial chemotherapy. A study of arterio-venous shunting and passage of a labeled marker. Med Oncol Tumor Pharmacother 4:87–96
20. Starkhammar H, Håkansson L, Sjödahl R, Svedberg R, Ekberg S (1987) Effect of portal blood flow and intra-arterially injected starch microspheres on the passage of a labeled tracer through the liver. Acta Oncol 26:217–221

21. Sterchi JM (1985) Hepatic artery infusion for metastatic neoplastic disease. Surg Gynecol Obstet 160:477–489
22. Teder H, Nilsson B, Jonsson K, Hellekant C, Aspegren K, Aronsen K-F (1983) Hepatic arterial administration of doxorubicin (adriamycin) with or without degradable starch microspheres: a pharmacokinetic study in man. In: Hansen H (ed) Anthracyclines and cancer therapy. Excerpta Medica, Amsterdam, pp 166–174
23. Thulin L, Tydén G, Nyberg B, Calissendorff B, Hultcrantz R (1986) Reduction of hepatic arterial flow by degradable starch microspheres in patients with liver tumour. Acta Chir Scand 152:447–451
24. Tuma RF (1984) The use of degradable starch microspheres for transient occlusion of blood flow and for drug targeting to selected tissues. In: Davis SS, Illum L, McVie JG, Tomlinson E (eds) Microspheres and drug therapy. Elsevier, Amsterdam, pp 189–203
25. Zeissman HA, Thrall JH, Tyves JW, Ensminger WD, Niederhuber JE, Tuscan M, Walker S (1983) Quantitative hepatic arterial perfusion scintigraphy and starch microspheres in cancer hemotherapy. J Nucl Med 24:871–875

Increasing the Uptake of a Low Molecular Weight Marker in Liver Tumours by Degradable Starch Microspheres: Possible Mechanisms of Action

T. Cooke and D. Chang

University Department of Surgery, Royal Infirmary, Glasgow G40 SG, United Kingdom

Introduction

The prognosis for patients with hepatic metastases remains poor despite the increasing number of treatments available to the physician. The results of recent trials show that there has been no benefit in terms of survival with systemic chemotherapy [12], irradiation [3] or hepatic dearterialisation [2]. However, there is a sound rationale for treating hepatic tumours by manipulating their arterial blood supply [8]. As the tumour grows, its nutritional and blood supply is derived almost wholly from the hepatic artery, whereas normal liver tissue has a dual blood supply dominated by the portal vein. The preliminary results from several prospective randomised trials of regional chemotherapy look to be promising [5, 6] but it is becoming clear that merely infusing the cytotoxic drug into the hepatic artery is inadequate and that further manipulation of the tumour's blood supply could potentially improve drug delivery to tumor [1]. A variety of methods have been employed to alter tumour blood flow, one such technique being temporary arterial embolisation with degradable starch microspheres (DSM; Spherex, Pharmacia, Sweden). These microspheres, with a mean diameter of 45 μm, consist of starch polymers cross-linked with epichlorhydrine. They are degraded in vivo by endogenous serum α-amylase and have a half-life in human serum of about 20–30 min. Therefore treatment with these microspheres is readily repeatable. Regionally delivered drugs given concomitantly with DSM are retained for longer in the liver than when the drug is given alone [10]. Furthermore, an increased regional concentration of drug to tumour has been seen [13]. It is not clear, however, how these microspheres produce this effect. In order to elucidate the underlying mechanisms of action of DSM we describe a series of experiments carried out using a rat liver tumour model to find the intrahepatic distribution of a low-molecular-weight marker similar in size to the commonly used cytotoxic drugs.

R. Jakesz/H Rainer (Eds)
Progress in Regional Cancer Therapy

Materials and Methods

Liver Tumour Model

Liver tumours were established in syngeneic Hooded Lister rats weighing 200–300 g by the intraportal inoculation of 5×10^5 HSN fibrosarcoma cells obtained from the Institute of Cancer Research at Sutton.

The animals were studied 18–21 days later, when four to seven overt tumours measuring 0.5–1 cm in diameter were observed scattered throughout the liver.

Vascularity of Tumour

In view of the heterogeneity of human hepatic metastases it was necessary to determine the vascularity of this particular tumour. This was assessed by histological examination and by the intrahepatic distribution and passage of 16.5 μm ^{57}Co non-degradable microspheres (Nen-Trac, New England Nuclear) which were injected intraportally ($n = 6$) or intra-arterially ($n = 6$). Each injection contained approximately 6×10^4 microspheres.

Microspheres

The serum amylase level of rats (2000–3000 IUl^{-1}) is much higher than in man, therefore human DSM are degraded within minutes after parenteral administration to rats. Consequently, for these studies microspheres with a greater number of cross-linkages were used so that their degradation time in the rat, at 20–30 min was similar to that of human microspheres in man.

Procedures

The rats, restricted to water overnight, were anaesthetised by means of an intraperitoneal injection of sodium pentobarbitone (6 mg per 100 g). A cannula was placed in the gastroduodenal artery with its tip lying at the junction of the coeliac and hepatic arteries.

Subsequent injections were given via this cannula in a volume of 50 μl, as this had previously been ascertained to be approximately the vascular volume of the rat liver. The only exception were the intraportal injections, which were given directly into the portal vein.

Optimising the Dose of DSM

A monitoring system has been developed by Pharmacia, Sweden for measuring the passage of low-molecular-weight substances through the liver after injection into the hepatic artery. By mixing different doses of DSM with the low-molecular-weight marker ^{99}Tc^{m}-methylene diphosphonate (^{99}Tc^{m}-MDP) the passage of MDP through the liver could be reduced in comparison to the initial dose of MDP given alone. A sodium iodide scintillation counter placed over the upper thorax was used to detect the radioactivity of the MDP passing into the systemic circulation. During the injections the passage of marker alone and in combination with DSM was continually observed with an operating microscope to ensure that all of the marker passed into the hepatic artery.

Low-Molecular-Weight Marker

The substance $^{99}Tc^{m}$-MDP was chosen because very little of it, about 1%, is actively retained in the liver [15]. Furthermore, it is similar in size to many commonly used cytotoxic drugs but has the advantage of being easily radiolabelled and counted.

Experimental Groups

The rats were randomized to either $^{99}Tc^{m}$-MDP alone or $^{99}Tc^{m}$-MDP + DSM. The animals were then killed by cervical dislocation at 1 min or at 90 min. The liver was immediately excised and washed with isotonic saline and then divided into sections of approximately 100 mg, each being weighed and its radioactivity counted in a well scintillation counter. A picture of $^{99}Tc^{m}$-MDP distribution in tumour and, normal liver tissue could then be constructed.

In a further series of experiments the portal vein was clamped prior to administration of $^{99}Tc^{m}$-MDP + DSM and the animals were killed after 1 min. A separate group again had their portal veins clamped before injection of marker and DSM, but the clamp was removed after 1 min and the animals not killed until 90 min after injection. Tissue concentrations of $^{99}Tc^{m}$-MDP were expressed in percentage injected dose per milligram of wet weight tissue.

Statistical Analysis

The difference between the concentration of MDP in normal liver tissue and in tumour was measured using the non-parametric Mann–Whitney test.

Results

Tumour Vascularity

Histologically the tumour was relatively hypovascular compared with the normal liver parenchyma. This histological appearance was confirmed by the intra-arterial and intraportal distributions of the ^{57}Co microspheres which produced normal liver to tumour ratios of 4:1 and 40:1 respectively. Of the total regionally injected microspheres less than 1% were counted in the lungs, indicating insignificant arteriovenous shunting.

DSM Optimisation

The dose of DSM maximally reducing the passage of $^{99}Tc^{m}$-MDP through the liver without causing overspillage of the microspheres into the splanchnic circulation was found to be 2 mg. This dose of microspheres was used in all the subsequent experiments.

Intrahepatic Marker Distribution

Intra-arterial injection of $^{99}Tc^{m}$-MDP assessed after 1 min resulted in a marker concentration of 3.55 ± 0.15 per cent of the injected dose per mg tissue $\times 10^4$ (mean $\pm$ SE) in normal liver tissue compared with 5.17 ± 0.55 in tumour, a difference significant at the 0.05 level. However, when DSM were given with MDP there was immediately a significantly greater ($p < 0.001$) retention of marker within the liver, with more MDP in tumour (26.03 ± 2.81) than in normal liver parenchyma (8.67 ± 0.81; $p < 0.001$) (Table 1). After 90 min the MDP was distributed throughout the body and very little remained within the liver. Also, at this stage over 95% of the DSM had degraded. This was reflected in the results of the MDP alone group, where there was no significant difference between normal liver and tumour (Table 1). The animals that received DSM with the MDP again had little MDP remaining in normal tissue (0.69 ± 0.08), but 14 times more marker was retained in tumor (11.11 ± 1.08; $p < 0.001$).

Portal Vein Clamping

The effect of clamping the portal vein on the marker's intrahepatic distribution when administered with DSM intra-arterially is summarised in Table 2. Under these

Table 1. Intrahepatic distribution of $^{99}Tc^{m}$-MDP

			Per cent injected dose/mg tissue $\times 10^{-4}$ (Mean $\pm$ SE)	
Injection	n	Time (min)	Normal liver	Tumour
MDP alone	10	1	3.55 ± 0.15	5.17 ± 0.55
MDP + DSM	10	1	8.67 ± 0.81	26.03 ± 2.81
MDP alone	10	90	0.61 ± 0.04	0.79 ± 0.07
MDP + DSM	10	90	0.69 ± 0.08	11.11 ± 1.08

Table 2. Intrahepatic distribution of $^{99}Tc^{m}$-MDP + DSM following portal vein occlusion

			Per cent injected dose/mg tissue $\times 10^{-4}$ (Mean $\pm$ SE)	
	n	Time (min)	Normal liver	Tumor
Portal vein clamped	7	1	25.54 ± 1.58	8.59 ± 1.34
Portal vein clamped temporarily for 1 min	8	90	2.21 ± 0.12	4.38 ± 1.16

conditions more marker is found in normal liver (25.54 ± 1.58) than in tumour (8.59 ± 1.34). In the second group temporary clamping of the portal vein again altered marker distribution, though the MDP now had time to be washed out of liver, leaving 2.21 ± 0.12 in normal liver and 4.38 ± 1.16 in tumour.

Discussion

Several previous studies have demonstrated that DSM influences uptake of coinjected substances [9, 13]. However, ours is the first animal model to reproduce the parameters that apply to human studies in a controlled physiological manner. Initially it was important to establish a liver tumour model that would represent the main vascular characteristics of a human colorectal liver metastasis, and the hypovascular, non-shunting nature of the HSN tumour reflected many of these features [4, 16].

By watching the flow of injected substance into the hepatic artery with the aid of an operating microscope it was possible to observe when backflow down the coeliac artery occurred. Injecting large amounts of DSM rapidly blocks the hepatic artery, forcing the microspheres into the splanchnic circulation, where they embolise splanchnic organs. Clinically this is heralded by epigastric pain and vomiting [14]. The optimal dose of DSM was taken to be the one that maximally reduced the passage of a coinjected marker without causing overspillage of microspheres, for this model 2 mg.

Our initial observation in the control group when MDP was injected alone was surprising. One would predict less marker in tumour than normal liver parenchyma due to the tumour's comparatively poor arterial supply. However, the insignificant portal venous flow to tumour reduces the portal venous washout of substances reaching the tumour circulation [11]. This appears to be borne out at 90 min, when the marker has had time to be washed out of the tumour so that there is now no significant difference between normal liver and tumour.

After coadministration of marker with DSM considerably more MDP is retained within the liver, predominantly in tumour, so the immediate effect of DSM appears to be directing more marker to tumour. Ninety minutes later, after DSM degradation, MDP is no longer retained within normal liver, but washed away and redistributed throughout the body. At this stage the amount remaining in tumour tissue had only dropped by just over half, being 14 times greater than if DSM had not been added. This prolonged retention of MDP in tumour can again be explained by the reduced portal washout effect.

Microspheres will have a tendency to follow the pathway of greatest flow and are an indirect mean of measuring organ blood flow [17, 18]. Similarly, the DSM will preferentially embolise in areas of high flow, which in this model is the more vascular normal liver parenchyma. The flow to these areas will therefore be blocked first. Coinjected substances distal to these microspheres will be washed out by the portal flow, whilst those following, including more microspheres, will be redirected to the initial areas of low flow, i.e. the hypovascular tumour.

Reducing portal flow produces a compensatory increase in hepatic arterial flow [7]. By stopping portal flow, much more marker was retained within the liver when given with DSM, but now the relative concentration in normal and tumour tissue were reversed. This alteration in intrahepatic marker distribution is seen again when the portal clamp is temporarily applied and portal washout is allowed to take place. These phenomena can be explained by the increased arterial flow to normal liver leading to an initial greater accumulation of microspheres and coinjected marker in normal liver than in tumour.

This study, which we designed to accurately reflect the clinical situation, has shown that DSM can increase the hepatic retention of a low-molecular-weight marker which is not normally actively held within the liver. Furthermore, there is preferential localisation of marker in a poorly vascularised tumour. DSM appears to produce an immediate haemodynamic alteration in blood flow by mechanical blockade with redirection of a coinjected substance away from areas of high flow to those of initial low flow. The marker then remains for a longer period in the tumour tissue because of the poor portal circulation to this area.

It would be expected that by adding cytotoxic drugs which are actively taken up by the liver an even greater effect would be achieved than with MDP. However, manipulation of the portal blood flow in attempts to reduce the portal washout may have a detrimental effect on localisation of cytotoxics in hypovascular tumours.

Summary

Degradable starch microspheres (DSM) appear to enhance the effect of regional chemotherapy for hepatic metastases. An animal tumour model was designed to examine the possible mode of action of DSM.

Overt hepatic tumour was induced in Lister rats by intraportal injection of HSN fibrosarcoma cells. The tumour was hypovascular as characterised by histology and the hepatic intra-arterial and intraportal distribution of 16.5-μm ^{57}Co non-degradable microspheres. The optimal dose of DSM to minimise the passage of a labelled marker through the liver was 2 mg. Combinations of DSM and this marker, ^{99}Tc^{m}-methylene diphosphonate (MDP), representing a cytotoxic drug, were regionally injected to determine intrahepatic distribution 1 min and 90 min after injection and following clamping of the portal vein.

The distribution, expressed in per cent injected dose/mg tissue $\times 10^4$, for MDP injected alone was 1.04 ± 0.10 in tumour compared to 0.77 ± 0.04 in normal liver. When given with DSM at 1 min there was significantly more ($p < 0.001$) marker in tumour (26.03 ± 2.81) than in normal liver (8.67 ± 0.81). Ninety minutes later, when DSM degradation was complete, more marker remained in tumour (11.11 ± 1.08) than in normal liver (0.69 ± 0.08). After occlusion of the portal vein, DSM increased marker retention in normal liver (2.21 ± 0.12), but now less so in tumour (4.35 ± 1.16).

These results show that DSM enhance the retention of a low-molecular-weight marker in a hypovascular hepatic tumour. This effect is immediate and appears to be due to a combination of redistribution of marker to tumour and reduced portal washout from tumour tissue.

References

1. Ackerman NB, Jacobs R (1988) Increased capillary flow in intrahepatic tumors due to alpha-adrenergic effects of catecholamines. Cancer 61:1550–1554
2. Almersjo O, Bengmark S, Rudenstom CM et al. (1972) Evaluation of hepatic dearterialisation in primary and secondary cancer of the liver. Am J Surg 124:5–9
3. Borgelt BB, Gelber R, Brady LW et al. (1981) The palliation of hepatic metastases: results of the radiation therapy oncology group pilot study. Int J Radiat Oncol Biol Phys 7:587–591
4. Healey JE (1965) Vascular patterns in human metastatic liver tumours. Surg Gynecol Obstet 120:1187
5. Hohn DC (1987) The NCOG randomized trial of intravenous vs. intrahepatic FUDR for colorectal cancer metastatic to the liver (abstract 333). Proc Am Soc Clin Oncol 6:85
6. Kemeny N, Reichman B, Oderman P et al. (1986) Update of randomised study of fluorodeoxyuridine in patients with liver metastases from colorectal cancer (abstract 345). Proc Am Soc Clin Oncol 5:89–93
7. Lautt WW, Greenway CV (1987) Conceptual review of the hepatic vascular bed. Hepatology 7:952–963
8. Lee Y-TM (1987) The rationale for intra-arterial chemotherapy. Eur J Cancer Clin Oncol 23:1265–1268
9. Lindell B, Aronsen K-F, Nosslin B et al. (1978) Studies in pharmacokinetics and tolerance of substances temporarily retained in the liver by microspheres embolisation. Ann Surg 187:95–99
10. Loffler T, Aigner K, Hausamen TU (1985) Cisplatin, mitomycin-C and 5-FU tissue concentrations in hepatic metastases after intra-arterial chemotherapy alone and with use of starch microspheres. Proc Annu Meet Am Assoc Cancer Res 26:156
11. Nott DM, Yates J, Grime S et al. (1988) The effect of portal venous flow on the washout of a regionally injected marker from the liver. Eur J Surg Oncol 14:359
12. Schwartz SI, Jones LS, McCune CS et al. (1985) Assessment of treatment of intrahepatic malignancies using chemotherapy via an implantable pump. Ann Surg 201:560–567
13. Sigurdson ER, Ridge JA, Daly JM (1986) Intra-arterial infusion of doxorubicin with degradable starch microspheres: improvement of hepatic tumour uptake. Arch Surg 121:1277–1281
14. Starkhammar H (1987) On the effect of degradable starch microspheres on intra-arterial chemotherapy. Thesis, Linkoping University, Linkoping
15. Subramanian G, McAfee JG, Blair RJ et al. (1975) Technetium-99m-methylene diphosphonate—a superior agent for skeletal imaging:comparison with other technetium complexes. J Nucl Med 16:744–755
16. Suzuki T, Sarumaru S, Kawabe K et al. (1972) Study of vascularity of tumors of the liver. Surg Gynecol Obstet 134:27–34
17. Utley J, Carlson EL, Hoffman JIE et al. (1974) Total and regional myocardial blood flow measurements with 25, 15, 9 and filtered 1–10 μm diameter microspheres and antipyrine in dogs and sheep. Circ Res 34:391–405
18. Yipintsoi T, Dobbs WA Jr, Scanlon PD et al. (1973) Regional distribution of diffusable tracers and carbonised microspheres in the left ventricle of isolated dog hearts. Circ Res 33:573–587

Dextrane Particle Use in Regional Chemotherapy; Problems of Monitoring

M. Burk, W.D. Schoppe, A.A. Miller, R.M. Jungblut, and W. Schneider

Abteilung Hämatologie, Onkologie und klinische Immunologie, Medizinische Klinik und Poliklinik, Heinrich Heine-Universität Düsseldorf, Moorenstraße 5, 4000 Düsseldorf 1, FRG

Introduction

Malignant liver tumors are vascularized primarily by the hepatic artery [1, 3]. Therapeutic approaches to nonresectable liver malignancies have therefore aimed at the arterial administration of cytostatic drugs to get a high therapeutic index. The systemic adverse effects of substances with a low hepatic clearance were diminished by a simultaneously reduced arterial hepatic blood flow [4].

The development of biodegradable starch microspheres allowed for a reversible blockage of hepatic arterial blood flow for 15–30 min, thus holding a simultaneously injected drug solution in the arterial capillary bed and providing a relatively high local drug concentration [2, 5–7, 9]. We started a pilot study to evaluate the clinical usefulness of the administration of microspheres in combination with the anthracycline derivative 4′-epirubicin. This substance belongs to an important group of cytostatic drugs but has a low hepatic extraction ratio, and therefore would profit from prolonged tumor exposure.

Methods

After informed, written consent 15 patients participated in the study. All had unresectable isolated liver tumors and no extrahepatic manifestations. Patients with anomalous hepatic arteries, liver failure, or a poor performance status were excluded from treatment. The eight male and seven female patients, mean age 60 years (SD 7 years), had had no prior treatment. One patient had hepatocellular carcinoma, in the remainder the tumors were metastases from colorectal cancer.

A subcutaneous port (Port-A-Cath, Pharmacia, Sweden) was implanted with the catheter placed through the gastroduodenal artery just ending at the hepatic artery. To prevent local complications small arterial vessels to the gastric wall were cut and a prophylactic cholecystectomy was done. The decrease of hepatic artery blood flow was monitored radiologically by means of digital subtraction angiography (DSA).

All treatment was administered through the implanted port. Drug and microspheres (Spherex, Pharmacia) were delivered simultaneously. The treatment protocol is listed in Table 1. Courses I and II alternated every 3 weeks until cessation

R. Jakesz/H Rainer (Eds.)
Progress in Regional Cancer Therapy

Table 1. Treatment protocol

Course I	
Days 1–4:	microspheres 450 mg IA and 4′-epirubicin 20 mg IA bolus (5 min, 10 ml)
Course II	
Day 1:	4′-epirubicin 20 mg IA bolus (5 min, 10 ml)
Days 2–3:	4′-epirubicin 60 mg IA continuously 48 h

or change of the therapeutic regimen. In eight patients venous blood was sampled at regular intervals for pharmacokinetic monitoring. Epirubicin concentrations in serum were analyzed using liquid chromatography with fluorescence detection, analogous to a previously published method [8].

Results

In most patients the angiographically determined blood flow of the hepatic arteries was diminished by simultaneous administration of microspheres. The reduction of the blood flow was dose dependent, with 150 mg microspheres being enough to have a significant effect (Fig. 1). In most cases 450 mg microspheres caused a sharp reduction in blood flow associated with retrograde flow along the common hepatic artery (flow of contrast 1.5 ml/s) (Fig. 2a–c). With a flow of contrast of 0.5 ml/s, this retrograde flow was minimized. In a small number of patients even 900 mg microspheres failed to stop blood flow. In these patients an early venous phase in DSA series was seen, probably a hint of extensive arteriovenous shunts (not shown).

Minor local complaints in the upper right abdomen (including vomiting in two patients) accompanied the administration of microspheres in about half of the patients. Patients whose blood flow was not reduced had no local adverse effects.

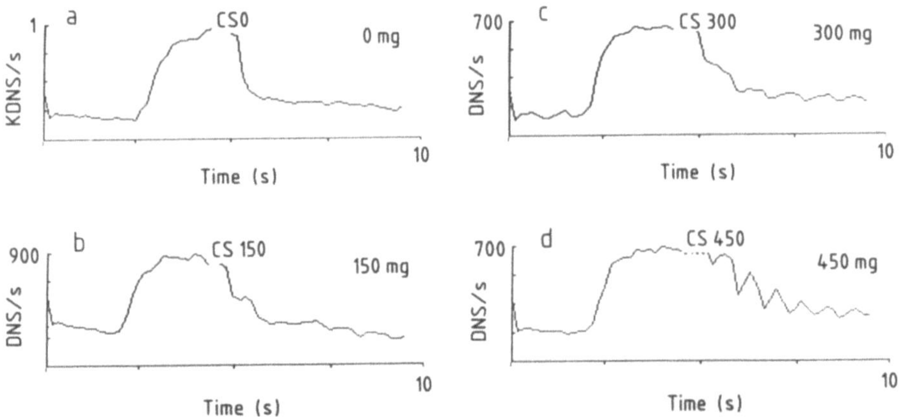

Fig. 1a–d. Course of radiographic density (DSA technique) of the proper hepatic artery after regional administration of **a** 0 mg, **b** 150 mg, **c** 300 mg, and **d** 450 mg microspheres. A widening of the contrast bolus is observed, correlated with the reduction of blood flow. Oscillations (**d**) indicate sharp reduction of orthograde blood flow through the hepatic artery

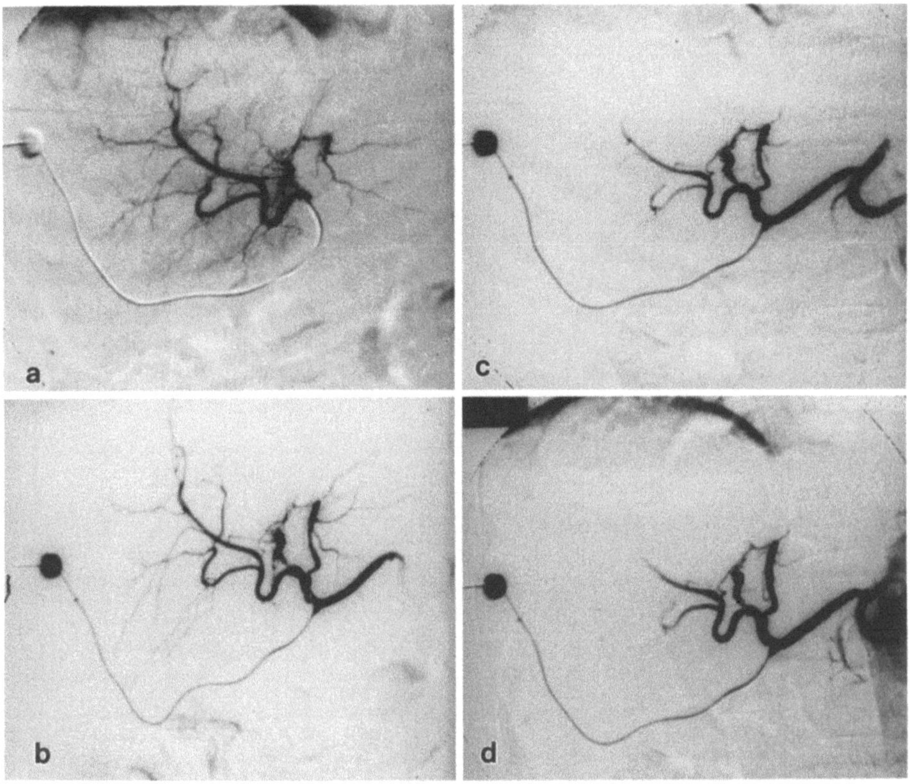

Fig. 2a–d. DSA series: hepatic arterial angiography using an implanted port. **a** Before application of microspheres, **b** after 300 mg, **c** after 600 mg, **d** after 900 mg microspheres

Angiographically normal blood flow was seen again 30–45 min after administration, indicating complete degradation of the starch microspheres.

A total of 58 courses of regional chemotherapy were given (mean four, range zero to eight). Whereas systemic adverse effects were minor and infrequent, there were extensive problems with local complications (Table 2). Thrombosis of the implanted catheter and postoperative subcutaneous infection of the bag were easily manageable. Complete thrombosis of the common hepatic artery and catheter dislocation required the discontinuation of regional therapy. In two patients an arteriobiliary fistula occurred after necrosis of tumor masses in association with thrombosis of the common hepatic artery (Fig. 3). Mean concentration time data for venous epirubicin revealed no significant difference in systemic drug exposure between epirubicin administration with and without microspheres. Only a tendency towards lower systemic drug levels could be observed with microspheres.

Discussion

The administration of biodegradable starch microspheres into the hepatic artery caused a reversible dose-dependent reduction of blood flow in most patients with only minor acute systemic effects.

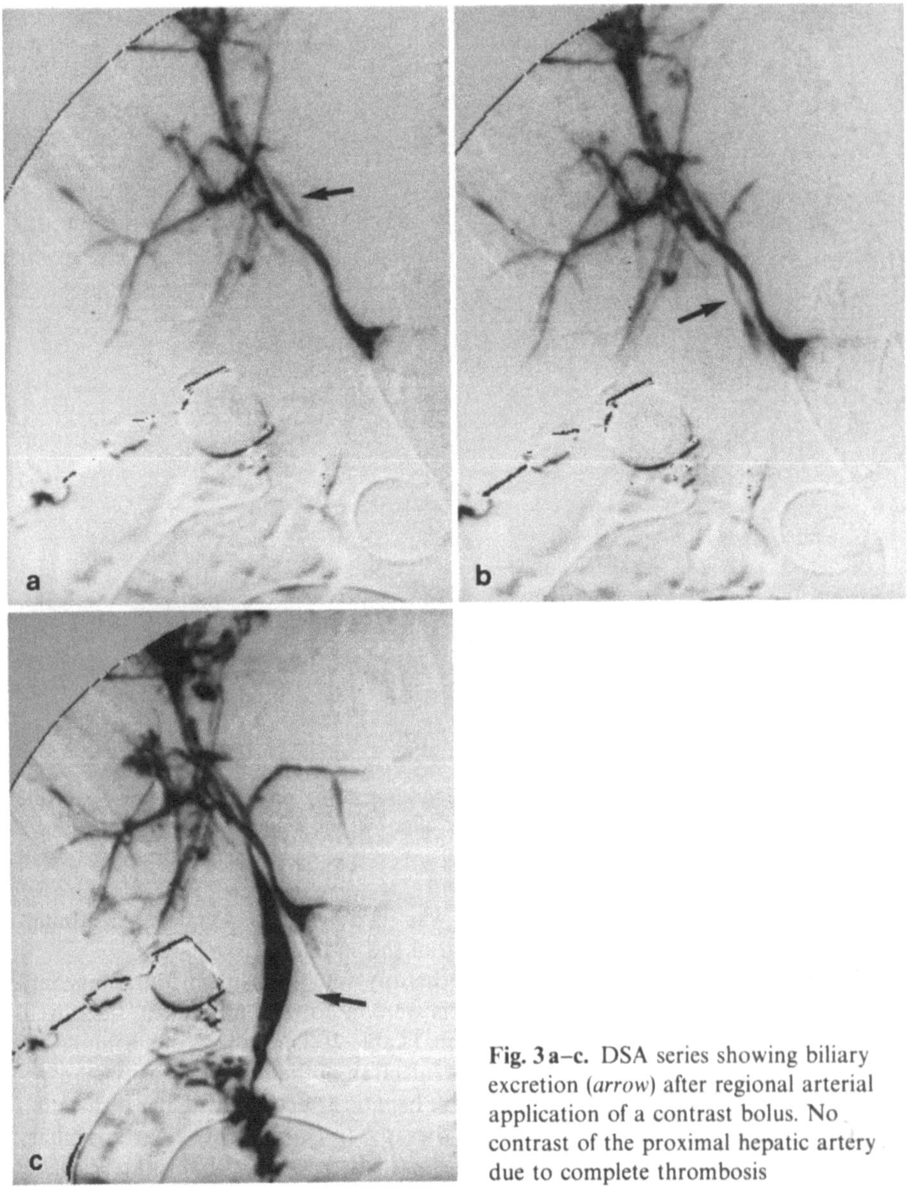

Fig. 3 a–c. DSA series showing biliary excretion (*arrow*) after regional arterial application of a contrast bolus. No contrast of the proximal hepatic artery due to complete thrombosis

With decreasing blood flow through the hepatic artery bed an increasing retrograde flow of the contrast bolus (flow 1.5 ml/s) was observed angiographically. The most striking finding was the high rate of local complications leading to discontinuation of treatment of our study. Thrombosis of the common hepatic artery was the most frequent complication and may have resulted from (1) the use of a (potent) drug with marked endothelial toxicity; (2) the low blood flow (and retrograde flow) along the hepatic artery caused by the administration of microspheres; and (3) surgical problems (one patient suffered from complete thrombosis of the hepatic artery before any treatment). Since in our hands local

Table 2. Complications of regional therapy (multiple entries)

Local complications	
1.	Thrombosis of common hepatic artery ($n = 6$)[a]
2.	Arterio-biliary fistula ($n = 2$)[a]
3.	Thrombosis of implanted catheter ($n = 2$)
4.	Extravascular dislocation of catheter tip ($n = 1$)[a]
5.	Postoperative infection of subcutaneous bag ($n = 1$)
Systemic effects	
1.	Alopecia ($n = 3$, WHO grade 2)
2.	Leukocytopenia ($n = 2$, WHO grade 1,2)

[a]Complications necessitating discontinuation of treatment.

therapy with epirubicin alone caused few local complications (data not shown), the combined use of epirubicin and microspheres is associated with difficulties in finding the optimal balanced blood-flow reduction along the hepatic artery. This is supported by simple analysis of peripheral blood concentration which was not influenced by intra-arterial administration of microspheres.

In summary, this study reports serious local problems of combined use of microspheres and epirubicin in hepatic artery chemotherapy. In our hands this regimen offers no clear advantages.

References

1. Ackerman NB, Lien WM, Kondi ES, Silverman NA (1969) The blood supply of experimental liver metastases I: The distribution of hepatic arterial and portal vein blood to "small" and "large" tumors. Surgery 66:1067
2. Aronsen KF, Hellekant C, Holmberg J (1979) Controlled blocking of hepatic artery flow with enzymatically degradable microspheres combined with oncolytic drugs. Eur Surg Res 11:99
3. Breedis C, Young G (1954) The blood supply of neoplasms in the liver. Am J Pathol 30:969–986
4. Chen HSG, Gross JF (1980) Intra-arterial infusion of anticancer drugs: theoretic aspects of drug delivery and review of responses. Cancer Treat Rep 64:31–40
5. Dakhil S, Ensminger W, Cho K, Niederhuber J, Doan K, Wheeler R (1982) Improved regional selectivity of hepatic arterial BCNU with degradable microspheres. Cancer 50:631–635
6. Gyves JW, Ensminger WD, Van Harken D, Niederhuber J, Stetson P, Walker S (1983) Improved regional selectivity of hepatic arterial mitomycin by starch microspheres. Clin Pharmacol Ther 34:259–265
7. Lindell BO, Aronsen KF, Nosslin B et al. (1978) Studies in pharmacokinetics and tolerance of substances temporarily retained in the liver by starch microsphere embolization. Ann Surg 187:95–99
8. Miller AA, Schmidt CG (1987) Clinical pharmacology and toxicity of 4'-o-tetrahydropyranyladriamycin. Cancer Res 47:1461–1465
9. Rothman U, Arfors KE, Aronsen KF, Lindell B, Nylander G (1976) Enzymatically degradable microspheres for experimental and clinical use. Microvasc Res 11:421

Chemoembolization of Hepatic Tumors with Degradable Starch Microspheres

M. Lorenz, C. Hottenrott, R.P. Baum, D. Liermann, and A. Encke

Klinik für Allgemeinchirurgie (Prof. Dr. A. Encke), Johann Wolfgang Goethe-Universität
Theodor-Stern-Kai 7, 6000 Frankfurt/Main, FRG

Introduction

The aim of regional treatment of cancer is to achieve increased tumor drug exposure, resulting in elevated response rates with reduced systemic toxicity [12]. Various forms of permanent or temporary central and peripheral artery occlusion are used to induce hypoxemia resulting in tumor retardation [3, 18]. However, procedures like hepatic artery ligation or embolization with nondegradable material induce rapid formation of collaterals [2].

Microparticles can be used to induce transient or permanent flow reduction by means of arteriole-capillary block resulting in different forms of tumor ischemia. This significantly affects the pharmacokinetics of simultaneously injected drugs. For coadministration of doxorubicin (Adriamycin), mitomycin C, BCNU and cisplatin a reduction of systemic concentration combined with increased hepatic drug exposure has already been demonstrated [5, 7–9, 15].

Dextran degradable starch microspheres (DSM; Spherex, Pharmacia, Sweden) have proved to be useful for repeated treatment because blood flow is restored after 15–30 min and no major side effects have been observed [7, 15]. The first clinical studies, however, differed on the appropriate doses for adequate reduction of blood flow, and the need for a monitoring system to avoid overflow and misperfusion became obvious. Furthermore, the concomitant right upper abdominal pain was difficult to treat [16].

The aim of this phase I study was therefore to determine the effect of repeated tumor blood flow reduction combined with mitomycin C in patients with various liver tumors. Due to the accelerated activation of mitomycin C under hypoxic conditions, a triple DSM embolizations was followed by additional mitomycin C chemoembolization in patients with liver metastases of colorectal cancer [14]. Further, the value of digital subtraction angiography (DSA) in individual determination of the appropriate DSM dosage was tested.

R. Jakesz/H Rainer (Eds)
Progress in Regional Cancer Therapy

Patients, Materials, and Methods

Patients

Twenty-one patients with liver malignancies were analyzed in a prospective study. In 15 patients prior treatment failed or biliary sclerosis due to sclerosing cholangitis occurred, in four patients primary embolization was considered because of extensive disease, and in two patients low perfusion of one lobe due to trifurcation of the hepatic artery was the indication for DSM treatment. In 19 patients a Silastic catheter was placed surgically up to 10 months before the start of the embolization according to Watkins et al. [12], and in two patients the catheter was placed percutaneously into the hepatic artery. Patients with arteriovenous shunt greater than 30% were excluded.

Materials

Cross-linked dextran DSM (Spherex, diameter $\pm 40\,\mu m$) are trapped at the arteriolar level and maintain their size during degradation (18, 19). The concentration of microspheres in solution was 6 million/ml (60 mg/ml).

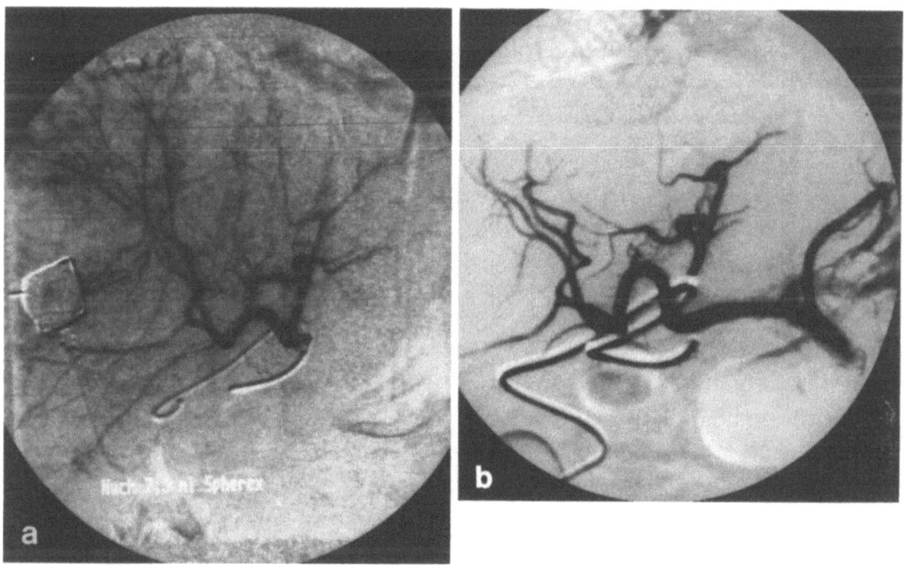

Fig. 1 a, b. Digital subtraction angiography in a patient with liver metastases of choroidal melanoma. **a** After 7.5 ml DSM: significant hepatic flow reduction with demonstration of all major hepatic vessels. **b** After 10 ml DSM: nearly complete occlusion of all minor liver vessels. Reversed flow in common hepatic artery led to perfusion of left gastric artery and demonstration of celiac trunk

Methods

DSM Titration. The appropriate individual DSM dosage was determined 1 day prior to treatment by means of DSA [19]. After angiographic control, DSM embolization was carried out in steps of 4–5 ml until retrograde flow in the common hepatic artery was observed (Fig. 1). DSA evaluation with DSM titration was repeated before each embolization.

Treatment. Treatment was carried out on the next day and consisted in 14 patients (groups I, II, Table 1) of four embolization cycles with 75% of the previous dosage every 2 h, the last DSM bolus being mixed with 10 mg mitomycin C. Embolization was repeated monthly. Treatment of hepatocellular carcinoma and liver metastases of choroidal melanoma (groups III, IV, Table 1) did not involve initial administration of DSM alone.

A previous pilot study had revealed that most patients suffered right upper abdominal pain and nausea [16]. Patients therefore received premedication consisting of buprenorphine 0.3 mg, metoclopramide 30 mg, and promethazine 30 mg IV with further buprenorphine sublingually on demand.

DSM and Labeled Monoclonal Antibodies. In three patients Tc-labeled monoclonal antibodies (MAB; BW 431/26, Behring-Werke, FRG), and mixed with DSM, were given. In one of these patients, after proven positive uptake radioimmunotherapy was performed 3-min intra-arterial bolus injection of 100 mCi of ^{131}I-labeled MAB BW 431/26 mixed with DSM (group V, Table 1) [1].

Results

Effect of DSM on Hepatic Vascular System

In 11 of 21 patients complete occlusion could be produced by DSM. The dose required to produce reversed hepatic artery flow was 2–3 times lower than that needed for complete occlusion, indicating that reduction of hepatic flow occurred before definitive occlusion. Blood flow began to be reestablished within 5–15 min and was normalized after 30 min. DSA proved to be an appropriate test for DSM dosage determination (Fig. 1). The amount of DSM needed to induce reversed flow within the hepatic artery ranged from 5 to 19 ml (i.e., 30–114 million microspheres).

Repeated DSA of the liver vessels revealed no effect on hepatic vascular pattern (Fig. 2). However, the adequate dose of DSM showed an average decrease of 30% from the first to the last chemoembolization cycle. In two patients with anatomic variations of the hepatic arterial supply, simple TC-MAA scans performed shortly after operation revealed reduced arterial perfusion of parts of the liver. Here, DSM induced distribution of arterial perfusion to previously less perfused liver segments. In two cases hepatic artery thrombosis occurred after the second or third cycle of chemoembolization. In these two patients infusion chambers were implanted, in contrast to seven patients who received Infusaid 400 pumps (Norwood, Mass., USA) and continuous heparin administration to the hepatic artery.

Table 1. Patient characteristics, treatment, responses and survival

Group	No. of patients	Responses	Primary tumor	Mode of embolization	Median no. of treatment courses	Median survival time (months)	Median survival time after embolization (months)
I	11	CR 1 PR 3 SD 2 P 5	Colorectal cancer	After triple DSM alone, 10 mg mitomycin + DSM in 1 day monthly	3 2–6	15 3–39	7 3–27
II	3	CR 1 PR 1	Carcinoid	After triple DSM alone, 10 mg mitomycin + DSM in 1 day monthly	3	27 17–31	15 12–21
III	4	SD 1 P 3	Hepatocellular carcinoma	DSM + doxorubicin 25 mg/day for 4 days monthly	2 1–3	7.5 2–11	2.5 2–3
IV	2	SD 2	Choroidal melanoma	3 × DSM + 25 mg cisplatin/day for 2 days monthly	2.5	3–11[a]	3–11
V	1	P	Colon cancer	DSM + 100 mCi ^{131}I MAB	1	> 6	> 6

CR, complete response; PR, partial response; SD, stable disease; P, progression.
[a] Primary embolization.

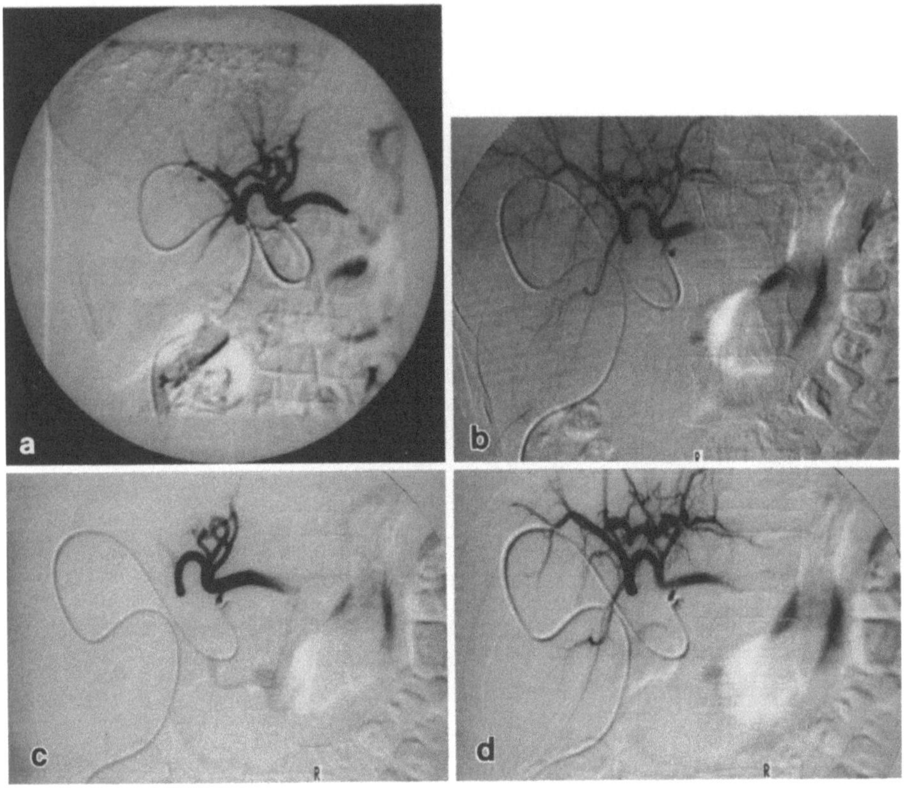

Fig. 2 a–d. Patient with liver metastases after curative anterior resection of a rectum carcinoma. **a** DSA after 5 ml DSM: nearly complete occlusion of all minor vessels. **b** Six months later. DSA before embolization after four cycles of mitomycin C chemoembolization: no variation or thrombosis of major or minor hepatic arteries. **c** DSA after 16 s embolization with 5 ml DSM. **d** DSA after 22 s embolization: significant flow reduction and reversed flow in common hepatic artery, no complete occlusion, minor liver vessels already visualized

Toxicity

No significant systemic toxicity was noted using mixed mitomycin C/DSM chemoembolization in groups I and II. Doxorubicin or cisplatin/DSM chemoembolization induced WHO grade II leukopenia and thrombocytopenia in two of five patients. Temporary elevations of liver enzymes up to 3 times the pretreatment values were observed in 10 of 21 patients. Chemical hepatitis was regarded as a result of transient lesions of liver parenchyma. Acute pain in the epigastrium and liver area was reported by nine of 11 patients in group I; duration ranged from 10 min to 7 days. In all but one case the pain appeared immediately after embolization. The character of the pain showed significant intraindividual fluctuation from treatment to treatment. Pain worsened from the first to the last chemoembolization cycle in four of 11 patients, and two patients refused further treatment. Dyspnea and nausea were less frequent and did not exceed 24 h in duration. Two patients had fever up to 39°C that resolved after 4 days.

Response

In six of 11 patients with colorectal liver metastases and failure of primary treatment tumor progression was halted. One patient showed complete response for 18 months. Their median duration of response was 6.5 months. In the case of primary progression after continuous FUDR treatment ($n = 2$) one partial response was noted. The median survival time from catheter implantation was 15 months, from first chemoembolization treatment, 7 months. All patients with carcinoid liver metastases are still alive at the time of writing without any evidence of hepatic progression. Hepatocellular carcinomas treated after failure of primary therapy did not respond to doxorubicin/DSM chemoembolization. Median survival time after the start of embolization treatment was 2.5 months. (Table 1). Choroidal melanoma liver metastases also failed to respond to DSM/cisplatin chemoembolization: tumor progression was delayed only for 2–3 months. One patient died 11 months after catheter implantation with generalized metastases.

Discussion

As chronic intra-arterial FUDR treatment rarely induces complete regression in liver metastases and the duration of response is only approximately 8 months, further second-line treatment alternatives are necessary [12]. In contrast to FUDR and 5-FU, other available cytostatics hitherto show low response rates in colorectal liver metastases and their extraction rate in the liver is – compared to FUDR – low. One way of enhancing tumor drug concentration is reducing blood flow. However, with permanent embolization and even more frequently with artery ligation, collaterals develop rapidly and impact on survival is low [2]. The administration of DSM does not alter the hepatic vascular pattern; blood flow is normal after 30 min. Additionally, microspheres are entrapped 3 times more within the tumor than in normal liver tissue, so simultaneously administered cytostatics will be selectively concentrated in the tumor tissue [20]. Up to now the appropriate mode of application remains unclear. Our preliminary study revealed the need for individual dosage of embolization [16]. Therefore, in contrast to most other studies, with their constant doses prior to every treatment the appropriate amount of microspheres was determined by DSA. In all patients flow reductions could be achieved and reversed flow was clearly demonstrated in the hepatic artery. As already reported, DSM proved to be effective in redistributing flow to the entire liver in cases of previously unilateral perfusion [4]. The hepatic vascular pattern remained unchanged after a total of over 40 embolizations. The required dose may be reduced by narrowing of arteries and arterioles due to thrombosis, endothelial cell proliferation, and scar formation after focal necrosis [11].

In contrast to the findings of previous studies, the subjective side effects of chemoembolization treatment were high despite morphine analgesia. Nine of 11 patients suffered from pain, in some cases long-lasting, in the right upper abdomen. Pain correlates with the histologically proven necrosis of nerves in the hilus of the liver observed in one patient 12 days after chemoembolization [11]. Therefore prevention with lidocaine as described by Dakhil et al. [5] may be insufficient. In order to induce optimal tumor hypoxemia, chemoembolization was combined with further DSM treatment. On the basis of the findings of Hansen et al. [10] and Eibl-Eibesfeld et al. [6] a triple embolization with DSM alone was performed before chemoembolization to produce cytostatic hypoxemia of tumor tissue. The repeated doxorubicin or cisplatin chemoembolization proved to be practicable, without major local side effects. The results, especially in hepatocellular carcinoma, were poor perhaps due to the reduced general performance status of the patients after previous intra-arterial chemotherapy. The benefit of DSM cisplatin chemoembolization was also slight in patients with metastases of choroidal melanoma, not comparable with the results of permanent embolization treatment using polyvinyl sponge and cisplatin [17]. Although the concentration of labeled MAB was higher after the combination of DSM and MAB than after injection of MAB alone, incorporation of labeled MAB into liver metastases was too low to achieve radiation dosage sufficient for tumor control: the dosage attained was < 1000 Gy. Reduced degradation, resulting in higher half-life of DSM, is perhaps one way to increase the duration of temporary stasis and to facilitate accumulation of drugs and labeled antibodies in the target areas.

Conclusion

Chemoembolization with mitomycin C and Spherex DSM proved to be a relatively effective second-line treatment for progressive liver metastases of colorectal cancer compared with further regional and systemic therapies [12]. The optimal sequence of mitomycin and DSM administration must be further evaluated in prospective phase II–III studies. Probably the DSM dose can be reduced and treatment performed more frequently, as there is almost no systemic toxicity. Coadministration of catecholamines should be evaluated, the aim being to increase the tumor: liver parenchyma ratio further [13]. DSA and dynamic scintigraphy with Tc-labeled MAB or cytostatics proved to be effective for determination of appropriate DSM dosage, prevention of malperfusion, and evaluation of retention time of the coadministered drugs.

References

1. Baum RP, Lorenz M, Hertel A, Hottenrott C, Hör G (1988) Flow-linked intraarterial radioimmunotherapy (FLIRT) by combined antibody and degradable starch microspheres infusion via the hepatic artery. Eur J Nucl Med 14:C3
2. Bengmark S, Rosengren K (1970) Angiographic study of the collateral circulation to the liver after ligation of the hepatic artery in man. Am J Surg 119:620–624
3. Bengmark S, Jeppson B, Lunderquist A, Tranberg K-G, Persson B (1988) Tumor calcification following repeated hepatic de-arterialization in patients – a peliminary communication. Br J Surg 75:525–526
4. Civalleri D, Scopiniaro G, Simoni G, Claudiani F, Repetto M, Decian F, Bonallumi U (1986) Starch microsphere-induced arterial flow redistribution after occlusion of replaced hepatic arteries in patients with liver metastases. Cancer 58:2151–2155
5. Dakhil S, Ensminger W, Cho K, Niederhuber J, Duan K, Wheeler R (1985) Improved regional selectivity of hepatic arterial BCNU with degradable microspheres. Cancer 50:631–635

6. Eibl-Eibesfeldt B, Pfeiffer KJ, Schweiberer L (1986) Regionale Therapie bei Lebermetastasen colorectaler Karzinome durch prolongierte temporäre Mikroembolisation. In: Hottenrott C, Nagel K, Lorenz M (eds) Regionale Chemotherapie der Leber und Extremitäten, Standortbestimmung. Kehrer, Freiburg
7. Ensminger WD, Gyves JW, Stetson P, Walker-Andrews S (1985) Phase I study of hepatic arterial degradable starch microspheres and mitomycin. Cancer Res 45:4464–4467
8. Fujimato S, Miyazaki M, Endoh F, Takahashi O, Okui K, Morimoto Y (1985) Biodegradable mitomycin C microspheres given intraarterially for inoperable hepatic cancer with particular reference to a comparison with continuous infusion of mitomycin and 5-fluorouracil. Cancer 56:2404–2410
9. Gyves J, Ensminger W, Vanharken D (1983) Improved regional selectivity of hepatic arterial mitomycin C by starch microspheres. Clin Pharmacol Ther 34:259–265
10. Hansen H (1984) Erste Ergebnisse der Therapie multipler Lebermetastasen durch passagere Leberdesarterisation und intraarterielle Chemotherapie. In: Koslowski L (ed): Chirurgisches Forum' 84 für Experimentelle und klinische Forschung. Springer, Berlin Heidelberg New York
11. Herrmann G, Lorenz M, Kirkowa-Reimann M, Hottenrott C, Hübner K (1987) Morphological changes after intraarterial chemotherapy of the liver. Hepatogastroenterol 34:5–9
12. Hottenrott C, Lorenz M (1987) Stellenwert der regionalen Chemotherapie der Leber. Z Gastroenterol 25:364–373
13. Iwaki A, Nagasue N, Kobayashi M, Inokuchi K (1978) Intraarterial chemotherapy with the concomitant use of vasoconstrictions for liver cancer. Cancer Treat Rep 62:145–146
14. Kennedy KA, Rockwell S, Sartorrelli AC (1980) Preferential activation of mitomycin C to cytotoxic metabolites by hypoxic tumor cells. Cancer Res 40:2356–2360
15. Lindell B, Aronsen KF, Nosslin B, Rothman U (1978) Studies in pharmacokinetics and tolerance of substances temporarily retained in the liver by microspheres embolisation. Ann Surg 187:95–99
16. Lorenz M, Hottenrott C, Kirkowa-Reimann M, Hecht M, Herrmann G, Rauber K, Encke A (1986) Temporäre Chemoembolisation von isolierten Lebermalignomen mit Mikrosphären und Mitomycin C. In: Nagel GA, Bach F, Bartsch HH (eds) Mitomycin 85. Zuckschwerdt, Munich
17. Mavligit C, Carasco N, Papadopoulos C, Charnsangavej C, Wallace S (1987) Regression of ocular melanoma metastatic to the liver after chemoembolization with cis-platinum (CDDP) and Polyvinyl sponge (PVS). Proc ASCO 830
18. Rauber K, Lorenz M, Kirkowa-Reimann M, Hottenrott C, Reimann H (1987) Digitale Subtrakionsangiographie zur Kontrolle subkutan implantierter Katheter zur regionalen Chemotherapie isolierter Lebermetastasen. Tumor Diagn 8:11–15
19. Watkins E, Khazei AM, Nahra KS (1970) Surgical basis for arterial infusion chemotherapy of disseminated carcinoma of the liver. Surg Gynecol Obstet 130:581–605
20. Ziessmann HA, Turall JH, Gyves JW, Ensminger WD, Niederhuber JE, Tuscan M, Walker S (1983) Quantitative hepatic arterial perfusion scintigraphy and starch microspheres in cancer chemotherapy. J Nucl Med 24:871–875

Cytostatic Treatment of Advanced Squamous Cell Carcinoma of the Maxillofacial Region

F. Scholz, K. Hollmann, J. Kühböck, W. Dobrowsky, and R. Scholz

Klinik für Kiefer- und Gesichtschirurgie, Universität Wien, Alser Straße4, 1090 Wien, Austria

Introduction

Squamous cell carcinomas of the maxillofacial region comprise 2% of all malignomas in Austria [1].

Up to now the best results in the treatment of maxillofacial tumors have been achieved by radical surgical intervention. In cases where the tumor affects the skull base or the vertebral column, however, radical surgery increase the operative risk or is not possible at all [2]. For these patients cytostatic therapy with or without radiation therapy is recommended.

Several studies have demonstrated that polychemotherapy is more effective than single-drug therapy [3, 4]. Accordingly, we used methotrexate + bleomycin (MTX + BLEO) and doxorubicin + cisplatin. The aims of our investigation were:

1. To establish the effectiveness of polycytostatic treatment in inoperable maxillofacial cancers
2. To ascertain whether intra-arterial administration of cytostatics has an advantage over intravenous application
3. To find out whether the changes in blood parameters differ between the beginning and the end of therapy in the treatment regimes used and whether any clues concerning prognosis can be derived from blood parameters, especially iron concentrations.

In order to achieve maximal drug concentration in the target area with minimal general toxicity [5, 7], we have been administering cytostatics intra-arterially since 1972. Because both the primary tumor and the draining lymph systems should lie directly in the area supplied by the artery with raised drug concentration, ligation of collaterals of the tumor artery was not carried out.

Baumgartner et al., using hyaluronidase as an adjuvant drug, reported tumor regression in 50% of patients previously treated unsuccessfully with cytostatics. They also observed a decreased recurrence rate when hyaluronidase was administered adjuvant to mitomycin [8, 9]. Khono found in vitro increased cell-killing activity and enhanced cell-wall penetration of doxorubicin in various squamous cell cancer lines when hyaluronidase was given as adjuvant drug [10]. In view of these

R. Jakesz/H Rainer (Eds.)
Progress in Regional Cancer Therapy

findings we have used adjuvant hyaluronidase in chemotherapy of far advanced tumors since April 1987.

Patients, Staging

The histories of 227 patients with 341 cycles of cytostatic treatment were reviewed retrospectively.

Regarding TNM staging, 81% of the intra-arterially treated (IA) patients and 61% of the intravenously treated (IV) patients had T4 tumors of different maxillofacial sites, and 92% (IA) and 76% (IV) had either T3 or T4 tumors. Clinically positive, homolateral, non fixed lymph nodes (N1) were found in 15% of the IA patients (123) and 24% of the IV patients (104). N2 nodes were observed in 6% of the IA patients and in none of the IV patients. N3 nodes in 6% of the IA patients and 21% of the IV patients. In summary, the IA patients had the more advanced tumors (Table 1). The findings concerning bone destruction point in the same direction. Eighty-six patients (70%) of the IA group and 62 patients (60%) of the IV group showed bone destruction before commencement of treatment (Table 2).

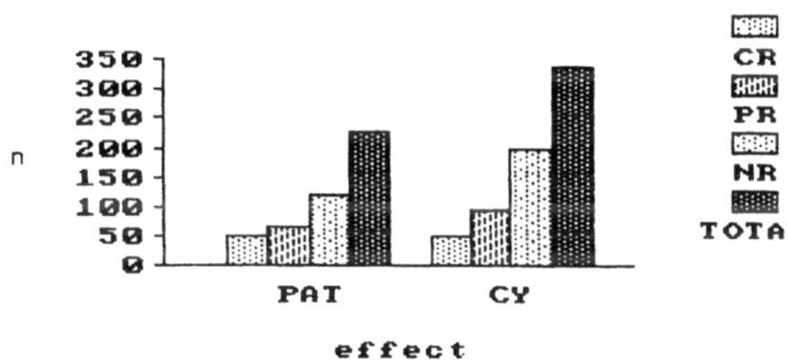

Fig. 1. Response to treatment. *PAT*, number of patients; *CY*, number of cycles

Table 1. TNM staging

Stage	Patients *n*	%
T4(IA)	99	81
T4(IV)	63	61
T4/T3(IA)	113	92
T4/T3(IV)	79	76
N1(IA)	19	15
N1(IV)	25	24
N2(IA)	7	6
N2(IV)	0	0
N3(IA)	7	6
N3(IV)	22	21

Table 2. Radiologically verified bone destruction

Treatment	Patients *n*	%
IA + RT	66	54
IV + RT	27	26
IA	20	18
IV	35	33
IA total	86	70
IV total	62	60

RT, radiation therapy.

Table 3. Average doses of cytostatics

Treatment	MTX/BLEO	DOX/DDP
IA + RT	495/280	120/60
IV + RT	539/198	134/166
IA	334/201	126/124
IV	716/183	108/210
IA total	464/264	121/73
IV total	643/189	119/192

Table 4. Hyaluronidase (HY) as adjuvant drug

	Cycles	RT
IA + HY	5	0
IV + HY	16	3
Total	21	3

Treatment

As already published (5–7) the average infused doses for IA patients were: MTX 464 mg + BLEO 264 mg, DOX 121 mg + DDP 73 mg. The IV patients on average received higher doses: MTX 643 mg + BLEO 189 mg, DOX 119 mg + DDP 192 mg (Table 3).

In the groups with radiation therapy the average radiation dose was similar in IA and IV patients (47 Gy and 46 respectively). In regard to hyaluronidase, 15 patients received an average of 1 366 000 units (Permease, Sanabo) intravenously per cycle over 12 h in advance of the cytostatics. Five of these patients received IA chemotherapy, 10 IV chemotherapy. All 15 were treated with DOX + DDP. Three of the IV patients were irradiated (Table 4).

Results

Altogether, 46 patients (20.3%) showed complete remission (CR), 64 (28.2%) partial remission (PR), and 117 (51.5%) no response (NR). For detailed analysis, the patients were divided into four groups corresponding to the different treatment regimes:

- IA patients with simultaneous RT (99 patients, 111 cycles of treatment)
- IV patients with simultaneous RT (43 patients, 67 cycles)
- IA patients without RT (24 patients, 33 cycles)
- IV patients without RT (61 patients, 130 cycles)

In the IA + RT group, 27 of 99 patients showed CR compared with four of 24 patients in the IA only group. Nine of 43 IV + RT patients and six of 61 IV only patients showed CR (Table 5).

Table 5. Distribution of complete remissions

	Patients	Cycles
IA + RT	27	28
IV + RT	9	10
IA	4	4
IV	6	6
Total	46	48

The average radiation dose was higher in patients with CR than in those with NR: 55 Gy vs 47 Gy (difference 20%) in IA patients and 46 Gy vs 42 Gy (difference 10%) in IV patients. Blood cell counts and protein and electrolyte values at the beginning, in the middle, and at the end of therapy and after therapy were reviewed. No significant differences in these parameters could be detected between the IA and the IV groups at the beginning of therapy. There were, however, more eosinophil granulocytes and fewer lobocytes in patients with CR than in those with NR. The level of iron (normal values: 80–150 ug/dl) at the beginning of therapy was 68 ug/dl (20 cycles) in patients with NR and 87 ug/dl (16 cycles) in patients with CR. After the end of therapy the iron level was 47 ug/dl (17 cycles) in patients with NR and 73 ug/dl (9 cycles) in patients with CR. With regard to the thrombocytes we observed an increase during the therapy in IA patients and a decrease in IV patients.

Discussion

The overall resopnse rate (CR + PR) of maxillofacial carcinomas after MTX + BLEO (159 patients) of DOX + DDP (30 patients) was 48.5%. Although, by tumor stage and bone destruction, the IA patients had more advanced tumors than the IV patients, the remission rate and the duration of survival time (Table 6) were clearly greater for the IA group. In both groups the carcinolytic effect of the chemotherapy was obviously patentiated by a radiation dose of at least 46 Gy. This is also true for patients treated with hyaluronidase as an adjuvant drug. Disappointingly, the blood parameters determined correlated poorly with the prognosis. The level of iron before the cytostatic therapy in both IA and IV patients who exhibited no tumor remission was already clearly below normal values, and by the end of cytostatic

Table 6. Duration of survival

Survival	IA		IV	
(years)	*n*	%	*n*	%
< 1	70	57	47	45
> 1	39	32	37	36
> 2	20	16	16	15
> 3	13	11	10	10
> 5	6	5	4	4

therapy it had decreased further to 70% of the initial value. In contrast, the level of iron at the beginning of therapy in IA and IV patients with complete tumor remission was still within the limits of normal, and decreased only slightly during treatment.

Conclusion

The two regimes MTX + BLEO and DOX + DDp in combination with high-dose radiation showed a carcinolytic effect in about 17% (CR) on nonoperable patients. Intra-arterially administered cytostatics were more effective than those given intravenously. The IA patients (who had the more advanced tumors) exhibited slightly longer survival (Table 6). Blood parameters yield no reliable clues for prognosis.

Summary

At the University Clinic for Maxillofacial Surgery in Vienna, 227 patients with advanced craniofacial tumors of different sites were treated with cytostatics; 142 of them underwent simultaneous radiation therapy. Complete remission was observed in 46 patients, partial remission in 64 patients, and 117 patients did not respond. Two cytostatic regimes were used: methotrexate + bleomycin and doxorubicin + cisplatin. These regimes were administered intravenously (104 patients) or intra-arterially (123 patients).

In so-called lost cases (those whose status is such that normally no further treatment is given; 15 patients, 21 cycles, all doxorubicin + cisplatin) hyaluronidase was administered as an adjuvant drug. The average infused dose of hyaluronidase was 1 366 000 units per cycle. Three of these patients were irradiated simultaneously. One complete remission and four partial remissions were observed. Ten patients did not respond.

References

1. Friedl HP (1986) Krebsstatistik 1984, Österreichisches Statistisches Zentralamt. Statistische Nachrichten 41:172–177
2. Kärcher H, Eskici A (1985) Ergebnisse bei der alleinigen operativen Behandlung von Karzinomen der Mundhöhle der letzten 10 Jahre. Zahn-Mund-Kieferheilkd 73:593–599
3. Bitter K (1977) Superadditive cytostatic effects after combined administration of vincristine, bleomycin ind methotrexate to Yoshida sarcoma. J Maxillo Fac Surg 5:115–117
4. Platz H, Engleder R, Fridric M, Hudec M, Schwarzl G (1988) Multimodale Therapie primär inoperabler Plattenepithelcarcinome des Mund-, Kiefer- und Gesichtsbereiches. Z Stomatol 85(6):359–370
5. Hollmann K, Mailath G, Kühböck J, Seitz W (1984) Die Kombinationsbehandlung orofacialer Malignome mit Strahlen und Zytostatika. Z Stomatol 81:171–177
6. Hollmann K, Kühböck J, Mailath G, Stadler B (1985) Surgical and oncological aspects of combined radio- and chemotherapy in the treatment of malignomas in the maxillofacial region (in Hungarian). Fogor Sz 78:268–273

7. Hollmann K, Kühböck J, Seitz W (1983) Combined intraarterial chemotherapy of methotrexate, bleomycin and radiation for advanced inoperable tumours of the head and neck region. Abstracts, 13th International Congress of Chemotherapy, Vienna, SE 12.1.11-5
8. Baumgartner G, Baumgartner M (1985) Ergebnisse einer Pilotstudie mit Hyaluronidase als Zusatz zur zytostatischen Therapie bei malignen Erkrankungen. Wien Klin Wochenschr 97:3
9. Baumgartner G, Fortelny A, Zähnker KS, Kroczek R (1988) Phase I study in chemoresistant locoregional malignant disease with hyaluronidase. Reg Cancer Treat 1:55-58
10. Khono N, Ohnuma T, Truog P, Biller H, Holland JF (1988) Effects of hyaluronidase (HYDase) on doxorubicin (DXR) penetration into multicellular tumor spheroids (MTS) and cell lethality. Proc Am Assoc Cancer Res 29:334

A Complex Chemotherapeutic Concept in the Treatment of Oral Carcinomas with Cisplatin and 5-Fluorouracil

H.P. Howaldt and K. Bitter

Klinik für Mund-, Kiefer- und Gesichtschirurgie, Johann Wolfgang Goethe-Universität, Theodor-Stern-Kai 7, 6000 Frankfurt/Main 70, FRG

Introduction

When the results of the prospective and retrospective observational studies of the German, Austrian, and Swiss cooperative Study group for oral and maxillofacial tumors (DÖSAK) are examined, no great difference in survival rates is seen between them, although they are separated by more than 20 years. The two studies embraced 1485 and 1021 patients respectively (Fig. 1). The 5-year survival rate improved by only 3% (see Fig. 1) over a period when surgical techniques improved substantially. Tumors can now be removed in a more radical manner using block resection and reconstruction of sizeable defects through microsurgical flaps, but this progress has not been reflected in the numbers of patients who survive long term.

Based on this we have arrived at the following conclusions: First, it seems possible to improve patient survival only in small steps. Hence large numbers of patients, good documentation, and long observation periods are required. Second, new treatment measures are needed to improve our results. Last, but not least, our efforts must be focussed on improving the patient's quality of life, as large increases in long-term survival rates due to any specific treatment appear to be out of reach.

In the attempt to fulfill these requirements we have started to treat patients suffering from squamous cell carcinomas of the oral cavity with chemotherapy in the following manner.

Materials and Methods

The chemotherapy regimen that we have now been using for 5 years consists of a 100 mg/m^2 bolus injection of cisplatin and 1000 mg/m^2 5-fluorouracil as a continuous infusion over 96 h. This regimen was first introduced at Wayne State University, USA [6], and has since become the most widely used chemotherapy for head and neck tumors in the United States.

Overall response rates of up to 89% for untreated tumors have been reported [11]. Several modifications of dose and number of treatment courses failed to improve the results [3]. In contrast to the group at Wayne State, we use this chemotherapy postoperatively. The first of three cycles is given 2 weeks after surgery

R. Jakesz/H. Rainer (Eds.)
Progress in Regional Cancer Therapy

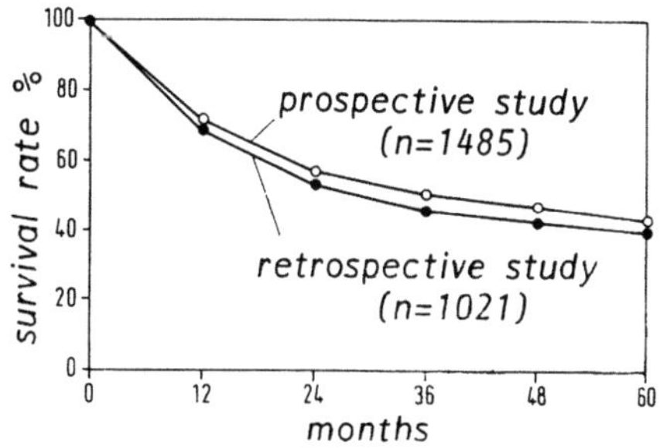

Fig. 1. Survival rates in the prospective and retrospective DÖSAK trials

intended as radical. Patients with unresectable disease are exposed to the same regimen as a neo-adjuvant treatment, followed by irradiation.

Chemotherapy is considered whenever an increased number of tumor-related risk factors – according to the therapeutic prognostic index (TPI) [7] – are evident. These risk factors are: tumor diameter over 4 cm, depth of infiltration exceeding 5 mm, evidence of clinically positive, fixed nodes, evidence of distant metastasis. The patient's age is also relevant. We have tried to apply chemotherapy whenever one of the first four risk factors is present except in the presence of one of more of the following contraindications: age above 75, active tuberculosis, renal dysfunction above WHO grade 2, severely impaired general condition.

A course of chemotherapy is stopped under any of the following circumstances: an attack of gout, white blood cell count below 2500, platelet count below 90 000.

Results

Since 1983 we have treated 109 patients suffering from primary squamous cell carcinomas of the oral cavity and oropharynx (see Table 1). The regimen was used 85 times postoperatively (group 1) and 24 times as a neo-adjuvant treatment

Table 1. Tumor stage, risk factors, and outcome

AJCC stage	Group 1 (postoperative)	Group 2 (neo-adjuvant)
I	5	0
II	7	0
III	26	2
IV	47	22
Total number of patients	85	24
Average number of risk factors (TPI)	1.1	2.5
Alive without tumor	59	4
Alive with relapse	6	4
Dead	20	16
No remission	—	3 (12.5%)
Partial remission	—	12 (50.0%)
Complete remission	—	9 (37.5%)

(group 2). The tumors were classified according to the TNM system [9, 10] and the American Joint Committee (AJC) system [1], as well as on the basis of the TPI [7].

The chemotherapy had to be stopped in two patients because of severe diarrhea, in four instances because of WHO grade 3 leukopenia, and once because of a gout attack. One patient's tuberculosis flared up again during chemotherapy. Two patients died shortly after treatment, one from general sepsis following untreatable diarrhea, the other from a lung embolism. Treatment complications of this kind have been reported previously [2].

In group 1 59 patients have suffered no tumor recurrence by the time of writing. Six are alive with recurrent disease, and 20 have died. In group 2 the overall

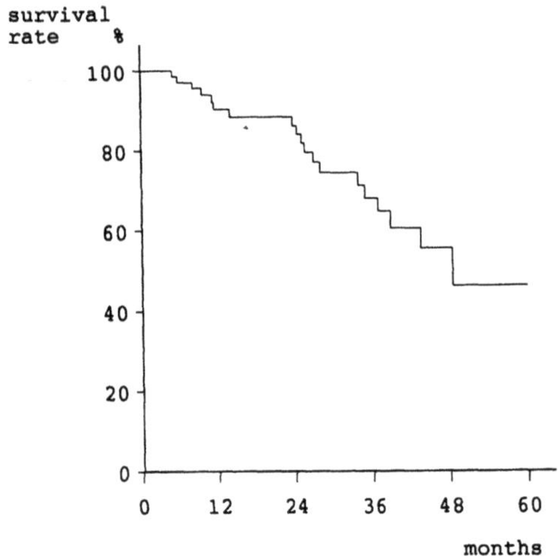

Fig. 2. Survival rate of all patients in Group 1 (postoperative treatment) n = 85

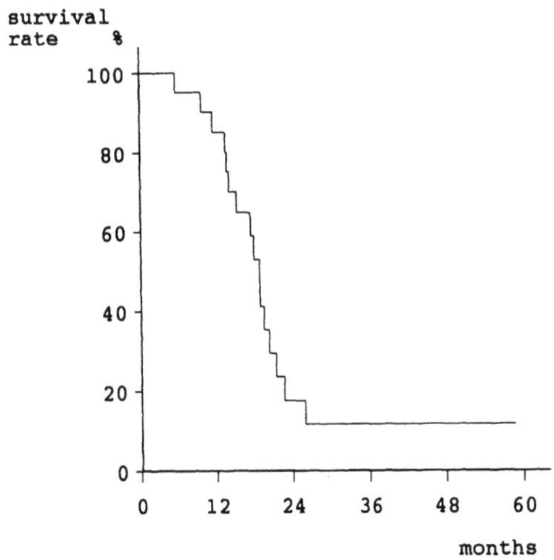

Fig. 3. Survival rate of all patients in Group 2 (neo-adjuvant treatment) n = 24

remission rate was 87.5%; partial remission was observed in 50% of patients and complete remission in 37.5%. One patient has remained free of disease for 4.5 years. So far 16 patients have died from their cancers. The survival curves of the two groups (see Figs. 2, 3) prove neither failure nor success of the treatment. The two curves, calculated according to the Kaplan–Meier method, differ substantially, as the two groups not only include various stages of tumor disease, but also differ in the average number of risk factors present (see Table 1).

In order to analyze the results, we applied the therapeutic prognostic index (TPI) [7], which is based on the data from approximately 1000 patients in the retrospective DÖSAK study. The patients were classified according to the TPI, and those in TPI groups which revealed the same prognostic index were grouped together. The resulting homogeneous samples were compared with the specific estimated survival rate of the TPI (see Fig. 4).

A sample of 24 patients from the 85 in group 1 was selected by this means. Visual comparison of the curves gives the impression that survival in our trial was better than in the control group (see Fig. 5).

In group 2 the survival of 10 patients having the same prognostic index was compared with the specific estimated survival rate of the TPI (see Fig. 6). Here, the duration of survival appears to have been extended, while the 5-year survival rate hardly differs from that of the control group.

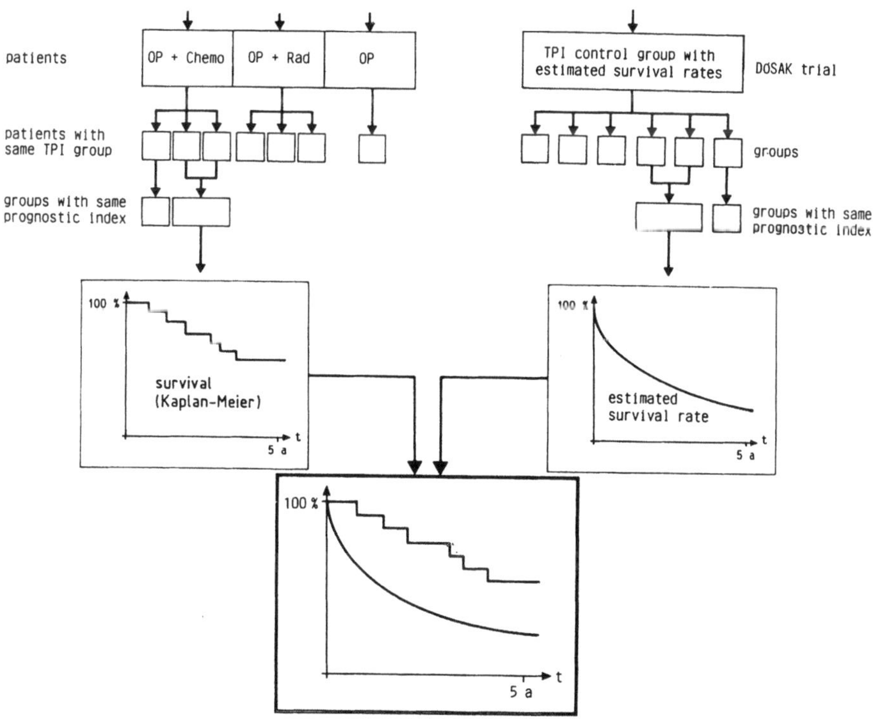

Fig. 4. Comparison of actual survival data with the therapeutic prognostic index (*TPI*)

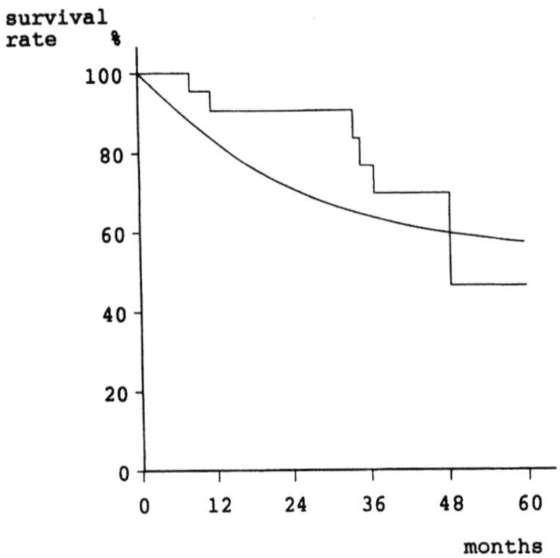

Fig. 5. Survival of 24 patients with TPI main groups E·14, E 37 (in group 1)

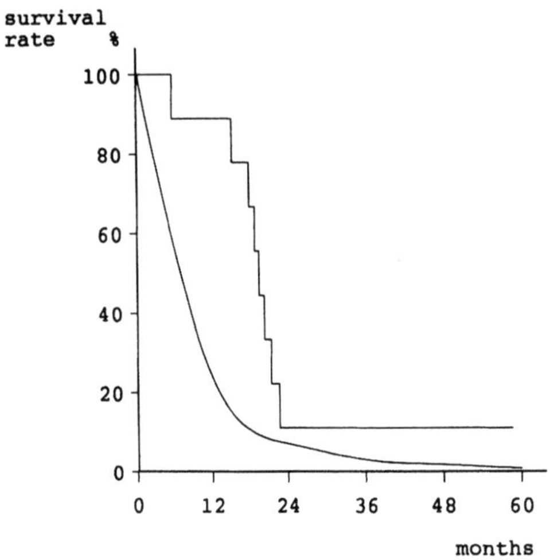

Fig. 6. Survival of 10 patients with TPI main groups EE 9, E 43 (in group 2)

Discussion

The chemotherapeutic concept described here includes a first-choice treatment for patients having a relatively good prognosis and a second-choice, palliative treatment for those with a poor prognosis.

There are good reasons for administering first-choice chemotherapy postoperatively. The more effective treatment, surgery, is carried out first, so that no side effects of chemotherapy can result in surgical complications. After surgery the full amount of drug acts on the few residual tumor cells, which is therapeutically advantageous. While many patients are reluctant to undergo surgery after experiencing a complete or partial remission following chemotherapy [5], noncompliance is not a problem with postoperative regimens. As second-choice treatment, chemotherapy is given prior to irradiation. Again, the more effective treatment is being given first. With the Wayne State protocol comprising cisplatin and 5-fluorouracil we achieved an overall remission rate of 87.5%, almost as good as those reported previously [4, 12] Dental care to prepare the patient for irradiation can be provided between chemotherapy cycles, thus shortening the overall time required for treatment. The final outcome for patients without operative treatment, as in group 2, is inevitably worse as such a course should be followed only in the case of unresectable disease.

Although we have treated more than 100 patients over a period of 5 years, it is not easy to assess the significance of the results. Only controlled randomized clinical trials, requiring a multicentric approach can produce fully reliable data.

In order to assess the results of this one-branch clinical trial performed at one single center, an appropriate control group is needed. We believe we have found an adequate equivalent in the TPI, which is based on the 1021 patients of the retrospective DÖSAK trial. When comparing the actual Kaplan-Meier survival curve with the mathematically calculated expected survival rate, one has to be very careful in interpreting the data. No significant difference in outcome between the trial group and the TPI control group can be proved. A difference may emerge, however, on comparison of the original data of the patients comprising the control group with those of the trial group, and we hope to present such a comparison soon.

References

1. American Joint Committee on Cancer (1988) Manual for staging of cancer, 3rd ed. Lippincott, Philadelphia
2. Decker DA, Drelichman A, Jacobs J, Hoschner J, Kinzie J, Loh JJK, Weaver A, Al-Sarraf M (1983) Adjuvant chemotherapy with cis-diamminodichloroplatinum II and 120-hour infusion 5-fluorouracil in stage III and IV squamous cell carcinoma of the head and neck. Cancer 51:1353–1355
3. Greenberg B, Ahmann F, Garewal H, Koopmann C, Coulthard S, Berzes H, Alberts D, Shimm D Slymen D (1987) Neoadjuvant therapy for advanced head and neck cancer with allopurinol-modulated high dose 5-fluorouracil and cisplatin. Cancer 59:1860–1865
4. Haas C, Byhardt R, Cox J, Duncavage J, Grossman T, Haas J, Hartz A, Libnoch J, Malin T, Ritch P, Toohill R (1985) Randomized study of 5-fluorouracil (F) and cisplatinum (P) as initial therapy of locally advanced squamous carcinoma of head and neck (LASCHN): a preliminary analysis. Proc Am Soc Clin Oncol 4:143
5. Hong WK, Wolf GT, Fischer S, Spaulding M, Endicott J, Hillmann R, Laramore G (1987) The VA cooperative studies program: a new strategy to preserve the larynx in advanced laryngeal cancer. Preliminary report. Proc Am Soc Clin Oncol 6:130
6. Kish J, Drelichman A, Jacobs J, Hoschner J, Kinzie J, Loh J, Weaver A, Al-Sarraf M (1982) Clinical trial of cisplatin and 5-FU infusion as initial treatment for advanced squamous cell carcinomas of the head and neck. Cancer Treat Rep 66:471–474
7. Platz H, Fries R, Hudec M (1986) Prognoses or oral cavity carcinomas. Results of a multicentric retrospective observational study. Hanser, Munich
8. Platz H, Fries R, Hudec M (1988) Einführung in die "Prospektive DÖSAK-Studie über Plattenepithelkarzinome der Lippen, der Mundhöhle und des Oropharynx". Dtsch Z Mund Kiefer Gesichtschir 12:293–302
9. UICC: (1979) TNM Klassifikation maligner Tumoren. 3. Aufl. Springer, Berlin Heidelberg New York

10. UICC: (1987) TNM Klassifikation maligner Tumoren. 4. Aufl. Springer, Berlin Heidelberg New York
11. Weaver A, Fleming S, Kish J, Vanderberg H, Jacob J, Crissman J, Al-Sarraf M (1982) Cisplatinum and 5-fluorouracil as induction therapy for advanced head and neck cancer. Am J Surg 144:445–448
12. Weaver A, Fleming S, Ensley J, Kish JA, Jacobs J, Kinzie J, Crissman J, Al-Sarraf M (1984) Superior clinical response and survival rates with initial bolus of cisplatin and 120 hour infusion of 5-fluorouracil before definitive therapy for locally advanced head and neck cancer. Am J Surg 148:525–529

Pathological Assessment of the Results of Intra-arterial Chemotherapy for Head and Neck Carcinomas by Serial Sections of the Whole Specimen

A. Carbone, L. Barzan, R. Volpe, S. Sulfaro, G. Caruso, S. Frustaci, S. Monfardini, and R. Comoretto

Division of Pathology, Cancer Center, Via Pedemontana Occidentale, 33081 Aviano, Italy

Introduction

The prognosis of patients traditionally treated by surgery and radiotherapy for advanced tumors of the head and neck may be improved with the introduction of chemotherapy [3]. Chemotherapy as primary treatment can be more effective because the tumor has an intact vascular supply and the cellular kinetics are favorable; besides, previously untreated patients have a better performance status (PS) and better tolerance of drug.

It is generally stated that the response to first treatment is a valid prognostic index for head and neck tumors: therefore, one of the most important research goals is to indentify a therapy able to obtain higher response rates with less toxicity. Intra-arterial chemotherapy (IAC) can achieve very high drug concentration in the area of the tumor and can therefore exploit the steep dose-response relationship showed by the majority of antineoplastic agents [1,2]. It is therefore reasonable to expect a higher response rate, but studies must be carried out to discover whether this means improvement in survival [6].

Based on our previous experience [5] we started a new protocol including IAC and subsequent radical surgery, aiming to increase the overall response rate to initial IAC and to reduce the treatment duration and therefore the catheter dwell time (the latter may increase the patient's compliance and reduce the risk of catheter complications) without delaying the definitive local treatment. In order to obtain reliable information on the impact of this therapeutic approach in terms of pathologically proven complete response, the protocol included a histopathological procedure for assessment of tumor regression based on the examination of large serial sections of the whole surgical specimen.

Material and Methods

From February 1985 to November 1987, 22 patients affected by advanced squamous cell carcinomas (SCC) of the head and neck were treated with IAC (cisplatin and bleomycin) and subsequent radical surgery. The eligibility criteria were: biopsy-proven SCC, tumor mass > 3 cm, nodal status N0–N1, no distant

R. Jakesz/H. Rainer (Eds.)
Progress in Regional Cancer Therapy

Table 1. Main clinical findings, toxicity, response to therapy, and follow-up of 22 patients with advanced head and neck carcinomas treated with intra-arterial chemotherapy and radical surgery

Case no.	Sex	Tumor site	TNM[a]	Performance status	Toxicity type (grade)	Response	Further treatment	Follow-up
I 01865	M	Tonsil	T3 N0	80	—	CR	—	Alive, NED
I 01866	M	FM	T2 N0	80	TCP (1), Creat. (1)	CR	—	Alive, NED
I 02341	M	Tongue	T2 N0	80	HL (3)	PR > 50%	RT	Dead, second esophageal tumor
I 03495	M	RA	T2 N1	80	—	PR > 75%	RT	Alive, NED
I 03508	M	Tongue	T2 N0	80	—	PR > 75%	—	Alive, NED
I 03518	F	BT	T2 N0	90	TCP (2), LP (4), A (1), HL (3)	PR < 50%	RT	Alive, NED
I 03564	M	Tongue	T2 N0	80	TCP (1)	PR > 75%	—	Second SCC of BT; third SCC of the contralateral tongue; fourth SCC of PY; alive, NED
I 03700	M	Tongue	T3 N0	100	A (1), pulmonary (1)	PR < 50%	RT	Relapse contralateral neck, surgical rescue; alive, NED
I 06018	M	Tonsil	T3 N0	80	TCP (1), LP (1), A (1)	PR > 75%	RT	Alive, NED
I 06285	M	Tongue	T2 N1	80	Creat. (1), LP (3), A (2), TCP(1)	CR	RT	Alive, NED
I 06539	M	Tonsil	T3 N1	80	Creat. (1), TCP (2), LP (3)	PR > 75%	—	Alive, NED
I 06553	F	C	T4 N0	70	Peripheral palsy, seventh cranial nerve	PR < 50%	RT	Alive, NED
I 06870	M	Tonsil	T2 N0	70	—	PR > 75%	—	Second primary lung tumor; alive
I 06925	M	Tonsil	T3 N1	90	—	CR	—	Relapse contralateral anterior pillar; second SCC of contralateral RA; surgical rescue; alive NED
I 07090	M	Tongue	T3 N0	90	—	PR > 50%	—	Postoperative death, cardiac failure

I 07579	M	BT	T3 N1	90	Creat. (1)	PR > 75%	—	Alive, NED
I 07638	F	RA	T2 N1	70	LP (4), A (1)	PR > 75%	—	Alive, NED
I 08001	M	BT	T2 N1	80	Peripheral palsy, twelfth cranial nerve	CR	RT	Relapse contralateral neck; surgical rescue; alive, NED
I 09547	M	Tongue	T3 N1	80	—	CR	—	Alive, NED
I 10744	M	Tonsil	T3 N0	90	—	PR > 75%	—	Relapse contralateral neck; surgical rescue; alive, NED
I 11019	F	C	T3 N1	80	—	PR > 50%	—	Alive, NED
I 11451	M	Tongue	T3 N1	80	HL (3)	CR	RT	Dead, intercurrent disease

Abbreviations: A, anemia; BT, base of tongue; C, cheek (skin); Creat., decrease in creatinine renal clearance; FM, floor of mouth; HL, hair loss; LP, leukopenia; NED, no evidence of disease; PY, pyriform sinus; RA, retromolar area; RT, radiotherapy; SCC, squamous cell carcinoma; TCP, thrombocytopenia.

[a]Clinical TN classification (UICC 1987).

metastases, life expectancy > 3 months, age < 75 years, PS > 70, no previous treatment, and adequate renal, pulmonary, and medullary function.

Patient Characteristics

The main characteristics of the 22 patients were: male/female ratio 18/4; median age 58 years; median PS 80 (70–100); stage II in six patients, stage III in fifteen, stage IV in one. The other data are shown in Table 1.

Treatment Modalities

The treatment consisted of cisplatin (CDDP) 25 mg in 100 ml normal saline plus 2500 IU heparin administered over a 4-h period, followed by bleomycin 15 mg in 100 ml normal saline plus 7500 IU heparin administered over a 20-h period. The treatment continued without modifications for 10 consecutive days. Clinical evaluation was performed after 2 weeks, at the time of maximum response; radical surgery was performed on the 15th day after chemotherapy ended. Surgical operations were: Commando in 10 patients, pull-through in seven patients, cheek resection with parotidectomy in two patients, subglossopharyngectomy in two patients, transoral hemiglossectomy in one patient. The limits of the surgical resection were based on the tumor extent before IAC. Mono- or bilateral neck dissection was performed in 21 of the 22 patients.

Criteria for Clinical Response Evaluation

Clinical responses were classified as follows: complete response (CR), total disappearance of tumor clinically; partial response (PR) > 75%, shrinkage of tumor by > 75% as measured by the product of the two greatest diameters; PR > 50%; PR < 50%.

Pathological Procedure

The surgical specimens were evaluated prospectively according to a standardized pathological procedure. Each specimen was grossly described, measured, and fixed in Bouin's solution. Thereafter, irrespective of the site of the primary tumor and of the presence of macroscopic residual tumor, the whole specimen was cut into serial large slices 0.3–0.4 cm thick, usually in the frontal plane, parallel to the minor axis of the involved region, and numbered in sequence. An average of 12 such tissue blocks (range 6–19) were obtained from each specimen. These blocks were processed, embedded in paraffin, sliced into large histologic sections 5–6 μm thick, and stained with hematoxylin and eosin.

Histological Evaluation

The effect of the treatment was evaluated histopathologically on the basis of the following parameters: (1) *residual tumor*: RO = no residual tumor; R1 = microscopic residual tumor (tumor residue detectable only at the microscopic level); R2 = macroscopic residual tumor (tumor mass detectable also on the fresh or fixed specimen and/or with the naked eye on the stained tissue sections); (2) *histological changes in the tumor cells:* presence of cytolysis or necrosis, large and bizarre mono- or multinucleated tumor cells with irregular hyperchromatic or pyknotic nuclei, islands of keratotic material without tumor cells; (3) *stromal changes possibly associated with tumor regression:* granulation tissue, foreign body granulomas, and fibrosclerosis, presence and type of the inflammatory reaction.

When feasible, the latter two parameters (2 and 3) were also evaluated in the metastatic lymph nodes.

Results

Clinical Findings

The clinical responses observed were: CR in seven patients (31.8%); PR > 75% in nine patients (41%); PR > 50% in three patients (13.6%); PR < 50% in three patients (13.6%). Therefore, an objective significant tumor regression was recorded in 19/22 patients (86.4%); the regression became apparent between the 8th and the 15th day after the end of IAC.

Surgery was deferred in two patients (9.1%) who experienced severe toxicity (leukopenia); we waited for spontaneous recovery without observing progression of the tumor. Two other patients had peripheral palsy of the seventh and twelfth cranial nerve respectively. As of September 1988, 19 patients were alive, 18 without evidence of disease (see Table 1).

Pathological Findings

Histopathologically, complete disappearance of tumor tissue (RO) was verified in four cases (18.2%) in which SCC of the tongue (two cases) and of the tonsil (two cases) had been diagnosed in biopsy specimens. Microscopic residual foci (R1) of SCC were found in eight cases (36.4%); it is remarkable that in all these cases microscopic residual tumor consisted of single or few carcinomatous strands surrounded by marked fibrosis (Fig. 1). Tumor residues were located either superficially or deeply in areas corresponding to the primary tumor site. In the remaining 10 cases (see Table 2) a tumor mass (R2) was detected grossly on the fresh or fixed specimen and/or on the stained tissue sections; the presence of SCC was confirmed on microscopic examination (Fig. 2).

Lymph vessel invasion was recorded in three cases (two in the R2 group and one in the R1 group); in one of these (the R1 case) endolymphatic emboli were the only microscopic residue found.

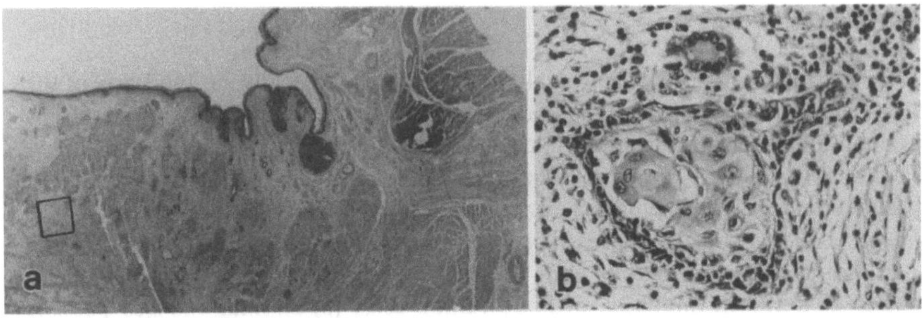

Fig. 1 a, b. Case no. I 8001: primary SCC of the base of the tongue. **a** In this large section of the specimen passing through the anterior faucial pillar, only microscopic residual tumor (R1) was found. Tumor residues were located deeply in the area corresponding to the primary tumor site (*square*). Original magnification 3×. **b** Microscopic detail of the square. Histologically, tumor residues consisted of few carcinomatous strands surrounded by fibrosis, lymphocyte infiltrate, and scattered foreign body multinucleated giant cells **b** H&E, original magnification ×250.

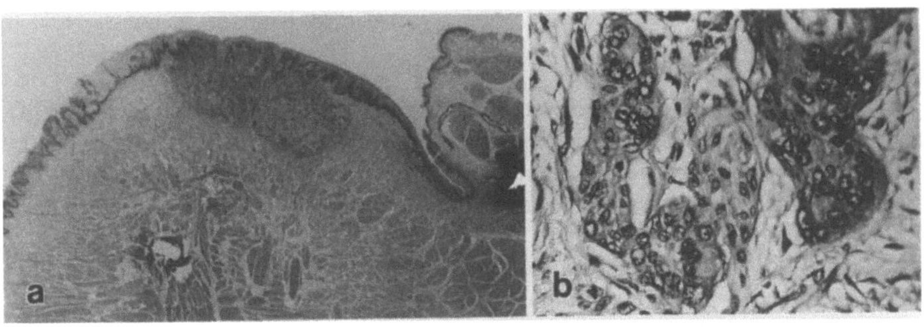

Fig. 2 a, b. Case no. I 10744: primary SCC of the amygdaloglossopalatine region. **a** Tumor residue (R2) is detectable in the stained tissue section; the residual tumor mass involving the lateral margin of the tongue, shows a well-defined border. Original magnification 3×. The presence of a SCC was confirmed at the microscopic level **b** H & E, original magnification ×250

Overall, cytological and/or stromal changes possibly associated with tumor regression were observed in 16/22 cases (72.7%).

As far as the histological changes in the tumor cells are concerned, bizarre and multinucleated cells were observed in six cases (27.3%): three in the R1 group (37.5%) and three in the R2 group (30%). Necrosis was never found. Islands of keratotic material without tumor cells were seen in 5 cases (22.7%): four in the R1 group (50%) and one in the R2 group (10%); the keratosis was invariably associated with multinucleated giant cells of the foreign body type (Fig. 3, Table 2).

In areas corresponding to the primary tumor site, stromal reaction features possibly associated with tumor regression were observed in 15 cases (68.2%): four in the R0 group (100%), eight in the R1 group (100%), and three in the R2 group (30%). Foreign body granulomas and a fibrosclerotic reaction were found in seven cases, (two in the R0 group and five in the R1 group), fibrosis alone in three cases, (two in the R0 group and one in the R2 group) and foreign body granulomas

Table 2. Residual tumor, lymph node status and pertinent histopathologic findings in 22 patients with squamous cell carcinoma of the head and neck treated with IAC and radical surgery

Primary site									Lymph nodes					
Case no.	Site	Tumor residue	Bizarre cells	Tumor necrosis	Keratotic material	Foreign body granulomas	Fibrosis	Granulation tissue	pN	Bizarre cells	Tumor necrosis	Keratotic material	Foreign body granulomas	Fibrosis
I 06285	Tongue	R0	–	–	–	–	+	–	N2b	+	–	+	+	+
I 07090	Tongue	R0	–	–	–	–	+	–	N2c	NE	NE	NE	NE	NE
I 06925	Tonsil	R0	–	–	–	–	+	–	N0					
I 06539	Tonsil	R0	–	–	–	–	+	–	N1	+	+	–	+	+
I 07579	BT	R1	+	–	–	+	+	+	N0					
I 08001	BT	R1	–	–	–	+	+	–	N0					
I 01866	FM	R1	+	–	+	+	+	–	N0					
I 03495	RA	R1	–	–	+	+	–	–	N2a	+	+	+	+	–
I 03508	Tongue	R1	–	–	–	+	–	–	N0					
I 03564	Tongue	R1	–	–	+	+	–	–	N0					
I 09547	Tongue	R1	–	–	+	+	+	–	N0					
I 01865	Tonsil	R1	+	–	–	+	+	–	N0					
I 03518	BT	R2	–	–	–	–	–	–	N0					
I 06553	C	R2	–	–	–	–	–	–	N1	–	–	–	–	–
I 11019	C	R2	+	–	–	–	–	–	N0					
I 07638	RA	R2	–	–	–	–	–	–	N2a	–	–	–	–	–
I 02341	Tongue	R2	–	–	–	–	–	–	N0					
I 03700	Tongue	R2	–	–	–	–	–	–	N2b	–	–	+	+	+
I 11451	Tongue	R2	+	–	–	–	+	–	N2b	+	+	–	+	+
I 06018	Tonsil	R2	–	–	–	–	–	–	N2b	–	–	+	+	–
I 06870	Tonsil	R2	–	–	+	+	–	–	N0			+[a]	+[a]	
I 10744	Tonsil	R2	+	–	–	+	–	–	N0					

Abbreviations: BT, base of tongue; C, cheek (skin); FM, floor of mouth; NE, not evaluated, embolic metastasis only in contralateral cervical lymph node; RA, retromolar area; R0, no tumor residue; R1, microscopic tumor residue; R2, macroscopic tumor residue.
[a] No tumor cells found.

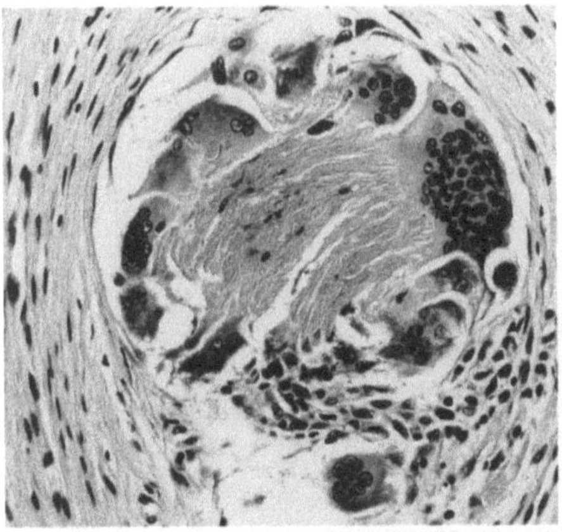
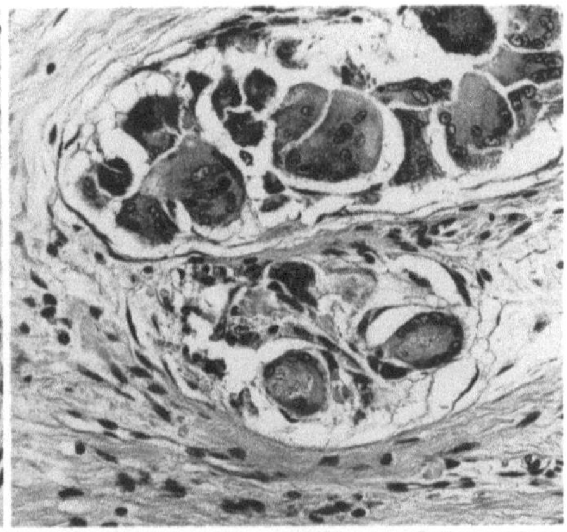
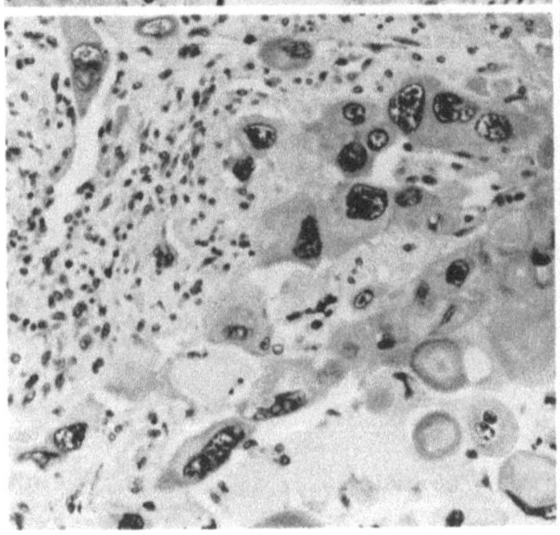
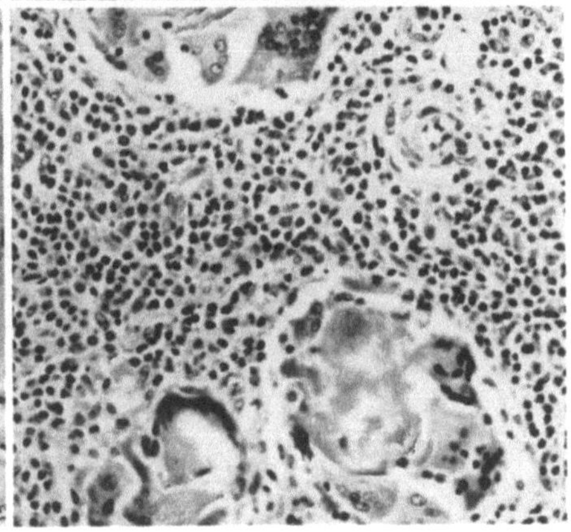

Fig. 3 (*upper left*). Foreign body multinucleated giant cells surrounding keratotic material H&E, original magnification × 250

Fig. 4 (*upper right*). A foreign body granuloma is surrounded by a stromal fibrosclerotic reaction H&E, original magnification × 250

Fig. 5 (*lower left*). Lymph node metastasis: carcinomatous squamous cells with bizarre and grotseque nuclear features H&E, original magnification × 250

Fig. 6 (*lower right*). A nonmetastatic lymph node in which keratotic material surrounded by foreign body multinucleated giant cells constituted the only pathologic feature, possibly testifying to tumor regression H&E, original magnification × 250

alone in the remaining five cases (three in the R1 group and two in the R2 group) (Fig. 4). Associated findings were a chronic inflammatory reaction in six cases, a xanthogranulomatous process in one case, and the presence of granulation tissue in one case.

Metastatic lymph nodes were found in 9 cases (40.9%): three in the R0 group (75%), one in the R1 group (12.5%), and five in the R2 group (50%). Excluding one R0 case in which only a metastasis of the embolic type was found, regression changes in lymph node metastases were observed in six out of the remaining eight cases (2/2 in the R0 group, 1/1 in the R1 group, and 3/5 in the R2 group) (Fig. 5). In another R2 case, keratotic material surrounded by granulomatous reaction in the absence of neoplastic residue (pN0), was found in two of the 43 lymph nodes dissected (Fig. 6); in this case, regression changes were seen in the primary site as well (Table 2).

Discussion

The present IAC protocol displayed good tolerability; severe and life-threatening toxicity (leukopenia) was encountered in only two patients (9.1%). The administration of CDDP caused two cases of peripheral cranial nerve palsy, clearly correlated with the high drug concentration in the perfused area; both nerves had to be resected during the surgical procedure to achieve oncological radicality.

The clinical response was impressive: 86.4% of the patients obtained an objective tumor regression; progression of the disease was never noticed. The specific advantage of this schedule was the high response rate achieved in a short period of time. This result is not matched by any of the many intravenous schedules [2, 3, 6].

The rapidity of tumor regression, without relevant persistent toxicity, meant that the definitive local treatment could be undertaken 4–5 weeks from the first outpatient visit. Compared with our previous experience employing CDDP [5] and regimens without CDDP, this schedule achieved the highest response rate in the shortest time and with acceptable and well-manageable toxicity.

Using a standardized and prospective histopathological procedure, tumor cell and/or stromal changes possibly associated with tumor regression were observed in 72.7% of cases. We were able to verify histological disappearance of the tumor in four of the 22 patients (18.2%). Interestingly, in a recent study [3] involving a series of 130 patients with advanced head and neck SCC treated with intravenous chemotherapy including methotrexate, CDDP, bleomycin, and vincristine, complete disappearance of tumor was observed in three of the 20 cases pathologically evaluated (15%). Moreover, the procedure we used permitted detection of histological persistence of microscopic tumor residue in eight cases (36.4%). The detection of small carcinomatous foci in this relatively large proportion of cases after a complete sampling of the surgical specimen strongly corroborates the contribution of such a procedure to careful and reliable evaluation of the tumor response to IAC. In a previous study on a superimposable series of patients treated with intra-arterial CDDP [7], complete disappearance was seen in 12/24 (50%) primary advanced head and neck cancers. The authors made no mention of the modes of response evaluation; however, the reported value is similar to that obtained in our series by adding the cases with complete disappearance of tumor and those showing microscopic persistence of tumor (12 R0 + R1/22, 54.6%). In another study on 129 cases of oral cavity carcinoma [8], tumor regression, including complete disappearance, was demonstrated in 39% of the pathologically evaluated cases. The patients were treated with intra-arterial methotrexate and subsequent radical surgery. The pathological evaluation was performed on the surgical specimens.

In the present study we also evaluated the possible effects of IAC on tumor cells and stromal components. Two main histopathological changes were noted: the appearance of bizarre and multinucleated tumor cells and the presence of islands of keratotic material associated with multinucleated giant cells of the foreign body type. This latter change, often combined with fibrosis, predominated in the R1 group of cases and could be related to the tumor regression [4, 9]. Interestingly, in one R2 case, keratotic material with granulomatous reaction in the absence of tumor cells (pN0) was found in two neck lymph nodes.

In conclusion, the percentage of overall (clinical and pathological) responses to IAC we observed suggests that the protocol reported here is one of the most effective in advanced head and neck carcinomas; nevertheless, the role of IAC has not yet been completely defined, and randomized trials have to be planned. The impact of the downstaging on local disease-free survival and overall survival has to be further evaluated with a larger number of patients and longer follow-up.

References

1. Baker SR, Wheeler R (1983) Intraarterial chemotherapy for head and neck cancer. 1: Theoretical considerations and drug delivery systems. Head Neck Surg 6:664–682
2. Baker SR, Wheeler R (1984) Intraarterial chemotherapy for head and neck cancer. 2: Clinical experience. Head Neck Surg 6:751–760
3. Cognetti F, Pinnaro P, Carlini P, Ruggeri EM, Ambesi Impiombato F, Del Vecchi MR, Giannarelli D, Perrino A (1988) Neoadjuvant chemotherapy in previously untreated patients with advanced head and neck squamous cell cancer. Cancer 62:251–261
4. Fajardo LF (1982) Morphologic changes in irradiated tumors. In: Fajardo LF (ed) Pathology of radiation injury. Masson, New York, pp 244–251 (Masson monographs in diagnostic pathology, vol 6)
5. Frustaci S, Barzan L, Tumolo S, Comoretto R, Quadu G, Galligioni E, Lorenzini M, Crivellari D, Caruso G, Piccinin G, Veronesi A, Tirelli U, Grigoletto G (1986) Intra-arterial continuous infusion of Cis-diamminedichloroplatinum in untreated head and neck cancer patients. Cancer 57:1118–1123
6. Molinari R (1983) Present role of intra-arterial regional chemotherapy in head and neck cancer. Drug Exp Clin Res 9:491–504
7. Mortimer J, Cummings C, Laramore G, Greenberg P (1986) Feasibility and efficacy of weekly intra-arterial cisplatin in locally advanced (stage III and IV) head and neck cancers. In: Proc Am Assoc Cancer Res 27:179 (abstr 710)
8. Richard J, Domenge C (1986) La chimiothérapie intra-artérielle d'induction dans les tumeurs des voies aéro-digestives supérieures. In: Jaquillat C, Weil M, Khayat M (eds) Neo-adjuvant chemotherapy. (Colloque INSERM vol 137) Libbey, London, pp 447–453
9. Shimosato Y, Oboshi S, Baba K (1971) Histological evaluation of effects of radiotherapy and chemotherapy for carcinomas. Jpn J Clin Oncol 1:19–35

The Bypass Method in Head and Neck Cancer

J. von Scheel and E.R. Kastenbauer

Hals-Nasen-Ohrenklinik, Allgemeines Krankenhaus Altona, Paul-Ehrlich-Straße 1, 2000 Hamburg 50, FRG

Introduction

Since the first attempts at intra-arterial (IA) antineoplastic infusion therapy by Biermann and Klopp in 1950, a few other investigators have performed some pilot studies using various techniques and cytostatic drugs. The results of these studies have been disappointing, because of either technical difficulties or insufficient effectiveness of the drug(s) employed. Long-term results have rarely been published. Moreover, many investigators have doubted the efficiency of the pharmacokinetic principle of IA infusion, i.e., delivery of greater fraction of the drug dose to the tumor region than to other tissues. From the literature and from our own experiments [4, 5], we have learned that the following prerequisites are crucial for the success of IA cytostatic drug infusion:

1. The infusion should be selective in order to enhance the first-pass effect. Infusion into the trunk of the external carotid artery would be of negligible advantage.
2. The infusion rate should be slow, as the percentage of drug extracted from the blood into the tissue during the first pass in the tumor region attenuates with extreme drug doses. Bolus injection is thus expected to be of lower pharmacokinetic benefit.
3. The treatment schedule should be independent of the technique of infusion employed. Our hypothesis was and is that intermittent infusion would enhance the advantage of IA infusion in parallel to the generally accepted principle of fractionation in radiation therapy.
4. Infusion of the superior thyroid artery should be possible in order to include tumors of the epiglottis and base of the tongue.

The "bypass" method described herein was created to fulfill these criteria by being as selective as necessary, allowing a slow infusion rate and intermittent infusion over several weeks (or even months), and being the only method permitting safe infusion of the superior thyroid artery.

R. Jakesz/H. Rainer (Eds.)
Progress in Regional Cancer Therapy

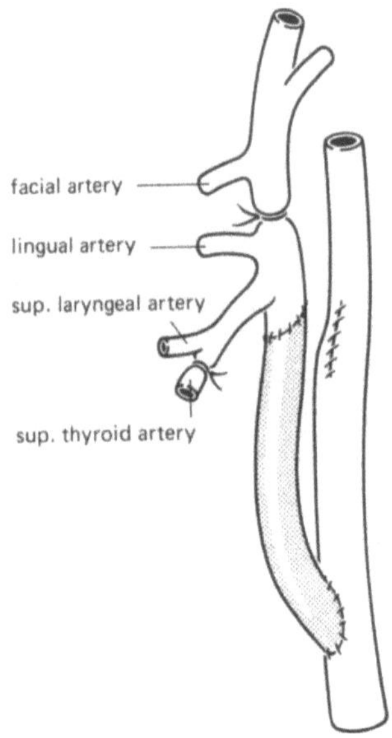

Fig. 1. Vascular surgical procedure in patients with tumors near or at the epiglottis. Note that the superior thyroid artery participates in the arterial perfusion of this area

Materials and Methods

The bypass method is described in detail elsewhere [2, 3]. In short, the first step is radical neck dissection: After exposure of the neck artery system, the external carotid artery is severed at its origin from the common carotid artery and is prolonged by an autogenous saphenous vein graft which is sutured end-to-side to the common carotid artery more proximally (Fig. 1). After wound healing the bypass is palpable through the skin and can be repeatedly punctured for IA infusion, somewhat similar to the Cimino shunt in hemodialysis.
The curative treatment protocol consists of:

1. Radical neck dissection with surgical preparation of the neck arteries (bypass)
2. After wound healing, intermittent IA chemotherapy of the (inoperable) primary tumor over 4–6 weeks
3. After completion of IA chemotherapy, full-dose irradiation (^{60}Co).

Such a bypass was constructed in 69 patients in Berlin. In three additional patients the origin of the external carotid artery was situated sufficiently far caudal for a bypass to be unnecessary. Sixty-five of the patients were previously untreated. The histology was squamous cell carcinoma in 66 cases, adenoid cystic carcinoma in three, transitional cell carcinoma in two, and undifferentiated carcinoma in one. Four consecutive patients had the bypass operation without subsequent IA infusion because of poor compliance. These patients died shortly thereafter despite alternative therapy.

The drug mostly used was cisplatin, 20 mg per day infused over 8 h. The normal dosage was 100 mg in the 1st week, followed by 60–100 mg per week in the second and subsequent weeks, aiming at a total dose of about 400 mg (less in light patients, over 500 mg in heavy patients). Hydration was only oral instead of IV; diuretics were not used. Side effects were detected by means of serial blood cell counts and monitoring of kidney function and hearing. Since in the first series of patients early thrombosis of the bypass proved to be a major problem, we started to perform anticoagulation with phenprocoumon, restricted to the period of IA infusion, i.e. 4–6 weeks. The response to IA chemotherapy was considered complete if there was complete clinical regression of the tumor. A partial response was defined as a reduction in the size of the tumor by half of more.

Results

The only intraoperative complication of vascular surgery was poor quality of the saphenous vein graft, in three cases. One patient died 3 days after operation of bleeding from a gastric ulcer.

Technical problems with IA infusion (early thrombosis of the bypass) occurred in six cases, including the three with poor-quality grafts. However, five of these were among the first 15 patients, only one among the following 50 patients. The frequency of early thrombosis of the vein graft with experience was thus about 2%.

Of 51 nonpretreated patients with adequate IA infusion over 4–6 weeks, 25 (49%) had a complete remission. A further 21 patients (41%) displayed a partial response, including some remissions that were almost complete. In five patients (10%) there was no change or progression of disease. These data refer to chemotherapy alone.

For the evaluation of the oncological advantage of IA infusion it is necessary to exclude the patients with previous treatment, as their IA treatment was palliative in nature. In four of five previously irradiated patients the response was poor. They died within 1 year postoperatively.

The 2-year survival rate of previously untreated patients with adequate IA infusion followed by full-dose radiation therapy was 50% (21/42). In nine patients the follow-up period at the time of writing was too short for evaluation; however, eight were alive with no evidence of disease. The 3-year survival rate was 51.5% (17/33), the 5-year survival rate 36% (8/22).

Discussion

The term "bypass" reflects the surgical technique. As in any kind of vascular surgery, thrombosis of the vein graft proved to be a handicap, especially in our first series of patients. However, by consistent use of phenprocoumon the frequency of early thrombosis was reduced to 2% (1/51). From the technical point of view, therefore, the bypass method of IA infusion has proven its usefulness and practicability. All four criteria mentioned in the introduction were fulfilled:

1. Selectivity was provided by ligation of branches of the external carotid artery not participating in the blood supply of the tumor region, with the effect that loss of hair occurred only in patients with maxillary tumors where the maxillary and the middle meningeal artery were infused. Induction of mucositis by cytostatic drug was observed only in the infused region, e.g., one half of the tongue.
2. The slow infusion rate and low daily dose led to low subjective toxicity: especially patients without infusion of the maxillary artery (and middle meningeal artery)

rarely experienced nausea or vomiting. Objective toxicity with a lethal outcome occurred in one case of cisplatin-induced kidney damage and one case of aplastic anemia. More subtle monitoring might have prevented these developments.
3. The infusion schedule was independent of the infusion technique. In the majority of cases IA therapy could be performed over about 6 weeks. In most cases the bypass remained open even after the discontinuation of chemotherapy and phenprocoumon, thus facilitating further IA infusion in case of recurrence. This is one of the advantages of the bypass method over retrograde cannulation of the superficial temporal artery.
4. One of the most problematic tumor regions from the surgical point of view is the base of the tongue and the epiglottis. The bypass method is the only IA technique facilitating safe infusion of the superior thyroid artery, which cannot be accomplished by any of the traditional or more recent catheter techniques. The oropharynx as the site of the primary tumor is therefore one of the most important indications for the bypass method.

In spite of the moderate toxicity the rate of complete remissions was high. The partial remission group contains 11 cases of 90% remission, including seven with a tumor-free interval of at least 2 years. In two of these eleven patients the follow-up period is too short for evaluation. The overall response rate is similar to that reported by Choi et al. [1], who also used the bypass method. A 2-year and 3-year survival rate of 50% means that use of the bypass method was worthwhile for these patients, as they had a relatively high quality of life in this period: swallowing was improved or normalized, and pain was reduced or eliminated. Moreover, about one third of patients survived 5 years or more (maximum 8 years), indicating that in some cases the treatment schedule can be expected to have a curative effect.

In conclusion, the bypass method has proven its usefulness and is of great value for at least half of the patients. It could be demonstrated that the pharmacological principle of IA infusion can be realized in the clinic situation. However, the oncological advantage of the method will have to be assessed in a prospective trial comparing IA chemotherapy plus irradiation with other treatment schedules. Moreover, a great variety of regimens of cytostatic drugs and drug combinations for IA antineoplastic chemotherapy of head and neck cancer via the bypass route will have to be evaluated.

References

1. Choi TK, Wei W, Lau WF, Lam KH (1987) Regional chemotherapy through a saphenous vein graft for the treatment of head and neck cancers. Cancer 60:1432–1438
2. Kastenbauer E, von Scheel J (1983) Gibt es in der Behandlung des Plattenepithelkarzinoms des Oropharynx Fortschritte? Laryngol Rhinol Otol (Stuttg) 62:542–547
3. von Scheel J (1981) Zur Methodik der intraarteriellen Chemotherapie maligner Tumoren im Kopf-Hals-Bereich. Laryngol Rhinol Otol (Stuttg) 60:275–277
4. von Scheel J, Golde G (1984) Pharmacokinetics of intra-arterial tumour therapy. An experimental study. Arch Otorhinolaryngol 239:153–161
5. von Scheel J, Golde G (1984) Ein Computer-Modell zur Simulation der intraarteriellen Tumortherapie im Bereich der A. carotis externa. Laryngol Rhinol Otol (Stuttg) 63:575–579

Intratumoral Treatment of Incurable Head and Neck Cancer with Recombinant Human Tumor Necrosis Factor-α

R. Pavelka, K. Hollmann, F. Scholz, and C. Schober

II. Universitäts Klinik für Hals-Nasen-Ohrenheilkunde,
Universitätsklinik für Kieferchirurgie Wien, Alser Straße 4, 1090 Wien, Austria

Introduction

As early as 1893 Coley [5] observed a patient whose sarcoma showed hemorrhagic necrotization in the course of an infection with erysipelas. Subsequent experiments revealed that bacterial polysaccharides might be the cause of this hemorrhagic tumor necrosis.

In 1975 Carswell et al. [4], in Lloyd Old's laboratories, showed that the ability to induce tumor necrosis could be transferred by serum obtained from mice in which tumor necroses were induced by lipopolysaccharide (LPS) after pretreatment with Bacillus Calmette-Guérin (BCG). Macrophages were found to produce this serum factor. When Pennica published the chemical structure of this tumor necrosis factor (TNF) in 1984 [6] identity was seen with cachexin, a substance responsible for endotoxic shock, as shown by Beutler et al. in 1985 [2].

Today TNF is available in almost pure form as a substance produced by recombinant genetic engineering in *E. coli.*

The antitumor activity of TNF is based mainly on its following three properties [8]:

1. Cytotoxic and/or cytostatic effect on several tumor cell lines, but not on normal cells in vitro.
2. Toxicity to endothelial cells, preferentially those of tumor vessels, leading to the formation of fibrin thrombi and thus causing ischemic necrosis with extravasation of erythrocytes.
3. Immunomodulation by activation of macrophages, resulting in endogenous production of TNF, interleukin-1 (IL-1), and granulocyte–colony-stimulating factor (G-CSF), activation of T lymphocytes (directly or via IL-1), stimulation of phagocytosis of the neutrophils, stimulation of response in mixed lymphocytes culture, and stimulation of antibody-dependent cellular cytotoxicity (ADCC).

In accordance with its pathophysiological function as cachexin, treatment with TNF is accompanied by a high rate of side effects [3, 7]:

- Fever and chill on the day of injection, headache, fatigue, anorexia
- Hypotension caused by capillary leakage with the danger of hypovolemic shock,

R. Jakesz/H. Rainer (Eds.)
Progress in Regional Cancer Therapy

metabolic disturbance, increase of glutamic oxaloacetic transaminase (GOT), hyperglycemia and hypertriglyceridemia, changes in blood counts, mild anemia, leukopenia, thrombopenia
- Local inflammatory reactions or induration after subcutaneous injection

In patients with metastatic tumors, isolated cases of severe and lethal toxicity to the kidneys, liver, heart, and lungs, thromboembolic complications, and epilepsy have been reported.

In early studies in man, the tumor response rate to TNF was about 10% after intravenous or intramuscular injections [3]. In 1986 Taguchi et al. [9] reported a tumor response in 11 of 24 patients (46%) after intratumoral injection of recombinant TNF (rTNF), while side effects were considerably decreased. Similar findings were published by Pfreundschuh et al. of Cologne [7] and Bartsch et al. of Göttingen [1].

Patients and Methods

Encouraged by these results, we set up a clinical trial in which rTNF-α is injected intratumorally, in patients with incurable head and neck carcinoma. The study protocol was approved by the local ethics committee. rTNF-α was produced by Genentech (San Francisco) and kindly supplied by Boehringer Ingelheim (Bender & Co., Vienna). TNF is injected into the tumor once a week with doses increasing every 2nd week, starting with 50 $\mu g/m^2$ and increasing to 300 $\mu g/m^2$ and more if tolerated. The total volume injected is 2 ml. Based on a complete dose escalation the duration of the treatment is 12 weeks. Only patients with incurable locoregional recurrences or persistent tumors are entered in the trial. Those with distant metastases or diseases of parenchymatous organs are excluded.

At the time of writing, treatment had been completed in four patients and a further patient was still undergoing treatment. Of these five patients, four had squamous cell carcinoma and one had a neck metastasis of an undifferentiated carcinoma; autopsy revealed a primary adenocarcinoma of the pancreas.

Results

The local injections of TNF were well tolerated in all but one case; this patient with a parapharyngeal tumor recurrence needed premedication with pethidine hydrochloride and diazepam and local anesthesia. The systemic toxicity was slight to moderate. A fever of 38–40°C on the day of injection was seldom associated with chills. Severe hypotension necessitating treatment occurred only in one patient, at the maximum dose of 400 $\mu g/m^2$. There were no noteworthy changes in blood counts or blood chemistry; specifically, no alterations in hepatic enzymes, fibrin degradation products (FDP), or lipid fractions.

Two patients died of their progressing cancer during treatment. Autopsy confirmed that these deaths were not related to the TNF therapy. Serum levels of TNF were measured by enzyme immunoassay (EIA). The peak blood TNF was reached a half hour after injection and was followed by a rapid decrease. The peak values were considerably lower than those measured by other investigators after intravenous or intramuscular injection [3].

Serum neopterin was measured as a parameter of the cellular immune reaction. Neopterin is a metabolite of activated macrophages and T lymphocytes. Neopterin production regularly peaked 2 days after TNF injection and decreased to baseline before the next injection.

Measurements of interferon-γ by radioimmunoassay (RIA) and β_2-microglobulin by EIA did not reveal any influence by TNF.

Tumor Reaction to TNF

The first patient suffered from a parapharyngeal recurrence of a squamous cell carcinoma of the larynx after laryngectomy with radical neck dissection and radiotherapy. The TNF was injected into the tumor under sonographic guidance. Hyperechoic inclusions of air demonstrated the correct siting of the injections within the tumor. Some of the injections were made transorally into the pharyngeal part of the tumor. Inflammatory reactions were regularly seen 2–3 days after injection but no necroses occurred. Computed tomography (CT) 1 month after the end of the therapy showed stable disease.

The second patient had extended, inoperable neck metastases of an undifferentiated carcinoma with progression of disease in spite of radiochemotherapy. TNF was injected into subcutanous metastases in the nonirradiated nape of the neck. As early as 16 h after the first injection of 50 $\mu g/m^2$, a hemorrhagic necrosis developed, with characteristic red and blue bleedings against a pale background. After 2 days the originally ischemic necrosis liquefied and formed an abscess, which perforated the skin. Following removal of the necroses a second injection was given to the margins. Two days later a second necrosis occurred, which liquefied after 2 days. Not all nodes reacted in the same manner, however, and new metastases appeared during therapy. The patient died within 4 weeks. Autopsy revealed that the primary tumor was an undifferentiated adenocarcinoma in the head of the pancreas.

The third patient had a squamous cell carcinoma of the tongue and the floor of the mouth with sublingual ulceration after extensive radiochemotherapy. He received TNF injections for 8 weeks. Each time, an ischemic necrosis was observed in the injected area after 20–24 h, with perforation of the subsequent abscess 2–3 days later. The ulceration in the floor of the mouth penetrated to a depth of several centimeters, and new ulceration occurred in the surrounding tumor tissue due to TNF treatment.

A CT scan after 6 weeks confirmed the clinical suspicion of undoubted progression of the tumor in spite of the marked necrotization in the center. Six weeks after discontinuation of TNF therapy the patient died of tumor cachexia. Autopsy revealed a huge area of destruction beneath the aponeurosis of the tongue surrounded by vital tumor.

The fourth patient, suffering from a huge recurrence of a squamous cell carcinoma of the whole pharynx and the tongue with penetration of the skin, was totally anergic and in very poor general condition. Neither inflammatory reactions nor tumor necroses were observed. The patient died of progressive tumor disease after the sixth injection.

Conclusions

Intratumoral administration was feasible. The mild nature of the side effects compared to intravenous or intramuscular application [3] could be explained by the low serum levels of TNF. General immunostimulation of serum neopterin, but no significant stimulation of interferon γ- and β_2-microglobulin, was measured.

In our first four patients, we observed no tumor response. One patient had stable disease lasting 4 months. Two other patients had progressive disease despite typical hemorrhagic tumor necroses at the injection site. We do not know whether the poor general condition of these heavily pretreated patients or a special reaction of head and neck tumors to TNF is the cause of this poor tumor response.

References

1. Bartsch HH, Golms R, Nagel GA (1988) Intralesional application of recombinant tumor-necrosis factor-alpha in patients with advanced malignancies. Workshop: Progress in Regional Cancer Therapy I, abstract 244, p 143
2. Beutler B, Greenwald D, Hulmes JD et al. (1985) Identity of tumor necrosis factor and the macrophage secreted factor cachectin. Nature 316:552–554
3. Blick M, Sherwin SA, Rosenblum M, Gutterman J (1987) Phase I study of recombinant tumor necrosis factor in cancer patients. Cancer Res 47:2986–2989
4. Carswell EA, Old LJ, Kassel RL, Green S, Fiore N, Williamson B (1975) An endotoxin-induced serum factor that causes necrosis of tumors. Proc Natl Acad Sci USA 72:3666–3670
5. Coley WB (1893) The treatment of malignant tumors by repeated inoculations of erysipelas; with a report of ten original cases. Am J Med Sci 105:487–511
6. Pennica D, Nedwin GE, Hayflick JS et al. (1984) Human tumor necrosis factor: precursor structure, expression and homology to lymphotoxin. Nature 312:724–729
7. Pfreundschuh M, Schaadt M, Steinmetz T, Tüschen R, Schenk V, Diehl V (1989) Phase-I-study of intratumoral application of recombinant human tumor necrosis factor. Int J Cancer (in press)
8. Ruff M, Gifford GE (1981) Tumor necrosis factor. In: Pick E (ed) Lymphokines vol 2. Academic, New York, pp 235–272
9. Taguchi T, Shiratori T, Kodama M, Takahashi T, Okajima K, Mori T et al. (1986) Clinical studies of recombinant human tumor necrosis factor (rHu-TNF: PT–050). Proceedings of the 14th International Cancer Congress, Budapest, abstract 4455, p 1159

Preoperative Local Immunotherapy with OK-432 (Picibanil) in Patients with Squamous Cell Cancer of the Oral Cavity

K.G. Vinzenz, N. Neuhold, H. Porteder, M. Matejka, G. Watzek, and M. Micksche

Klinik für Kiefer- und Gesichtschirurgie, Universität Wien, Alser Straße 4, 1090 Wien, Austria

Introduction

Lymphocytes of normal experimental animals and human subjects are able to kill in vitro, without presensitization, a variety of virus-infected and tumor-derived target cells. This natural killer (NK) cell activity can be detected in peripheral blood (PB) as well as in lymphoid organs such as spleen, tonsils, lymph nodes (LN), and bone marrow of both rodents and human [1]. Recently a minor subpopulation of lymphocytes, according to their morphologic characteristics designated large granular lymphocytes (LGL), have been demonstrated to act as NK cells. It has been suggested that natural cytotoxicity plays an important role in immune surveillance against nascent tumors and virus infection in experimental animals and humans [2]. Furthermore, there is evidence that NK cells are actively involved in the destruction of circulating tumor cells and thus in the inhibition of hematogenous metastatic spread [2]. In cancer patients, especially in those with widely disseminated disease, NK cell activity has been found impaired in PB, suggesting that NK activity is influenced and/or regulated by tumor burden [4]. Assuming that NK cells are actively involved in defense mechanisms at the tumor site, one might expect high levels of NK activity in the peri- and intratumoral area as well as in the draining LN. However, lymphocytes isolated from human solid tumors and also from malignant exsudates have been found to express low or almost no NK activity. Similarly, lymphocytes derived from LN draining human tumors – breast, lung, and colon cancer – have been found to express variable levels of NK activity [3, 6]. Data so far available suggest that NK cells, although present in regional LN, are functionally depressed. There is no evidence that macrophages-monocytes and/or lymphocytes, which have been found to suppress NK activity in PB and malignant effusion, influence NK activity in tumor-draining LN. The possibility that soluble factors such as prostaglandins or cytokines are released by growing tumors and modulate NK activity at the tumor site and also in PB has been proposed.

R. Jakesz/H. Rainer (Eds.)
Progress in Regional Cancer Therapy

Subjects and Methods

Patients

Thirteen patients (12 males, one female, age 44–70 years, mean 55 years) with cancer of the mouth floor or tongue were included in this study. Regarding histopathological staging, one patient was classified T2 NO, one T3 NO, one T2 N1, six T3 N1, and four T4 N1. After clinical staging and confirmation of malignant disease by biopsy, patients gave informed consent and were admitted to therapy.

OK-432 Pharmaceutical Preparation

OK-432 is a heat-killed and penicillin-treated preparation of the Su strain of *Streptococcus pyogenes* (generously supplied by Chugai Pharmaceutical, Tokyo, Japan) available in the form of vials continaining 0.1 mg (= 1 KE; Klinische Einheit, used to express the strength of the preparation) of lyophilized streptococci powder. Before use, the content of the vial was dissolved in sterile saline and adjusted to the desired dose and injection volume.

Regional Therapy

Patients were given increasing doses of OK-432 – 0.2, 0.5, 1.0, 1.5, 2.0, and 2.5 KE – injected by a hypodermic needle into small perilesional deposits around the tumor. Injection volumes were 0.1 ml at each site, and the total volume was 1.0 ml. Doses were individually adapted according to the side effects observed.

Recording of Side Effects

Local inflammatory response, regional LN swelling, and fluctuations in body temperature were evaluated during and after therapy for determination of side effects.

Preparation of Effector Cells

Heparinized PB was diluted, and the mononuclear cell fraction was separated by Ficoll-Hypaque (Lymphoprep. Nyegaard, Oslo, Norway) gradient centrifugation. Cells in the interphase were washed and resuspended in RPMI 1640 supplemented with 25 m*M Hepes, 2 mM L*-glutamine, 100 U penicillin/ml, 100 μg streptomycin/ml and 10% heat-inactivated fetal calf serum (FCS; Gibco Biocult, Glasgow, UK) (complete medium), and subsequently adjusted to the required cell number as previously described. LN were obtained during surgery of the primary tumor by radical neck dissection, trimmed of connective tissue and fat, and single-cell suspensions were prepared as described previously [5]. The mononuclear cell fraction was obtained by gradient separation as described for PB. Preparations of individual LN were never pooled, and were used for further studies only when viability (trypan blue exclusion) exceeded 90%. LN were free of metastases as verified by histology and/or cytology.

Treatment with Interferon and Staphylococcus Protein A

Mononuclear cells (5×10^5) were incubated for 18 h in complete medium with or without addition of 1000 IU/ml of purified natural IFN-α (Kindly supplied by Dr. Bodo, E. Boehringer Institute, Vienna, Austria) and/or 50 μl/ml *Staphylococcus aureus* protein A (SPA, Pharmacia, Upsala, Sweden). After incubation, cells were washed and resuspended in complete medium and tested in the cytotoxicity assay in the respective Effecter:Target ratios.

Cytotoxicity Assay

NK activity was determined in a 4-h ^{51}Cr release assay using K562 targets as described previously [5]. Briefly, 100 μl (1×10^4) of ^{51}Cr-labeled (Na_2- $^{51}CrO_4$, specific activity 100–350 μCi/μg; Amersham, UK) K562 cells and 100 μl effector cells were transferred to microwells of round-bottomed microtiter plates (NUNC 1482, Denmark), centrifuged, and incubated for 4 h at 37 °C in a humidified CO_2 atmosphere. After incubation, plates were centrifuged and supernatants (100 μl) were transferred to counter vials; radioactivity was counted in an autogamma scintillation counter (Beckman Instruments, Vienna, Austria). Spontaneous release (never exceeding 15%) was determined in wells containing targets alone, and maximum release by addition of Triton X-100. Percentage of specific cytotoxicity for triplicate samples was calculated by the formula

$$\text{Specific cytotoxicity} = \frac{\text{mean cpm test} - \text{mean cpm spont.}}{\text{mean cpm max.} - \text{mean cpm spont.}} \times 100$$

Statistical analysis was performed using Student's t-test and the χ^2 test.

Immunohistochemistry

LN samples obtained from patients with head and neck cancer (HNC) receiving OK-432 therapy preoperatively were also investigated for follicular reaction and the expression of HNK-1 phenotypes, detected on a certain proportion of NK cells by the immunoperoxidase method. Paraffin-embedded LN from both OK-432-treated and untreated patients were coded and prepared for analysis by an independent pathologist as described previously [9].

Results

Preoperative peritumoral immunotherapy led to local inflammatory reactions together with a rise of body temperature and swelling of regional LN. In PB, there was an increase of NK activity during preoperative immunotherapy (Table 1). In six patients NK activity was investigated in PB before initiation of immunotherapy and 2–3 days after surgery. In all of them regional immunotherapy prevented the induction of suppression of NK activity by surgery (Table 2).

In previous investigations we found that tumor-draining LN obtained at the time of primary tumor surgery from patients with HNC had low but significant NK activity. LN of 13 patients who had received preoperative OK-432 therapy showed significantly higher values of cytotoxicity (> 10%) than the controls (Table 3). Some 84% (11/13) showed significant levels of NK activity, in contrast to only 43% (10/23) of the controls (Table 3).

Moreover, we tested the in vitro reactivity of LN after OK-432 therapy in response to interferon (IFN) and the SPA. LN cells of individual patients were incubated overnight with IFN and SPA, and tested for NK activity. Without IFN (incubation in medium) at E:T 40:1, mean levels were 23.2% ± 16.2%, whereas with IFN they were 28.2% ± 16.1%. A significant increase was detected in three of nine samples, no change was observed in four, and there was a decrease in two LN; the latter samples had higher spontaneous reactivity than those that could be

Table 1. Effect of 7 days' preoperative IK-432 therapy on NK activity in peripheral blood

Therapy	*n*	Mean % cytotoxicity (E:T 20:1)	
None	13	35.2 + 12.2	
OK-432	13	49.3 ± 15.5	$p < 0.05$

Table 2. Influence of OK-432 therapy on NK activity in peripheral blood monoclear cells

	Mean % cytotoxicity (E:T 20.1) Before surgery	After surgery	*f*
Controls ($n = 9$)	45.1 ± 7.7	27.6 ± 5.8	0.05
OK-432 ($n = 6$)	49.3 ± 6.5	40.2 ± 5.3	n.s.

Table 3. Effect of preoperative OK-432 therapy on NK activity of draining LN

Treatment	LN/patients	Spontaneous cytotoxicity Mean % cytotoxicity (E:T 40:1)	No. with positive cytotoxicity (%)
None	23/14	11.2 ± 7.6	10/23 (43)
OK-432	13/6	20.8 ± 14.7 *	11/12 (84)

* $p < 0.01$.

Table 4. Influence of IFN on in vitro reactivity of lymph nodes (LN)

Treatment	LN/patients	No IFn	Mean % cytotoxicity IFN		Significant augmentation (%)
None	23/14	11.2 ± 7.6**	20.0 ± 12.6		9 (39)
OH-432	9/6	23.2 ± 16.2*	28.2 ± 16.1	$p < 0.005$	3 (33)

* $p < 0.1$.
** $p < 0.01$.

Table 5. Effect of preoperative OK-432 therapy on the number of HNK-1$^+$ cells in lymph nodes

Treatment	n	Follicular reactions +1	+2	+3	HNK-1$^+$ cells +1	+2	+3
None	11	8	3	0	7	4	0
OK-432	11	7	4	0	2*	1	8$^+$

x^2 test: * $p < 0.1$; $^+ p < 0.005$.

augmented (Table 4). For SPA too, no differences were detected concerning the stimulatory capacity on LN NK activity (results not given due to lack of space).

Previously we demonstrated that about 7% of cells in cell suspensions of LN draining cancer of the oral cavity react with the monoclonal antibody HNK-1 which identifies a certain proportion of cells mediating NK activity. Using immunoperoxidase staining, we investigated fixed and embedded LN material obtained from 11 patients who had received OK-432 therapy and compared it with samples from 11 patients treated only by surgery. Eight LN samples were found to contain an increased number of HNK-1$^+$ cells (grade + 3) in the OK-432 therapy group, in contrast to none in the untreated group. The latter had staining patterns classified grade 1 in seven LN, and grade 2 in four LN (Table 5).

These results suggest that OK-432 therapy leads to an increase in a population of cells in regional LN which is able to mediate NK killing, as has also been observed in cytotoxicity assays.

Summary

OK-432 is a pharmaceutical preparation of a low virulent Su strain of *streptococcur pyogenes* which has been developed in Japan by Okamoto and is produced by the Chugai Pharmaceutical Company, Tokyo.

Preclinical studies have clearly demonstrated that OK-432 is active in preventing primary and metastatic tumor growth in a variety of tumor models. Beside this, evidence exists that OK-432 is a potent immunomodulating agent which has an augmenting effect on T-lymphocyte, natural killer (NK) cell and also monocyte-macrophage functions. Lymphocytes derived from tumor-draining lymph nodes (LN) and from tumor infiltrates express minimal or no cytotoxic activity against autologous and/or allogeneic tumor cells in vitro. We previously documented that NK cell activity in draining neck nodes of patients with oral cavity cancer is significantly lower than that in peripheral blood (PB) of identical donors.

Additionally, the NK cell activity in PB showed a significant stage dependence according to the systemic immunosuppression of increasing tumor burden in extensive head and neck cancer.

After perilesional OK 432 therapy, a significant increase in cytotoxicity was observed in PB preoperatively. Postoperative suppression of PB NK cell activity was less pronounced in these patients. In tumor-draining LN, NK activity was significantly higher in patients receiving OK-432 than in those treated by surgery alone. Concerning the in vitro stimulatory capacity of IFN and/or Staphylococcus protein A on LN NK activity, no differences were detected between the OK-432-treated and -untreated groups. By the immunoperoxidase technique, LN of OK-432-treated patients were found to express a higher number of cells reacting with the monoclonal antibody HNK-1 than LN of the untreated patients. These results suggest an increase in the number and function of NK cells in regional LN together with an increase of NK activity in PB during OK-432 perilesional therapy.

References

1. Antonelli P, Stewart W II, Dupont B (1981) Distribution of natural killer cell activity in peripheral blood, cord blood, thymus, lymph nodes and spleen, and the effect of in vitro treatment with interferon preparations. Clin immunol Immunopathol 19:168–172
2. Bancroft G, Shellam G, Chalmer J (1981) Genetic influences on the augmentation of natural killer (NK) cells during murine-cytomegalovirus infection: correlation with pattern of resistance. J Immunol 126:988–994
3. Eremin O, Coombs RRA, Ashby (1981) Human natural cytotoxicity in the blood and lymphoid organs of healthy donors and patients with malignant disease. Int J Cancer 21::35–41
4. Kadisch AS, Doule AT, Steinhauer EH, Ghossein NA (1981) Natural cytotoxicity and interferon production in human cancer: dificient natural killer cell activity and normal interferon production in patients with advanced disease. J Immunol 127:1817–1822
5. Micksche M, Vinzenz K, Kokoschka EM, Kokoschka R (1985) Natural killer cell activity in tumor draining lymph nodes: investigations in patients with malignant melanoma and head and neck cancer. Nat immun Cell Growth Regul 4:315–327
6. Moore M, Vose BM (1981) Extravascular natural cytotoxicity in man: anti K562 activity of lymph node and tumor-infiltrating lymphocytes. Int J Cancer 27:265–272
7. Vinzenz K, Micksche M (1986) Immunotherapy in patients with head and neck cancer. Int J Immunother II (1):37–49
8. Vinzenz K, Micksche M (1987) Natural cytotoxicity in draining lymph nodes of squamous cell cancer in the maxillofacial region. J Oral Maxillofac Surg 45:42–47
9. Vinzenz K, Matejka M, Watzek G, Porteder H, Neuhold N, Micksche M (1987) Modulation of NK activity in regional lymph nodes by preoperative immunotherapy with OK-432 in patients with cancer of the oral cavity. Cancer Detect Prev [Suppl 1]:463–475

Intra-arterial Chemotherapy, Preoperative and Postoperative Radiotherapy, and Surgery for Primary "Unresectable" High-Grade Soft Tissue Sarcomas of the Extremities

H.J. Hoekstra, H. Schraffordt Koops, J. Oldhoff, W.M. Molenaar, D.T. Sleijfer, and D.M. Mehta

Division of Surgical Oncology, Groningen University Hospital, P.O. Box 30001, 9700 RB Groningen, The Netherlands

Introduction

The prognosis of soft tissue sarcomas of the extremities is determined by the location, size, histology, stage, and prior treatment of the tumor. Prevention of local recurrence and limb saving are two major considerations in the treatment of extremity sarcomas. Without adequate surgery, the risk of local recurrence is 30%–50%. Extensive surgery, compartment excision when possible, combined with 50–60 Gy postoperative external-beam radiotherapy (EBRT) in the case of marginal resections has reduced the local failure rate to 5%–20% [5]. Is it possible to increase the limb-saving rate in high-grade soft tissue sarcomas of the extremities without increasing the local failure rate or decreasing disease-free survival?

In an attempt to do just this, combined preoperative intra-arterial chemotherapy, preoperative radiotherapy, surgery, and postoperative radiotherapy were used in the treatment of primary "unresectable" tumors.

Patients and Methods

From 1983, 11 patients with primary "unresectable" high-grade soft tissue sarcomas of the extremities were treated at the Groningen University Hospital with combined intra-arterial chemotherapy, preoperative radiotherapy, surgery, and postoperative radiotherapy in the case of marginal resections. None of the patients received postoperative adjuvant chemotherapy.

An intra-arterial catheter was introduced into the contralateral extremity, using the Seldinger technique, and so positioned in the common iliac, external iliac, femoral, or axillary artery that the tumor in the involved extremity was optimally perfused with the cytostatic agent. The drug used was doxorubicin, given via the intra-arterial catheter by continuous infusion with the aid of an IVAC pump (IVAC

R. Jakesz/H. Rainer (Eds.)
Progress in Regional Cancer Therapy

Table 1. Clinical data, histologic type, tumor stage, therapy, tumor destruction, complications, and follow-up

Patient	1	2	3	4	5	6	7	8	9	10	11
Age (years)	27	63	66	35	24	70	48	52	61	43	47
Sex	M	M	M	M	M	M	M	F	F	M	M
Tumor site	Left thigh	Left lower leg	Left knee	Left thigh	Right wrist	Left thigh	Right thigh	Left thigh	Left knee	Left thigh	Left thigh
Histology	Epithelioid malignant schwannoma	Leiomyo-sarcoma	Synovial sarcoma	Liposarcoma	Synovial sarcoma	MFH	Liposarcoma	Liposarcoma	MFH	Myxoid liposarcoma	MFH
Stage	IIIB	IIIB	IIIB	IIIB	IIIA	IIIB	IIIB	IIIB	IIIA	IIIB	IIIB
IA chemotherapy, preoperative 35 Gy EBRT	+	+	+	+	+	+	+	+	+	+	+
Surgery	Upper leg amputation[a]	Marginal resection	Marginal resection	Marginal resection	Radical resection	Nonradical excision	Marginal resection	Marginal resection	Marginal resection[b]	Radical resection	Marginal resection
Postoperative EBRT	—	28 Gy	20 Gy	20 Gy	—	20 Gy	26 Gy	30 Gy	—	—	30 Gy
Tumor destruction	Indeterminate	Yes	Yes	Yes	No residual tumor	Indeterminate	Yes	Yes	Yes	Yes	Yes
Complication(s)	—	Chemoreaction, skin, left groin	—	Flexion contracture, knee	Chemoreaction, skin, elbow; wound dehiscence	Chemoreaction abdominal skin wound dehiscence	Neuropathy, sciatic nerve, 8 months	—	Wound dehiscence	—	—
Recurrence	Pulmonary metastasis, 15 months	Pulmonary metastasis, 31 months	Pulmonary metastasis, 24 months			Pulmonary metastasis, 3 months	—	—	Pulmonary metastases 3 months	—	—
Follow-up	DOD, 20 months	DOD, 40 months	DOD, 44 months	NED, 36 months	NED, 29 months	DOD, 3 months	NED, 24 months	NED, 22 months	AWD, 19 months	NED, 12 months	NED, 12 months

MFH, malignant fibrous histiocytoma; NED, no evidence of disease; AWD, alive with disease; DOD, dead of disease; marginal resection, narrow margin of normal tissue; nonradical excision, gross disease remaining.

[a] Local resection impossible due to involvement of sciatic nerve.

[b] No postoperative EBRT due to wound disturbances.

Corporation, San Diego) at a daily dose of 20 mg/m^2 for 3 consecutive days. To prevent thrombosis, heparin (2 × 5000 U) was given subcutaneously. Within 24 h of completion of the intra-arterial chemotherapy treatment, the preoperative EBRT started. The entire tumor compartment was irradiated with 10 doses of 350 cGy for a total of 35 Gy over 12–14 days. Surgical resection was performed immediately after completion of the preoperative irradiation. Wide local excisions were performed when possible, compartment excisions when necessary. Resections with a margin of less than 2 cm unaffected tissue were classified as marginal resections. If tumor resection was marginal, postoperative EBRT was started immediately after wound healing was complete and within 6 weeks after the initial surgery. The radiotherapy was given in daily fractions of 200 cGy to an individually adapted dose of 20–30 Gy.

The clinical data, histologic tumor type, tumor stage, type of resection, postoperative radiotherapy, tumor destruction due to the combined treatment, complications, and follow-up are listed in Table 1. All sarcomas were classified and staged according to the guidelines of the American Joint Committee on Cancer. To ascertain the effect of the combined modalilty therapy on the tumor, the pretreatment and post-treatment histology were investigated by one pathologist (WMM).

Results

The introduction and the positioning of the intra-arterial catheter caused any problems or complications; in particular no arterial thrombosis was diagnosed. Although the outflow from the catheter was studied with the aid of a contrast medium, three patients (27%) developed a red discoloration of the skin: in two patients (nos. 2 and 6) the outflow in the drainage area of the epigastric artery was too high and a mild to severe skin reaction due to the doxorubicin was found, and in one patient (no. 5) a mild discoloration of the elbow was noticed due to too much flexion of the elbow during the intra-arterial chemotherapy course. In one patient (no. 2) the severe skin necrosis required surgical excision. None of these skin complications influenced the primary therapy.

A limb-saving resection of the tumor was feasible in 10 patients (91%). In the first patient a limb-saving procedure was not performed because the sciatic nerve was surrounded by viable tumor.

A disturbance in wound healing was diagnosed in three patients (27%). In two patients (nos. 5 and 6) surgical intervention was necessary: in patient 5 a skin defect on the wrist had to be repaired with a pedicled abdominal skin flap, and the wound dehiscence in patient 6 required surgical drainage. One patient (no. 7) developed a motor and sensory neuropathy of the sciatic nerve 8 months after the primary treatment. There were no clinical signs of a local recurrence and on surgical exploration no abnormalities were found. A flexion contracture of the knee was diagnosed in one patient (no. 4). The total morbidity rate was 55%.

During a median follow-up of 30 months (range 12–68 months) no local recurrences were diagnosed. Lung metastases were diagnosed in five patients after 3 (2 ×), 15, 24, and 31 months (Fig. 1). In all patients except patient 5 an incisional biopsy of the tumor was performed prior to any treatment. Therefore the histological reaction of the tumor after the initial treatment could be analyzed in ten

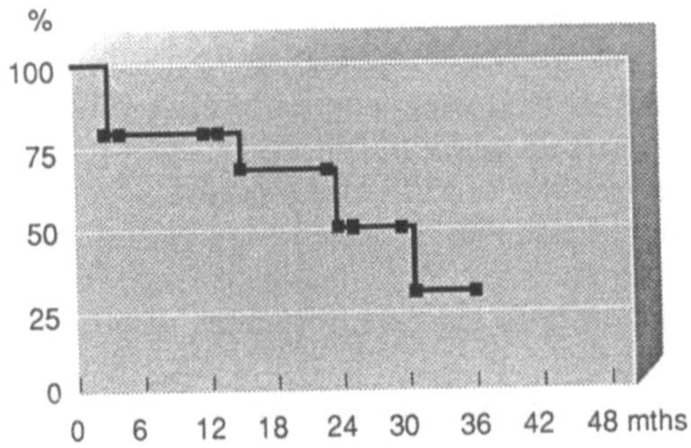

Fig. 1. Disease-free survival

Table 2. Histological effect of therapy

Patient	Tumor	Stage	Tumor destruction
1	Epithelioid sarcoma	IIIB	Indeterminate
2	Leiomyosarcoma	IIIB	Yes
3	Synovial sarcoma	IIIB	Yes
4	Liposarcoma	IIIB	Yes
5	Synovial sarcoma	IIIA	No residual tumor
6	MFH	IIIB	Indeterminate
7	Liposarcoma	IIIB	Yes
8	Liposarcoma	IIIB	Yes
9	MFH	IIIA	Yes
10	Myxoid liposarcoma	IIIB	Yes
11	MFH	IIIB	Yes

patients. Such analysis is difficult because a small biopsy specimen had to be compared with, in general, a large resected tumor. In addition, necrosis of the tumor occurring naturally has to be distinguished from tumor necrosis initiated by the therapy. There was judged to be a therapeutic effect if a definite decrease in cellularity and necrosis was observed in the immediate vicinity of nonthrombosed vessels. No grading of effect was undertaken. The effect is summarized in Table 2. Although this patient population is too small to allow any conclusions, both patients in whom chemotherapy failed to cause tumor destruction developed lung metastases, in contrast to only three of the other eight patients.

Discussion

Treatment with a combination of intra-arterial doxorubicin and EBRT was initiated by Eilber et al. [2] in the management of malignant soft tissue sarcomas and bone sarcomas. The idea was to achieve a high concentration of doxorubicin in the tumor. Doxorubicin is fairly effective in soft tissue sarcomas, with a response rate of 30%–50%, and also potentiates the effect of radiation therapy [6]. To increase the resectability rate, this approach was introduced in the treatment of "primarily unresectable" soft tissue sarcomas of the extremities. If still no radical resection could be performed after doxorubicin, patients were treated with postoperative EBRT. Amputation was only performed when neurovascular structures were involved with tumor. A limb-saving resection rate of 91% (10/11) could be achieved without any local recurrence. The morbidity rate was high (55%), but the complications did not necessitate amputation or any other major surgical procedures. Although several methods of investigating the distribution of the chemotherapeutic agent have been described, we do not believe that any of these techniques would have reduced the number of skin reaction to the chemotherapy. No conclusions may be drawn from the correlation found between tumor response to treatment and disease-free survival. Although Azarelli et al. [1] found significantly better survival in patients with extremity soft tissue sarcomas treated by intra-arterial chemotherapy, this was not confirmed by Eilber et al. (this volume).

It is questionable whether the same results in "primarily unresectable" soft tissue sarcomas of the extremities could be achieved with intravenous doxorubicin or with hyperthermic isolated regional perfusion. The experience with isolated regional perfusion is very limited, and the drug generally used is melphalan, which is not the first choice for sarcoma treatment [3]. Isolated regional perfusion with doxorubicin is contraindicated due to the severe toxicity [4]. Based on the results achieved, it may be concluded that the combined treatment modality described here increased the limb-saving rate for soft tissue sarcomas of the extremities which were primarily not amenable to curative resection.

References

1. Azzarelli A, Quagliulo V, Colella G, Agabiti E, Gennari L (1987) Pre- and postoperative procedures and limb salvage for soft tissue sarcomas of the extremities (abstract). Proceedings ECCO-IV, p 235
2. Eilber FR, Morton DL, Eckhardt J, Grant TT, Weisenburger T (1984) Limb salvage for skeletal and soft tissue sarcomas. Multi-disciplinary preoperative therapy. Cancer 53:2579–2584
3. Hoekstra HJ, Schraffordt Koops H, Molenaar WM, Oldhoff J (1986) Results of isolated regional perfusion in the treatment of malignant soft tissue tumors of the extremities. Cancer 60:1703–1707
4. Kroon BBR, Klaase JM, van Geel AN, Albus-Lutter ChE, Benckhuijsen C (1988) Perfusion for soft tissue sarcoma of the limbs. Progress in Regional Cancer Therapy I, Vienna, p 98 (abstr 168)
5. Chang AE, Rosenberg SA, Giatstein EJ, Antham KH (1989) Sarcomas of soft tissues. In: Devita VT, Hellman S, Rosenberg SA (eds) Cancer principles and practice of oncology, 3nd edn. Lippincott, Philadelphia, pp 1345–1398
6. Trott K (1986) Radiation-chemotherapy interactions. Int J Radiat Oncol Biol Phys 12:1409–1413

Regional Induction Chemotherapy Followed by Radiotherapy and/or Surgery in Management of Large and Aggressive Sarcomas in Shoulder, Pelvis and Limbs

F.O. Stephens, W. Marsden, and M.H.N. Tattersall

Department of Surgery, University of Sydney, Sydney, NSW 2006, Australia

Introduction

In treating large and histologically aggressive sarcomas mutilating surgery, often requiring radical amputation became standard practice because of a high risk of local recurrence after less radical surgery. However, in spite of radical local surgery, many patients with sarcomas still developed distant metastatic disease, so that less radical approaches have been investigated for control of local tumour, at least until the period of greatest risk of metastatic disease becoming manifest has passed. Cade [1] used radical local radiotherapy for this purpose, and if after 6 months there was no evidence of metastatic disease, he then proceeded to amputation. In this way, amputation was only carried out in those patients most likely to be cured by the procedure.

In attempts to avoid amputation, adjuvant radiotherapy used either pre- or postoperatively in combination with local surgical resection of the tumour only has been tried. This approach is still an option in Ewing's sarcoma, which is usually highly radiosensitive, but the incidence of local recurrence is high in tumours which are not radiosensitive. Small and moderate sized soft tissue sarcomas may be controlled by local surgery in which the whole muscle or tissue compartment is removed, but this is not applicable to large sarcomas.

Systemic chemotherapy given before or after local treatment by surgery and/or radiotherapy is also under investigation in some centres [6–8] and is commonly used in chemosensitive sarcomas, e.g., Ewing's sarcoma and embryonal rhabdomyosarcoma.

Regional chemotherapy delivered prior to definitive radiotherapy and/or surgical resection has been studied with the goal of rendering advanced or aggressive cancers more "curable" by the subsequent standard local treatments. This concept is based on the hypothesis that the local tumour is exposed to a greater concentration and somewhat greater total dose (concentration × time) of the agents used than with systemic administration [10]. Encouraging results using this approach have been reported in advanced cancers of the head and neck, limbs, breast and stomach [4, 11].

In the present report, patients with large, rapidly growing and/or histologically aggressive sarcomas, referred initially to the surgical oncology service at Sydney

R. Jakesz/H. Rainer (Eds.)
Progress in Regional Cancer Therapy

Hospital and more recently to the combined orthopaedic oncology service at the Royal Prince Alfred Hospital, were treated with one of two regimens of intra-arterial (IA) chemotherapy initially and subsequently with external radiotherapy and/or surgical resection. The objective was to shrink the sarcomas to dimensions where radiotherapy and/or surgical resection might be locally curative, and so to avoid radical mutilating surgery, especially forequarter or hindquarter amputation.

Materials and Methods

Twenty-two patients with advanced sarcomas of the buttock, lower limb, shoulder or upper limb were treated by one of two regimens of IA chemotherapy as follows:

1. *Continuous regimen (10 patients)*
   Day 1: doxorubicin 15 mg/m^2 IA in 500 ml saline over 8 h
   Day 2: hydroxyurea 2 g orally
   Day 3: vincristine 0.6 mg/m^2 IA in 500 ml saline over 8 h
   Day 4: actinomycin D 0.25 mg/m^2 IA in 500 ml saline over 8 h
   Then 3 rest days: dextrose/saline only
   Cyclophosphamide 50 mg each day by mouth. Between four and seven cycles were given depending upon tumour response, toxicity and patient tolerance. Heparin 5 000 units was added to each infusion container except in the case of doxorubicin infusion.

External radiotherapy 5 000 rads over 4–5 weeks was given to two of the 10 patients, commencing 3 weeks after chemotherapy had been completed. In one of these, a residual fibrous lump was surgically excised 6 weeks after radiotherapy was completed.

2. *Intermittent regimen* (12 patients)
   Day 1: cisplatin 100 mg/m^2 IA in 500 ml saline over 4h
   Day 2: doxorubicin 50 mg/m^2 IA in 500 ml saline over 8 h

This two-day cycle was repeated at intervals of 3 weeks.

On some occasions, for reasons of convenience, doxorubicin was given on day 1 and cisplatin on day 2. A minimum of three cycles and a maximum of seven cycles was given depending upon response, toxicity and patient tolerance. Heparin 5 000 units was added to each infusion container except in the case of doxorubicin infusion.

After completion of IA treatment, and depending on response and primary tumour site, either external radiotherapy or surgical resection was then performed. Radiotherapy (between 5000 and 6000 rads) was given to three patients, in two of whom local surgical excision was carried out approximately 4 weeks after completion of radiotherapy. In the third patient no local surgery was carried out as pulmonary metastases had become manifest. In the other nine patients no radiotherapy was given, but surgical resection of the residual tumour was performed.

The primary sites and histology of the sarcomas in both treatment groups are shown in Table 1. The 22 patients consisted of 14 men and 8 women with ages ranging from 13 to 63 years.

Table 1. Primary site, histology and treatment regimen of 22 patients treated with intra-arterial chemotherapy

Regimen	Primary site Buttock	Pelvis	Groin	Thigh	Shoulder	Elbow	Hand	Knee
Continuous	1	—	2	4	1	1	1	—
Intermittent	—	2	1	5	2	—	—	2

Regimen	Histology Malignant fibrous histiocytoma	Liposarcoma	Fibrosarcoma	Spindle cell carcinoma	Synovial sarcoma	Osteogenic sarcoma	Extraosseous Ewing's sarcoma
Continuous	4	4	1	1	—	—	—
Intermittent	3	1	—	1	1	5	1

Results

All patients except one, whether treated by the continuous or the intermittent regimen, showed at least partial response to IA chemotherapy. The exception was a patient with spindle cell sarcoma of the calf treated by the continuous regimen – this tumour was stabilised but was otherwise apparently unaffected by chemotherapy.

Continuous Regimen

Five of ten patients treated with the continuous regimen showed no histological evidence of residual tumour after completion of the primary chemotherapy; thus the complete response rate was 50%. One of the 10 patients refused surgery and received radiotherapy. (He had presented with an incompletely excised malignant fibrous histiocytoma of the hand and was treated with IA chemotherapy followed by radiotherapy because he had refused amputation.) He remains well with good use of his hand more than 2 years later.

Three patients showed clinical partial regression. These included two patients with liposarcoma, and at subsequent surgery, the periphery of the tumour appeared to be free of viable tumour in each case, but there were viable cells in the centre of the resected tumour. In one 17-year-old girl with malignant fibrous histiocytoma of the hand with bone involvement, no residual tumour was detected in the soft tissue, but tumour cells were found in bone. The last patient with spindle cell sarcoma of the calf showed no change in the primary tumour after 5 weeks of treatment. He was therefore treated by amputation, after which viable tumour was found in the deep calf veins. He later died of pulmonary metastases.

Intermittent Regimen

All 12 patients treated with the intermittent regimen showed evidence of tumour regression, but in only four cases was no evidence of residual tumour detected in biopsies or resections after chemotherapy (complete response rate 33%). In one of two patients with soft tissue sarcoma irradiated after chemotherapy, a positive biopsy was converted to negative. In six patients, after IA treatment the tumour was found to be largely replaced by necrotic or fibrous tissue, but some viable malignant cells were detected, especially at the sites of bone involvement.

In one patient, pulmonary metastases became manifest during IA treatment, so that no further biopsy or surgery was carried out. The primary tumour had responded partially, and the residual sarcoma (spindle cell) was then treated and well controlled with local radiotherapy.

Salvage of Limbs

Local tumour control was achieved without amputation in 9 of 10 patients treated with the continuous regimen, and in 10 of 12 treated with the intermittent regimen. The patient with spindle cell sarcoma of the calf treated with the continuous regimen underwent amputation because of poor response to chemotherapy. One patient with osteosarcoma of the pelvis who achieved a partial tumour response with the intermittent regimen eventually required a hindquarter amputation for locally recurrent tumour, and one patient with partial regression of a large osteosarcoma of the tibia and partial regression of a metastatic mass in the groin nodes still required hindquarter amputation. Amputation was avoided in the remaining 19 of 22 patients.

Long-Term Survival

The patients have now been followed up for a minimum of 18 months and a maximum of 13 years. Three of the 10 patients treated with the continuous regimen developed pulmonary metastases. These were the patient who had amputation for uncontrolled spindle cell sarcoma, a patient who had a locally controlled MFH of the thigh, and a patient with a locally controlled liposarcoma of the shoulder. Seven of the 12 patients treated by the intermittent regimen developed pulmonary metastases. These included the two patients who eventually underwent hindquarter amputation and the patient who developed pulmonary metastases whilst having treatment for his primary spindle cell sarcoma of the thigh. The patient with locally controlled extraosseous Ewing's sarcoma of the thigh, a patient with locally controlled synovial sarcoma of the thigh, a patient with locally controlled osteosarcoma of the humerus and a patient with a locally controlled malignant fibrous histiocytoma of upper tibia were the other four to develop pulmonary metastases.

Toxicity

Nausea and vomiting was moderate to severe in 8 of the 12 patients treated with the intermittent regimen, and about half of the patients in each group suffered moderate to severe (but temporary) alopecia. Three patients in each group also suffered a significant but temporary erythematous reaction in the skin of the extremity infused. In one patient on the intermittent regimen, skin damage resulted in ulceration over the site of the neoplasm.

Time in Hospital

The patients on the continuous regimen spent an average of 39 days continuously in hospital, whilst the patients on the intermittent regimen spent an average of 20 days in hospital spread over a period of 16 weeks.

Discussion

Patients with large, rapidly growing and histologically aggressive sarcomas in the buttock, shoulder or limbs have in the past had quite a dismal outlook. The incidence of local tumour recurrence after attempts at local surgical resection was high, and radiotherapy rarely achieved local control. Combinations of local surgery with pre- or postoperative radiotherapy were employed by some, but the results were still not obviously improved [7]. For these reasons, amputation became standard practice, and for large sarcomas near the hip or shoulder joints hindquarter or forequarter amputation was often required. Although radical and mutilating surgery may have offered the only prospect of cure, in some patients metastatic disease in the lungs or elsewhere later became manifest, making the mutilating surgery seemingly of no avail. The dying patient had the added burden of coping with a major amputation which had not cured the disease.

Approaches using induction (or preoperative) chemotherapy with or without radiotherapy to reduce the size and viability of the tumours have been reported with the goal of tumour eradication by subsequent aggressive local surgery, avoiding the necessity of amputation. Successful use of such techniques has been reported especially when the chemotherapy is given by regional IA infusion into an artery supplying the tumour site [8].

These tumours are uncommon, and properly randomised trials to confirm the value of such treatment have not been undertaken. Similarly, it is not known whether the results of the more complicated IA chemotherapy are significantly different from those of intravenous systemic chemotherapy. Moreover, the most effective agents for particular tumours are not known, and the best combinations, drug sequences or doses have not been determined. Experience with preoperative "induction" chemotherapy given IA as the first modality of treatment of advanced cancers in the head and neck, advanced breast cancers and gastric cancers [11] caused one of us (FOS) in 1975 to use a continuous IA regimen of agents in a similar manner for patients with sarcomas otherwise only resectable by radical amputation. Details of the techniques used have been described elsewhere [4, 12, 13].

More recently, intermittent IA infusion of doxorubicin, reported by Eilber et al. [3] and Jaffe et al. [5], and cisplatin [2, 9], especially in the case of osteosarcoma, has yielded encouraging results. These reports stimulated us to use a combination of doxorubicin and cisplatin given by IA infusion in management of osteosarcomas.

In general we tended to offer intermittent cisplatin and doxorubicin treatment to patients with osteosarcoma who could be reasonably considered potential candidates for limb salvage. Some patients with soft tissue sarcomas who for family, economic or social reasons preferred not to be admitted to hospital for a continuous period of several weeks, as is required for patients having the continuous chemotherapy regimen, were also selected for intermittent doxorubicin and cisplatin.

The number of patients treated to date is not large, but both regimens have shown encouraging results in patients whose standard care would have required amputation, in some cases hindquarter for forequarter amputation. As in patients having radical surgery, pulmonary metastases ultimately developed in some of our patients – in three of those treated by the continuous regimen and seven of those treated with the intermittent regimen. However, in all but three patients, local tumour control was achieved and major amputation was avoided.

There are certain advantages and disadvantages of the continuous and intermittent regimens of treatment, apart from any possible difference in results. The patients in this study were certainly not selected in any type of randomised fashion, but rather by historical accident. The continuous regimen treatment was first introduced along the lines of more established management of carcinomas in other situations, and the intermittent regimen was not developed until cisplatin had become available some years later. Also, the ability of cisplatin and doxorubicin to affect osteosarcomas was not known until the continuous regimen of treatment had been used for some years in treating soft tissue sarcomas.

Continuous Regimen

The continuous regimen requires about 6 weeks of uninterrupted inpatient care. It also requires the continuous services of a team of nursing and medical staff familiar with administration of IA chemotherapy, cannulas, pumps, and other aspects or potential complications of treatment. However, overall treatment is completed over a shorter period of time than with the intermittent regimen.

Intermittent Regimen

The intermittent regimen is more simply administered but is protracted over a period of between 3 and 4½ months. It requires the services of a skilled interventional radiologist, but patients stay only short periods in hospital and spend most of the time at home and, in some cases, at work. The treatment, however, is associated with a greater incidence of severe nausea and vomiting than is the continuous regimen.

Systemic Adjuvant Chemotherapy

Whether further chemotherapy should be given after completion of primary care of the sarcoma to control micrometastic deposits is controversial in soft tissue sarcomas, although its value in osteogenic sarcomas is accepted. In both the regimens of chemotherapy the patients are receiving systemic chemotherapy from day 1 of treatment. There is a flow-off of the IA drugs from the regional into the systemic circulation, so that micrometastases, if present, become exposed to chemotherapy from the outset of treatment. Also, in the continuous regimen oral cyclophosphamide is given to augment this effect at the time of primary treatment.

Summary

In treating patients with large, rapidly growing, and histologically aggressive sarcomas in the pelvis, shoulder or limbs, two regimens of IA chemotherapy have been used as the first modality of treatment. The objective has been to reduce the size, extent and viability of the tumours in order to make them more likely to be controlled by subsequent local radiotherapy and/or limb-preserving surgical resection.

Ten patients were treated with the continuous IA regimen, and local tumour eradication was achieved in nine of these without amputation. However, three patients subsequently developed pulmonary metastases, including the one who was treated by amputation because of poor tumour response to the IA treatment given.

Ten of the 12 patients treated with the intermittent IA regimen also avoided amputation with locally controlled disease. However pulmonary metastases developed in seven of these 12 patients, including the two who subsequently had an amputation. The remaining five patients remain well with no evidence of either local or systemic residual neoplasm.

The two regimens of treatment have been effective in allowing local tumour eradication to be achieved without amputation in the great majority of patients. Although the development of pulmonary metastases appears to be different in the two regimens, the patient groups are quite heterogeneous. All tumours were advanced when first treated, but different types of tumours were treated in the two groups, so that no direct comparisons can be made.

References

1. Cade S (1955) Osteogenic sarcoma: study based on 133 patients. J R Coll Surg Edinb 1:79–111
2. Calvo DB, Patt ZY, Wallace S et al. (1980) Phase I–II trials of percutaneous intra-arterial cisdiamminedichloroplatinum (II) for regionally confirmed malignancy. Cancer 45:1278–1283
3. Eilber FR, Mirra JJ, Grant TT et al. (1980) Is amputation necessary for sarcomas? A 7 year experience with limb salvage. Ann Surg 192:431–438
4. Ensminger WD, Gyves JW (1984) Regional cancer therapy. Cancer Treat Rep 68:101–115
5. Jaffe N, Robertson R, Ayala A et al. (1985) Comparison of intra-arterial cisdiamminedichloroplatinum II with high dose methotrexate and citrovorum factor rescue in the treatment of primary osteosarcoma. J Clin Oncol 3:1101–1105
6. Kinsell TJ, Loeffler JS, Fraass BA, Tepper J (1983) Extremity preservation by combined modality therapy in sarcomas of the hand and foot: an analysis of local control, disease-free survival and functional result. Int J Radiat Oncol Biol Phys 9:115–119
7. Lawrence W Jr, Neifeld JP, Torz JJ (1983) Egdahl RH (ed) Manual of soft-tissue tumor surgery. Springer, Berlin Heidelberg New York, pp 167–171
8. Lokich JJ (1979) Preoperative chemotherapy in soft tissue sarcoma. Surg Gynecol Obstet 148:512–516
9. Mavligit GM (1981) Intra-arterial cisplatin for patients with inoperable skeletal tumours. Cancer 48:1
10. Stephens FO (1983) Pharmacokinetics of intra-arterial chemotherapy. Recent Results Cancer Res 86:1–12
11. Stephens FO (1983) Clinical experience in the use of intra-arterial infusion chemotherapy in the treatment of cancers in the head and neck, the extremities, the breast and stomach. Recent Results Cancer Res 86:122–127
12. Stephens FO, Stevens MM, McCarthy SW, Johnson N, Packham NA, Ritchie JD (1987) Treatment of advanced and inaccessible sarcomas with continuous intra-arterial chemotherapy prior to definitive surgery or radiotherapy – a possible alternative to amputation or disabling radical surgery. Aust NZ J Surg 57:435–440
13. Stephens FO, Tattersall MHN, Marsden W (1987) Regional chemotherapy with the use of cisplatin and doxorubicin as primary treatment for advanced sarcomas in shoulder, pelvis and thigh. Cancer 60:724–735

Neo-adjuvant Chemotherapy for Osteosarcoma of the Extremities: The Experience at the Rizzoli Institute in 210 Patients Treated with Two Successively Activated Preoperative Protocols Using High-Dose or Moderate-Dose Methotrexate + Cisplatin or High-Dose Methotrexate + Cisplatin + Doxorubicin

G. Bacci, P. Picci, M. Mercuri, M. Avella, M. Fontana, A. Mancini, F. Gherlinzoni, A. Brach del Prever, A. Ferraro, A. Ferruzzi, P. Caldora, and M. Campanacci

Bone Tumor Center & 1st Orthopaedic Clinic, Istituto Ortopedico Rizzoli, Bologna, Italy

Introduction

The prognosis of localized osteosarcoma of the extremities (LOE) treated by surgery alone is very poor. In our experience, in spite of amputation, the disease-free survival rate for these patients is only 10%. This percentage seems unchanged in the last 20 years, at least at the Rizzoli Institute (Table 1).

Adjuvant chemotherapy (AC) has considerably improved the prognosis of these patients. At the Rizzoli Institute, we started to treat LOE with AC in 1972. Of the 238 patients treated between 1972 and 1982 with five different successively activated protocols, 105 (44.1%) were cured. However, it must be stressed that there were five treatment-related deaths (doxorubicin cardiotoxicity) and that more than 80% of these patients underwent amputation.

First Study

On the basis of the good results achieved by Rosen et al. [1] in LOE with preoperative chemotherapy in 1983, we started our first study of neo-adjuvant chemotherapy. The aims of the study were (a) to increase the cure rate for these patients; (b) to increase the percentage of limb salvage procedures; (c) to avoid, at least in some patients, the use of doxorubicin (ADM); and (d) to compare in multidrug therapy, the effect of high doses and moderate doses of methotrexate (HDMTX, MDMTX).

Study Design

Patients were considered eligible for the study if they fulfilled the following criteria: (a) typical clinical and histological features of primary, central, and high-grade osteosarcoma (OS); (b) tumor located in the extremities; (c) no prior history of cancer

R. Jakesz/H. Rainer (Eds.)
Progress in Regional Cancer Therapy

Table 1. Results achieved at the Rizzoli Institute in patients with LOE treated by surgery alone

Period	No. of cases	CDFS	Amputations
1959–1971	107	10.2%	96.2%
1972–1982	58	8.6%	87.9%

CDFS, continuously disease-free survival.

and no prior treatment elsewhere; (d) age under 50 years; (e) no evidence of metastases. Diagnostic procedures carried out to exclude metastatic disease were whole lung tomograms, CT scan of the chest, and total body bone scan with technetium.

Between March 1983 and August 1986, 234 newly diagnosed cases of OS were observed at the Rizzoli Institute. Sixty-six of these patients were not eligible (metastatic disease, 22; OS varieties, 29; previous tumor, 3; tumor not located in the extremities, 10; age > 50 years, 2). Of the 168 eligible patients, 30 refused to enter the trial and of the remaining 138 randomized patients, 12 were not evaluable (five refused surgery after preoperative chemotherapy, six refused further chemotherapy after the first cycle, and one died of pulmonary embolism after surgery). Of the remaining 126 patients, the subject of this report, 66 were randomized to receive HDMTX and 60 to receive MDMTX.

Preoperative chemotherapy consisted of two cycles of MTX and cisplatin (CP). MTX was given intravenously (IV) on day 1 in different doses on a randomized basis: 750 mg/m^2 in 30 min vs 7500 mg/m^2 in a 6-h infusion. In both cases, citrovorum factor (CF) rescue was started 24 h after the beginning of MTX. The patients receiving HDMTX had serum MTX levels monitored 24, 36, and 48 h after the end of MTX infusion. Further determinations were made if necessary, and CF rescue as well as hydration and alkalinization were protracted and increased in the case of delayed elimination of the drug. Following an interval of 6–7 days, 120–150 mg/m^2 CP was administered intra-arterially (IA) via a 72-h continuous infusion. A second cycle of both drugs was given after a 14-day interval. Surgery was performed 2 weeks after the end of chemotherapy. The choice between limb salvage procedures and ablative surgery was made taking into account the size of the tumor, the involvement of major neurovascular structures, and the residual expected functional activity. In all cases a wide surgical margin of clearance was intended. While chemotherapy was performed in three different institutions (Rizzoli Institute, 75% of the cases; Department of Pediatric Oncology in Bologna, 10%; Department of Pediatric Oncology of Turin, 15%, surgery was always carried out at the Rizzoli Institute by the same surgeons with expertise in the treatment of bone tumors.

After surgery, all the specimens were studied by the same pathologists, and necrosis was evaluated on at least two entire sections of the two major diameters of the tumor. Necrosis was graded "good" if greater than 90%, "fair" if between 60% and 90%, and "poor" if less than 60%.

Postoperatively, the treatment depended on the grade of necrosis observed. For good necrosis, the same treatment as given preoperatively was given IV at the same doses for two cycles. For fair necrosis ADM 45 mg/m^2 per day for 2 days was added to MTX and CP. The postoperative treatment started with ADM and continued after 21 days with three cycles of MTX and CP. Another dose of ADM was given at the end of the third cycle. For poor necrosis the treatment consisted of five cycles of ADM (45 mg/m^2 per day for 2 consecutive days), alternating with five cycles of BCD (bleomycin 15–20 mg/m^2 per day + cyclophosphamide 600 mg/m^2 per day + dactinomycin 0.6 mg/m^2 per day for 2 consecutive days). In December 1983, after four early metastatic relapses had been observed in the group of good responders, this arm of the study was discontinued. The good responders were then treated using the scheme for fair responders.

Rationale for Preoperative Chemotherapy with MTX-CP

ADM, HDMTX, and CP represent the most active drugs in OS. In metastatic disease, as well as in adjuvant and neo-adjuvant treatment, the combinations MTX + ADM and ADM + CP have been widely investigated. Few studies have been dedicated to MTX + CP, in spite of the fact that experimental data have shown a synergistic effect of CP with antimetabolites, both in vitro and in animal studies. The Children's Cancer Study Group [2], using vincristine (VCR) + HDMTX alternating with CP (given in a 6-h infusion), obtained a very high response rate (56%) in 29 patients with metastics OS. However, the toxicity of this regimen was significant (three deaths possibly related to the treatment). In addition, Crom et al. [3] demonstrated that the administration of CP increases the risk of delayed clearance of MTX. To reduce the toxicity of the combination HDMTX + CP, Gasparini et al. [4] in Milan devised a regimen where CP was delivered over a 72-h period. This long infusion period was warranted by previous observations that prolonged exposure to this drug at a low dose resulted, in laboratory experience, in a greater cell kill. In a pilot study [4] on a small number of patients with localized and metastatic OS, this regimen gave a high response rate (66%) with only moderate toxicity.

We tried this regimen at our Institute in a pilot study on a small group of patients with localized OS [5]. On the basis of the good results achieved by Jaffe et al. [6] and Benjamin et al. [7] in OS using CP intra-arterially, CP was delivered IA in some patients and IV in others. The percentage of good necrosis was considerably higher in the group that had received the drug IA (5/7) than in the IV group (0/6). For this reason we chose to deliver CP IA in this first study of neo-adjuvant chemotherapy.

We decided to employ two different doses of MTX because even though this drug has always been used at high doses in OS, the alleged superiority of these over moderate doses in multidrug regimen has never been demonstrated in adjuvant or neo-adjuvant treatment. In fact, the only randomized study performed in this regard [8] has shown that high and moderate doses of MTX used in addition to ADM in the adjuvant treatment of OS achieved the same results.

Results

In all but two cases, response of the tumor to preoperative chemotherapy was observed. It consisted in the disappearance of pain, if present; reduction of the tumor, with increasing density, on X-ray and CT scan; decreased vascularity on angiograms; and normalization of serum alkaline phosphatase, if evaluated. In two patients, amputation was performed after the first cycle of chemotherapy because of tumor progression.

Ninety patients (72.5%) were surgically treated with limb salvage procedures, 33 (26.1%) with amputation, and three (2.3%) with rotation plasty. In spite of the high number of resections performed, only six local recurrences (LR) (4.7%) were observed, five in patients treated with limb salvage procedures (5.5%) and one in an amputated patient (2.7%). In all but one of these patients the necrosis had been fair or poor. According to surgical margins, the percentage of LR was 2.1% (2/95) for wide surgery, 21.4% (3/14) for marginal surgery and 50% (1/2) for intralesional surgery. No LR was observed in the 15 patients treated with radical surgery.

The necrosis achieved by preoperative chemotherapy was "good" in 52% of cases, "fair" in 36% and "poor" in the remaining 12%. The percentage of "good" necrosis was higher in the patients treated with HDMTX than in patients treated with MDMTX (62% vs 42%) ($P < 0.04$).

At follow-up after 4.5–5 years, of the 15 good responders treated postoperatively with only two cycles of MTX + CP, only four (26%) remained continuously disease free (CDF), 10 developed metastases, and one had metastases and a local recurrence. This local recurrence was due to a skip metastasis erroneously not detected preoperatively. These 15 patients were no longer considered, and the following evaluation refers only to the remaining 111 patients, all postoperatively treated with ADM. At 3-year follow-up, 63 of these patients (56.7%) remained CDF, 43 had metastases, and five had both metastases and local recurrence.

The proportion of continuously disease-free survival (CDFS) was 65% for those treated with HDMTX and 48% for those treated with MDMTX ($P < 0.05$; Table 2, Fig. 1).

Analyzing the results in terms of necrosis induced by preoperative chemotherapy (Table 2, Fig. 2) CDFS was 78% for good responders, 43% for "fair" responders, and 20% for "poor" responders. The difference between "good" and "fair" responders is highly significant ($P < 0.001$), while the difference between "fair" and "poor" responders is not significant. It must be stressed that the "fair" responders among these 111 patients had the same postoperative treatment as the "good" responders, while postoperative chemotherapy was performed with alternative agents in poor responders.

Table 2. Disease-free survival according to the dose of MXT and the grade of necrosis

Necrosis	HDMTX	MDMTX	Total
Good	26/32 (81%)	14/19 (73.6%)	40/51 (78.9%)
Fair	10/20 (50%)	10/26 (38.4%)	20/45 (44.4%)
Poor	1/6 (16.6%)	2/9 (22.2%)	3/15 (20%)
Total	37/57 (64.9%)	26/54 (48.1%)	63/111 (56.7%)

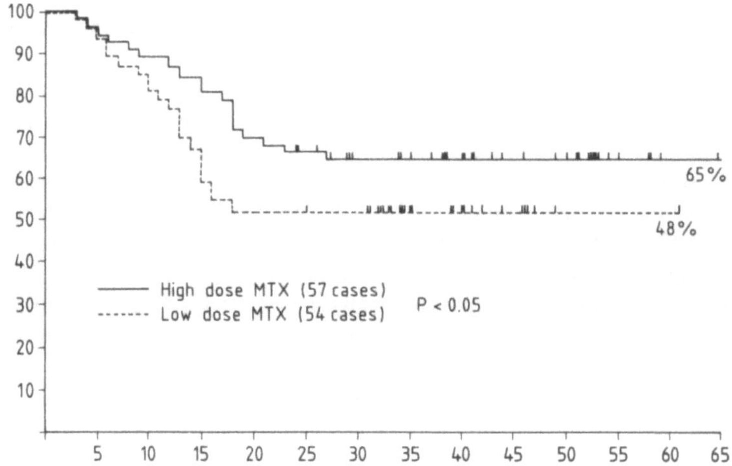

Fig. 1. Disease-free survival of patients treated with HDMTX and MDMTX

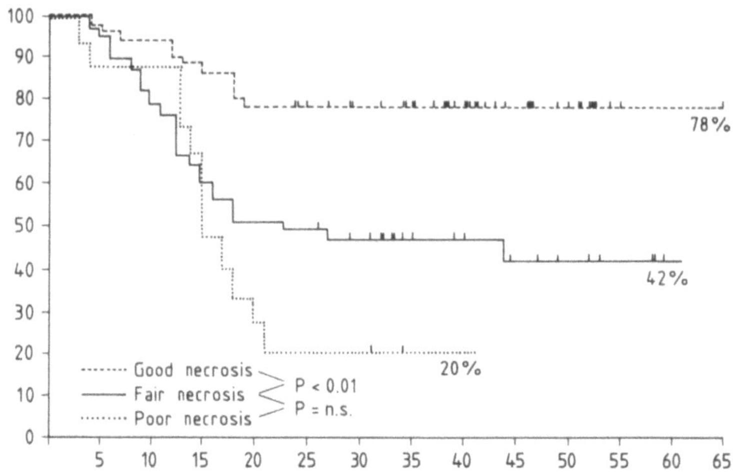

Fig. 2. Disease-free survival of patients according to necrosis induced by preoperative chemotherapy

No statistically significant difference in CDFS was observed between patients treated with limb salvage and those treated with amputation (60.5% vs 48.5%), nor were differences found according to age (64% for patients under 14 years old vs 50% for older patients), sex (50% for males vs 65% for females), or site of tumor (53% for tumors in the femur vs 60% for tumors at other sites).

If we compare these results with the results obtained in the 108 patients treated at our Institute between 1980 and 1982 with adjuvant chemotherapy (MTX + ADM), [9] there is only a slight advantage for the patients of the present study (56.7% vs 44.4% DFS). This difference is not statistically significant. However, it must be considered that the amputation rate was 78% in the group of patients treated with adjuvant chemotherapy vs 31% in the group treated with neo-adjuvant chemotherapy.

Toxicity

Toxicity in both arms of this study was moderate and never life-threatening, with the exception of two cases of delayed clearance of HDMTX, which was resolved without permanent sequelae by means of adequate hydration and CF rescue; in no case was impairment of renal function observed.

Conclusions

1. With neo-adjuvant chemotherapy, limb salvage is possible and safe in about 70% of the patients with LOE.
2. Patients who histologically have good necrosis also have a good prognosis. This has been reported by many authors [1, 10, 11], but our study yields the first confimation with preoperative chemotherapy partially delivered by the IA route.
3. The break point between good prognosis and poor prognosis is probably 90% necrosis.
4. Even in good responders, postoperative chemotherapy must be sufficiently protracted and must include ADM. Our attempt, in good responders, to reduce the postoperative treatment and to avoid the use of a toxic drug such as ADM failed.
5. In poor responders the prognosis remains poor even when changing the drugs in the postoperative treatment.
6. In our multidrug regimen, high doses of MTX are more effective than moderate doses.
7. Toxicity in both arms of this study was moderate. Particularly, administering CP over a long period of time, it was possible to combine this drug with MTX without impairment of renal function. This lack of significant toxicity makes up for the disadvantage of the prolonged hospital stay.

Second Study

Based on the results of the first study, a new protocol was instituted in September 1986. The aims were to increase the number of good responders to preoperative chemotherapy and to increase the DFS in poor and fair responders by means of more aggressive postsurgical chemotherapy. For this reason, ADM was given at a dose of 60 mg/m^2 IV in 8 h together with CP IA as preoperative chemotherapy, in addition to the previous scheme, on the 3rd day. The dose of MTX was established in all patients at 8 g/m^2. A second cycle was given after 28 days, and surgery was performed 2 months after the beginning of treatment. The postoperative treatment for good responders was the same as in the first study, with the exception of MTX, which in all cases was given at the dose of 8 g/m^2. Fair and poor responders were treated with ADM (45 mg/m^2 per day in 8 h for 2 days), followed after 21 days by ifosfamide (2 g/m^2 per day in 1 h for 5 days with MESNA uroprotection), followed after 21 days by MTX and CP given IA as in the preoperative treatment, except that CP was combined with etoposide (100 mg/m^2 per day for 3 days). This cycle was repeated three times, and one more cycle of ADM was given at the end of treatment.

By September 1988, 164 new cases of osteosarcoma had been observed, of which 119 were eligible for the study. Of these patients, 101 agreed to enter the trial and 89 were evaluable for surgery and necrosis at the time of writing, the remaining 12 being in preoperative treatment. Limb salvage was performed in 79 (88.7%), rotation plasty in four (4.4%), and amputation in the remaining six cases (6.7%). Although it is obviously too soon to report the results of this second study, necrosis was found to be "good" in 72 patients (80.7%), "fair" in 12 (13.4%), and "poor" in only five (5.6%). This rate of good necrosis in significantly higher than that obtained in the previous study. Up to now, patients with LOE and a good histological response to preoperative chemotherapy have had a very good prognosis [1, 10, 11], even when chemotherapy was delivered IV [6, 7]. We hope that a substantial improvement in DFS will be obtained with this new scheme of treatment.

References

1. Rosen G, Marcove RC, Caparros B et al. (1979) Primary osteogenic sarcoma: the rationale for preoperative chemotherapy and delayed surgery. Cancer 43:2163–2177
2. Morgan E, Baum E, Bleyer WA et al. (1984) Treatment of patients with metastatic osteogenic sarcoma: a report from the Children's Cancer Study Group. Cancer Treat Rep 68:661–664
3. Crom WR, Pratt CB, Gree AA et al. (1984) The effect of prior cisplatin therapy on the pharmakinetics of high-dose methotrexate. J Clin Oncol 6:655–661
4. Gasparini M, Fossati-Bellani F, Rottoli L et al. (1983) Remission induction by chemotherapy (VCR, HDMTX, CDP) in osteosarcoma. Proc ASCO 2:239
5. Bacci G, Springfield DS, Capanna R et al. (1987) Neoadjuvant chemotherapy for osteosarcoma of the extremity. Clin Orthop 221:268–276
6. Jaffe N, Knapp J, Chuang W et al. (1983) Osteosarcoma: intra-arterial treatment of the primary tumor with cisdiammine-dichloroplatinum (CDP). Cancer 51:402–408
7. Benjamin RS, Chawla SP, Carrasco CH et al. (1987) Primary chemotherapy of patients with osteosarcoma of an extremity. Proc ASCO 6:139
8. Krailo M, Ertel I, Makley J et al. (1987) A randomized study comparing high dose methotrexate with moderate dose methotrexate as component of adjuvant chemotherapy in childhood nonmetastatic osteosarcoma: a report from the Children's Cancer Study Group. Med Pediatr Oncol 15:69–77
9. Bacci G, Gherlinzoni F, Picci P et al. (1986) adriamycin-methotrexate high dose versus adriamycin-methotrexate moderate dose as adjuvant chemotherapy for osteosarcoma of the extremities: a randomized study. Eur J Cancer Clin Oncol 22:1337–1344
10. Winkler K, Beron G, Kotz R et al. (1984) Neoadjuvant chemotherapy for osteosarcoma: results of a cooperative German/Austrian study. J Clin Oncol 2:617–624
11. Winkler K, Beron G, Delling G et al. (1988) Neoadjuvant chemotherapy of osteosarcoma: results of a randomized cooperative trial (COSS-82) with salvage chemotherapy based on histological tumor response. J Clin Oncol 6:329–337

Neo-adjuvant Therapy of Soft Tissue Sarcomas of the Extremities with Intra-arterial Chemotherapy and Radiation

F.R. Eilber, J.F. Huth, G. Rosen, and M. Selch

Division of Surgical Oncology, University of California, Leconte Avenue, Los Angeles, CA 10833, USA

Introduction

The optimal treatment for patients with soft tissue sarcomas of the extremities remains controversial. The relative rarity of the tumor has made it difficult to perform randomized clinical trials comparing one treatment with another in order to determine the best primary therapy. In addition, the tumors have numerous histological variants, vary considerably in size, making standardized surgical procedures difficult, and present in different anatomic sublocations within the extremity.

From a historical perspective surgery was, and remains, an integral component of the primary treatment. Radiation therapy either pre- or postoperatively has proven to be a valuable adjunct, and chemotherapy has recently been shown to be beneficial in certain circumstances.

Historical Perspective

The primary treatment for patients with soft tissue sarcomas of the extremities has been surgical excision. In 1977, the American Joint Committee on Staging End Results reported the results of treatment following primary surgical therapy of 437 patients with soft tissue sarcomas of the extremities [1]. They clearly showed, in this retrospective review, that tumor grade was a major determinant of overall prognosis. That is, patients with grade 1 tumors enjoyed an approximately 75% 5-year survival rate, whereas patients with high-grade (grade 3) tumors had only a 26% 5-year survival rate. It is to be noted that all patients were treated by surgery alone, and that the local recurrence rate, in this retrospective review, was approximately 30%. The primary surgical technique has been compartment resection, which is based on the principle that the tumors spread up and down fascial planes and involve the entire compartment. Therefore, successful surgery involves resection of the compartment where the tumor originates. Several investigators adhering to this principle have utilized surgery as a single treatment modality. Their results are given in Table 1, which shows that this approach results in variable end results both in terms of local tumor control and the necessity for

R. Jakesz/H. Rainer (Eds.)
Progress in Regional Cancer Therapy

Table 1. Reported results of surgical excision

Authors	No of cases	Local recurrence rate	Amputation rate
Enneking et al. [2]	40	15%	50%
Markhede et al. [3]	97	21%	18%
Bertoni et al. [4]	78	37%	17%

amputation. Local tumor failure varies from 15% to 37% and the amputation rate from 50% to 70% [2–4]. The problem with this principle is that amputation, although it may be appropriate for the large majority of the tumors, is unacceptable to most patients, and in the case of very large proximal tumors does not achieve a very satisfactory margin of clearance. Moreover, the compartment resection concept is not universally applicable because many tumors are extracompartmental, such as in subcutaneous fat or in such anatomic spaces as the groin, popliteal space, or foot, and many tumors are in fact located in more than one compartment. Thus, employing compartment resection as a primary treatment method results in the necessity for amputation in 35%–50% of cases and is not applicable to many patients whose tumors do not fit into a specific compartment.

In the early 1970s, several investigators reported the results of complete excision of the tumor and postoperative radiation therapy at a dose of 5000–7000 cGy. This treatment was based on the concept that these tumors were not radioresistant, and that microscopic residual disease (which must be present following a wide excision) was in fact sensitive to high doses of radiation therapy. Table 2 lists the reported trials of high-dose postoperative radiation therapy following wide local excision [5–7]. It should be noted that these wide local excisions were not based on compartment principles but were predicated upon the premise that en bloc excision of all gross tumor had been accomplished. The amputation rate was relatively low (less than 10%) in all these studies, but the local recurrence rate varied from 13% to 29%. All authors used approximately the same radiation equipment, voltages, fields, and treatment techniques. This variability is difficult to understand from a pure radiation-biology standpoint, but may in fact be due to the different qualities of surgical excision. Although excision of all gross disease was said to have been achieved in all cases in these three studies, it is clear that the amount of surgical resection, and thereby the amount of residual microscopic disease, was extremely variable. This variable, then, is difficult to control adequately in a postoperative setting.

Table 2. Reported results of surgical excision and postoperative radiation therapy

Authors	City	No. of cases	Local recurrences
Lindberg et al. [5]	Houston	299	40 (13%)
Suit et al. [6]	Boston	148	22 (15%)
Lattuda and Kenda [7]	Milan	146	43 (29%)

The results of treatment at UCLA from 1971 to 1978, surgery followed by postoperative radiation, were similar – the amputation rate was 33%, the local failure rate 24%.

Neo-adjuvant Therapy

Beginning in 1974, based on a review of the literature and our own results with postoperative radiation, we began a series of trials of treatment including preoperative therapy [8]. The rationale was administration of chemotherapy and/or radiation to a nondisturbed tumor bed, and we hoped that if the therapy was effective, it would allow shrinkage of the tumor, or at the very least allow a clarification of the margin of the tumor by increasing the tumor pseudocapsule. The treatment scheme employed was intra-arterial chemotherapy with doxorubicin (Adriamycin). A percutaneous catheter was placed in the groin vessel, the catheter fed to the opposite side, and the tip placed in a high-flow vessel such as the common femoral or axillary artery. Doxorubicin 30 mg/day was instilled through the catheter continuously at a constant rate for consecutive days, for a total of 90 mg. Following this, the catheter was removed and patients were treated with radiation therapy in 350-cGy fractions through AP and PA opposed ports per day. Each extremity was treated daily for 5 days per week, sparing a portion of the skin opposite the major tumor mass. The doses of radiation therapy varied in the various protocols: 10 × 350 cGy, 5 × 350 cGy, and, most recently, 8 × 350 cGy. The protocol also followed the shrinking field concept, that is, the largest field, treated first, was the entire extremity, a second radiation field was smaller, and, finally, the proposed surgical resection constituted an even smaller field.

Results

A total of 77 patients were treated according to our first protocol, utilizing intra-arterial doxorubicin and 3500 cGy of radiation. Table 3 gives the results of treatment. Among the 77 patients treated there have been five local recurrences (6%). The minimum follow-up for this group of 77 patients is 7 years, and the protocol ran from 1974 to 1981. However, complications of this treatment were severe. Thirty-three (42%) of the patients developed a complication, and 18 (20%) of them required reoperation to correct it. The complications included wound slough (17 patients) fracture of adjacent long bones (eight patients), seroma, edema, nerve palsy, hematoma, etc. The most disturbing complication was that of fracture. All eight of

Table 3. Results of first protocol: preoperative doxorubicin, 3500 cGy radiation, and excision

	Amputation		Local	Complications	
n	Primary	Secondary	recurrence	Total	Surgery
77	2	1	5 (6%)	33 (42%)	18 (20%)
	(4%)				

the patients affected had open reduction of the fracture. No tumor was found in any of these cases, but presumably the preoperative therapy had resulted in osteoradionecrosis of bone.

Because of this, a second protocol was begun in 1981, involving identical use of doxorubicin (intra-arterially 30 mg/day × 3 days) followed by a reduced dose of radiation therapy of 1750 cGy (350 cGy × 5). A total of 137 patients were treated according to this protocol: to date 20 (15%) have developed a local recurrence (Table 4). The complication rate of this treatment was only 25% (35 patients), and only eight (5%) of the entire series required reoperation. Therefore, reduction of the radiation dose did reduce the complication rate but also increased the local failure rate.

As a consequence a third protocol was begun in 1984, and involving preoperative chemotherapy and radiation therapy at the higher dose of 2800 cGy (350 cGy × 8) (Table 5). To date, 103 patients have been treated according to this protocol. The local recurrence rate is 7% and only two patients have had amputation. Complications have occurred in 26 patients, only seven of whom required reoperation. In addition, a second randomization was carried out in this protocol: intra-arterial vs intravenous doxorubicin. Forty-eight patients received intra-arterial and 55 intravenous chemotherapy. The local recurrence rate is identical in the two groups, as is the complication rate.

Finally, since 1987, a fifth protocol has been employed, utilizing intra-arterial cisplatin followed by intravenous doxorubicin and 2800 cGy of radiation (Table 6).

Table 4. Results of second protocol: preoperative doxorubicin, 1750 cGy radiation, and excision

	Amputation		Local	Complications	
n	Primary	Secondary	Recurrence	Total	Surgery
137	7 (5%)		20 (14%)	35 (25%)	8 (5%)

Table 5. Results of third protocol: preoperative doxorubicin, 2800 cGy radiation, and excision

	Amputation		Local	Complications	
n	Primary	Secondary	Recurrence	Total	Surgery
103	2 (2%)		8 (7%)	26 (25%)	7 (7%)

Table 6. Results of fourth protocol: preoperative doxorubicin, cisplatin, 2800 cGy radiation, and excision

	Amputation		Local	Complications	
n	Primary	Secondary	Recurrence	Total	Surgery
30		1 (3%)	1 (3%)	11 (36%)	7 (23%)

To date, 30 patients have been treated according to this protocol: no primary amputations have been carried out, local failure has occurred in one patient, and complications requiring reoperation in seven patients.

Pathological Assessment

Careful pathological assessment was made of the resected tumor specimen following preoperative therapy. Figure 1 illustrates the median tumor cell necrosis. In our first protocol (3500 cGy), involving both grade III and grade II tumors, the median tumor cell necrosis was 78%. The median tumor cell necrosis in the grade II patients was 50%. When the radiation dose was reduced to 1750 cGy, the median tumor cell necrosis decreased from 78% to 58%. When the radiation dose was increased to 2800 cGy, regardless of whether the patient received intra-arterial or intravenous drugs,

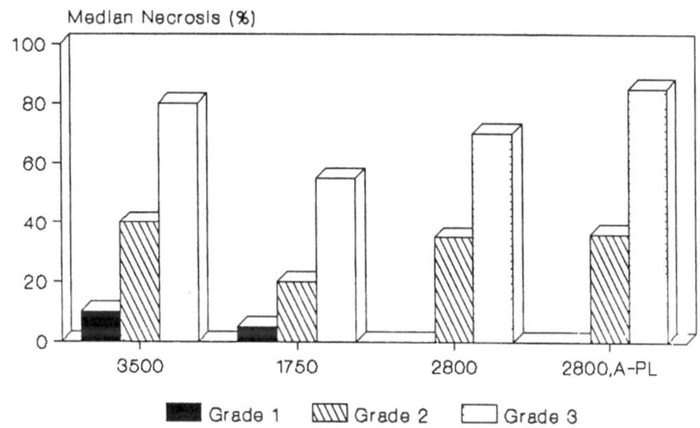

Fig. 1. Effect of preoperative therapy on tumor histology (by tumor grade). *A-PL*, doxorubicin + cisplatin

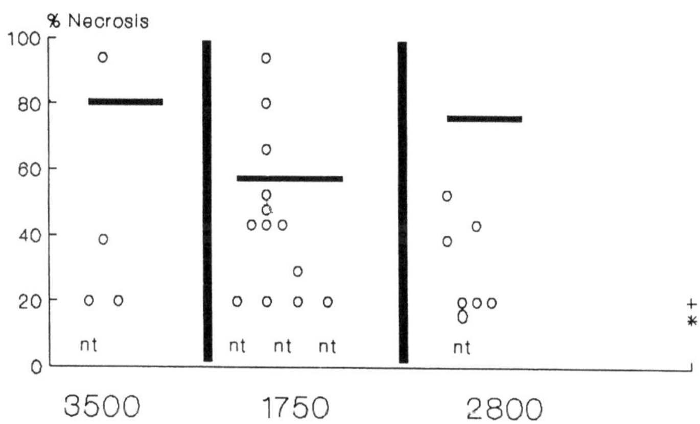

Fig. 2. Relationship of local tumor recurrence to effect of preoperative therapy. *nt*, no tumor; ○, local recurrence; ——, median

median necrosis went up to 70%, and finally, with intra-arterial cisplatin and doxorubicin followed by 2800 cGy, median tumor cell necrosis increased again to 85%. It should be noted, however, that there was a wide range in tumor cell necrosis: even in patients with identical-grade tumors given exactly the same preoperative therapy, the amount of necrosis can vary from 5% to 100%.

There is evidence that tumor cell necrosis as assessed by pathological examination does correlate with local recurrence. Figure 2 shows the percentage necrosis noted in the patients who subsequently developed local recurrence. In the first protocol, with median tumor cell necrosis of 80% after 3500 cGy, four of the five patients who developed local recurrence had tumor cell necrosis of less than 30%. Similarly, in the 1750-cGy protocol, 17 of the 20 patients with local recurrences had necrosis in the specimen below the median. Finally, in the 2800-cGy group all patients who developed local recurrence had displayed less than 30% tumor cell necrosis.

Discussion

The results of this trial, as well as of others using similar concepts, indicate that with preoperative therapy, limb salvage is possible in a very high proportion (greater than 90%) of patients with soft tissue sarcoma of the extremities [6, 8, 9]. From our sequential trials it is apparent that the radiation dose is important in local tumor control. The rapid 350 cGy fraction for a total dose of 1750 cGy are inadequate for local tumor control, and 3500 cGy is adequate but has a high complication rate, but the dose of 2800 cGy in eight 350-cGy fractions appears to be satisfactory regarding both local tumor control and complication rate. The results of the randomized intravenous and intra-arterial chemotherapy indicate that, at least in this treatment scheme, there is no difference between the two routes in terms of local tumor control and histologic tumor cell necrosis.

We also feel that neo-adjuvant or preoperative therapy is an ideal clinical model system for investigating treatment effect in a preoperative fashion. It is possible to evaluate not only the effect of altering one variable in the preoperative scheme on local tumor control and disease-free survival, but also the histologic effect of adjuvant therapy on the tumor in vivo.

It appears from our latest study that cisplatin is a valuable adjunct, at least in terms of increasing the amount of necrosis in preoperative fashion. Therefore, it seems reasonable that sequential use of different chemotherapeutic agents in this model will allow objective assessment of their potential effect in the treatment of this disease.

Summary

The rarity of soft tissue sarcomas and their variability in terms of size, grade, and anatomic location makes a universal treatment scheme unlikely and, in fact, probably undesirable. Patients with low-grade tumors are probably best treated by surgery alone or surgery with low-dose postoperative radiation. Patients with larger and/or high-grade tumors, however, require additional therapy.

Surgery followed by high-dose postoperative radiation therapy is a very acceptable treatment method. Preoperative radiation therapy and surgery also achieve excellent local tumor control and excellent functional results. Any protocol that calls for surgery first eliminates the potential to evaluate the effectiveness of preoperative therapy on the tumor in vivo. The protocol of chemotherapy, radiation, and subsequent surgical excision has been very successful in terms of local tumor control, amputation rate, and complication rate. In our view, total surgical excision is a key factor in these equations. Pathological confirmation of tumor-free margins at the time of surgery is, in fact, essential. Although difficult to compare across protocols, the end functional result of patients with a salvaged limb is also very important. With the higher-dose radiation therapy, approximately 30% of our patients had chronic lymphedema, which although amputation was avoided was not ideal. With the lower doses of radiation therapy, function was much improved.

Finally, the results of treatment including intra-arterial cisplatin are also encouraging. It is hoped that with the continued use of preoperative or neo-adjuvant chemotherapy, irradiation, and surgery, more effective combinations of drugs and sequences of drugs and radiation will be identified. This will allow a greater percentage of patients to achieve good tumor cell necrosis, thereby defining more effective treatment methods. It is also hoped that evaluation of primary tumor response will help to prevent pulmonary metastases by ascertaining the degree of necrosis in the primary tumor prior to surgery, and also enable the initiation of effective systemic chemotherapy prior to local treatment.

References

1. Russell W, Cohen S, Enzinger F, Hajdu S, Heise H, Martin W, Miller W, Schmitz R, Suit H (1977) A clinical and pathologic staging system for soft tissue sarcomas. Cancer 40:1562–1570
2. Enneking W, Spanier S, Malawer M (1981) The effect of the anatomic setting on the results of surgical procedures for soft part sarcoma of the thigh. Cancer 47:1005–1022
3. Markhede G, Angervaoll L, Stenner B (1982) A multivariant analysis of the prognosis after surgical treatment of malignant soft tissue tumors. Cancer 49:1721–1733
4. Bertoni F, Capanna C, Biagini C, Baccini P, Guerra A, Ruggieri P, Present D, Campanacci M (1985) Malignant fibrous histiocytoma of soft tissue: an analysis of 98 cases located and deeply seated in the extremities. Cancer 56:356–362
5. Lindberg R, Martin R, Rhomsdahl M, Barkley T (1981) Conservative surgery and postoperative radiotherapy in 300 adults with soft tissue sarcomas. Cancer 47:2391–2397
6. Suit H, Mankin HJ, Wood WC (1985) Preoperative, intraoperative, and postoperative radiation in the treatment of primary soft tissue sarcoma. Cancer 55:2659–2667
7. Lattuada A, Kenda R (1981) Postoperative radiotherapy of soft tissue sarcoma. Tumori 65:191
8. Eilber F, Morton D, Eckardt J, Grant T, Weisenburger T (1984) Limb salvage for skeletal and soft tissue sarcomas: multidisciplinary preoperative therapy. Cancer 53:2579–2584
9. Goodnight J, Burger W, Voegeli T, Blaisdell F (1985) Limb-sparing surgery for extremity sarcomas after preoperative intraarterial doxorubicin and radiation therapy. Am J Surg 150:109–113

MELANOMA

Isolation Perfusion for Malignant Melanomas: Established Facts and Parameters to Be Clarified

W. Hohenberger

Chirurgische Universitätsklinik, Maximiliansplatz, 8520 Erlangen, FRG

Introduction

The history of isolation perfusion for malignant melanomas dates back to the 1950s, when Creech, Ryan, and Krementz [1] were the first to publish their experience. Later, Cavaliere et al. [2] introduced hyperthermia as another effective technique in isolation perfusion. Stehlin et al. [3] found that chemotherapeutic perfusion yielded better results under hyperthermic than under normothermic conditions.

The technique of isolation perfusion is now well standardized, though with some variations. Whatever the version employed, however, the rate of relevant complications should not exceed 5%.

Indications for Isolation Perfusion

The advantages of hyperthermic isolation perfusion are:

- Isolated use of antineoplastic drugs at high concentrations without systemic side effects
- Enhancement of the effects by hyperthermia
- Treatment of possible or established dermal tumor spread in the limb involved

The treatment may be prophylactic in patients at high risk of developing locoregional skin metastases, therapeutic, for satellitosis, in-transit metastases, and local recurrences.

*Prophylactic Isolation Pe*ı

The impact of prophylactic perfusion on in-transit metastases is not clearly established. These lesions are potentially present in up to 8% of cases in stage I disease [4]. Even after isolation perfusion, follow-up revealed in-transit metastases in 14 (6.9%) of a group of 204 patients treated in our department. Nevertheless, all retrospective studies of isolation perfusion demonstrate its superior effect regarding

R. Jakesz/H Rainer (Eds)
Progress in Regional Cancer Therapy

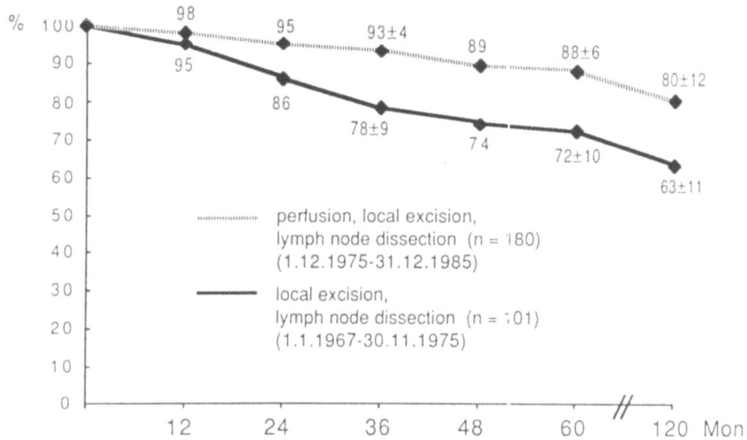

Fig. 1. Age-adjusted cumulative survival in stage I melanoma of the extremities, Breslow thickness > 0.76 mm (Erlangen 1967–1985/31.12.86)

survival and local recurrences. Data of the Surgical Department of the University of Erlangen also clearly document this superiority (Fig. 1). However, like in all historical comparisons, various factors subject to change during the periods concerned may have been at work. Therefore, definitive conclusions are some what problematic. The same is true for different studies including and not including perfusion.

Mixed pairs studies may elucidate this conflict, but will not solve it completely (Schraffordt-Koops, this volume). In situations like this, prospective randomized studies are recommended. Presumably, 500 patients in each group will be necessary to settle this question. Thus, in 1984 a prospective study was inaugurated by the WHO Melanoma Project and the EORTC. Up to now, about 600 patients have entered the study, with no significant benefit of adjuvant isolation perfusion shown so for. The only completed prospective study from one single institution was performed by Ghussen et al. [5, 6]. They seemingly proved the additional benefit of isolation perfusion. However, local recurrences occurred in 21 of 54 patients in the control group (39%), an exceedingly high proportion, suggesting factors of negative selection and severely reducing the value of this study.

Altogether, there is not yet any clear indication for prophylactic perfusion. But even if any particular current study fails to endorse prophylactic perfusion, some patients might still profit from it (for example, those with satellitosis or other factors increasing the risk of in-transit metastases).

Therapeutic Isolation Perfusion

In-transit metastases and local recurrences are an established indication for isolation perfusion. Even though it may take several weeks until these tumors disappear, no other therapy is as effective.

Complete response is reported at rates of between 7% and 82% [7, 8, 12-15]. In our experience, complete response occurred in 49% of cases (20/41 patients), with longstanding complete remission in 12 patients. The age-adjusted 10-year survival rate was 48%.

The Role of Hyperthermia

Without any doubt, hyperthermia may destroy malignant tumors completely without any adjuvant therapy. In contrast to radio- or chemotherapy, hyperthermia is effective even in hypoxic or nonmitotic cells (G_0 cells) [9].

The scale of clinical application of hyperthermia is limited by:

- Ineffectiveness of insufficiently high temperatures
- High rate of complications of excessively high temperatures

In this context, the terms "mild" (39°–40°C), "moderate" (40°–41°C) and "high" (more than 41°C) are commonly used to describe hyperthermia by surgeons dealing with hyperthermic perfusion [10]. However, in experimental research these categories may be misleading, as they are derived from complication rates and not from cell killing effect. Earlier studies clearly indicated that only above 43°C can cells be killed by hypothermia alone [11], and that no killing occurs below 41.5°C.

On the other hand, Cavaliere found severe postoperative complications with high temperatures of more than 41.5°C: six postoperative deaths and four additional amputations in 22 patients [2]. So, for widespread clinical use, safe hyperthermia is limited to 41.5°C or (from personal experience) 42.0°C. Complete responses have been reported, however, from several studies using lower temperatures [7, 8, 12–15].

These results question the need for hyperthermia at all, and they focus attention on the additional effects of cytostatic drugs. However, even these effects are temperature-dependent in various ways (Table 1) [16].

Table 1. Hyperthermia and interaction with drugs [from 16]

1. Drugs with no temperature threshold (increased effect with increased temperature):
   - Thiotepa
   - Nitrosourea group
   - Cisplatin
2. Drugs with a temperature threshold, about 43°C, before major potentiation is observed:
   - Bleomycin
   - Doxorubicin
   - Actinomycin
3. Drugs not normally cytotoxic at 37°C but which cause considerable cell kill above a threshold temperature:
   - Alcohols
   - Amphotericin
   - Cysteamine
   - AET (2-amino-ethyl-isothiourea)
   - Cysteine

Finally, these considerations indicate the need for further reassessment. For practical purposes and for comparison of different studies, some basic standards are necessary: first, the exact temperature applied and the duration of hyperthermia must be clearly identified. The impact of isolation perfusion is on the potential route of tumor spread, which in melanomas means skin and subcutaneous tissue, but not muscle. Thus, the only relevant parameters to be examined and reported are the dermal and subcutaneous temperatures.

As potential cure can be hoped for only in the case of complete response, and as complete response is a very clear-cut event, nothing else but the rate of complete responses should be considered when comparing the therapeutic effects of different (hyperthermic) isolation perfusion protocols.

The results recently compiled by Kroon [7] are more confusing than convincing, because there is no apparent temperature-dependent effect. There is unanimous agreement, however, that in the past, hyperthermic perfusions at temperatures less than 37°C have been performed more often than suspected. It is generally agreed that perfusions ought to be performed at a minimum of 37.0°C, because otherwise reduced or even no effect is to be expected.

Duration and Timing of Perfusions

Assuming that hyperthermia is an effective adjuvant to perfusion, the question remains: how long should it be applied? Most surgeons prefer 1 h and an additional 15 min for warming up. This time has proved to be safe concerning tissue damage. Irrespective of the rate of complications, durations of up to 6 h are reported [2]. However, experimental studies demonstrated increased survival after hyperthermia at a steady temperature of 41.5°C applied for only 4 min adjuvant to chemotherapy [17]. Thus, for the administration of heat, a perfusion shorter than 1 h may suffice. However, heat effects are only one aspect; the other also in terms of duration, is the administration of cytostatics. In this context, tumor cells are affected by peak effects and by integral effects. Whether the integral effect is less relevant in the presence of excessive peaks is not known. Thus, the uncertainty concerning the adequate duration of perfusion is apparently due more to the drugs than to the hyperthermia. There are various schedules for drug administration: bolus injection, fractionation, administration early in the beginning of the perfusion or, at the peak temperature. The influence of these regimens on the rate of eventual complications and on the maximal effect is not known. Some theoretical considerations argue for drug administration at lower temperatures.

Cytostatics are less effective in hypoxic cells, but not at less than 37°C. Hyperthermia induces cellular hypoxia, which might, however, be reversed by high oxygen tension, which is known to increase the effect of alkylating agents [18].

Peak levels of melphalan in the perfusate of up to 115 μg/ml were reached [8], up to 100 times higher than serum peaks in normal intravenous use. An increased rate of complications is attributed to these high levels if the temperature exceeds 40°C. We found no increased negative side effects with tissue temperatures of up to 42.0°C at drug levels of 33 μg/ml in the perfusate. Thus, these differences too are still a matter of discussion.

Drugs as Single Agents and in Combinations

Up to now, at least 11 chemotherapeutic agents have been used for isolation perfusion: melphalan, actinomycin, TSPA, thiotepa, mitomycin C, cisplatin, nitrogen mustard, etoposide, dacarbazine, methotrexate, and vincristine. Melphalan is still the drug most widely used and best examined, and appears superior to all the other cytostatics used alone or in combination [7]. As there are still so many imponderables surrounding isolation perfusion, we should concentrate our research on this one drug to evaluate the true benefit of isolation perfusion in melanomas.

Perspectives

Aside from clinical studies, current research is focused on in vitro sensitivity of melanomas in clinical stages II and III, tissue and oxygen concentrations during perfusion, and perfusion studies in animal models using microsurgical techniques. Thus, we can hope that many of the problems discussed here will be solved within the next 10 years.

References

1. Creech O Jr, Krementz ET, Ryan RF, Winblad JN (1958) Chemotherapy of cancer: regional perfusion utilizing an extracorporeal circuit. Ann Surg 148:616–632
2. Cavaliere R, Ciogatto E, Giovanella BC, Heidelberger C, Johnson R, Margottini M, Mondovi B, Moricca G, Rossi-Fanelli A (1967) Selective heat sensitivity of cancer cells. Cancer 20:1351–1381
3. Stehlin JS Jr, Giovanelli BC, Ipolyi PD, Muena LR, Anderson RF (1975) Results of hyperthermic perfusion for melanoma of the extremities. Surg Gynecol Obstet 14:339–348
4. Vaglini MM, Santinami M (1987) Rationale for prophylactic isolation perfusion in malignant melanoma of extremities. In: Veronesi U, Cascinelli N, Santinami M (eds) Cutaneous melanoma. Status of knowledge and future perspective. Academic, London pp 581–588
5. Ghussen F, Nagel K, Groth W, Müller JM, Stützer H (1984) A prospective randomized study of regional extremity perfusion in patients with malignant melanoma. Ann Surg 200:764–768
6. Ghussen F, Krüger I, Groth W, Stützer H (1987) Hypertherme Extremitätenperfusion mit Melphalan bei Melanompatienten. Spätergebnisse einer prospektiven Studie. Acta Chir Austriaca 19:365–366
7. Kroon BBR (1988) Regional isolation perfusion in melanoma of the limbs; accomplishments, unsolved problems, future. Eur J Surg Oncol 14:101–110
8. Minor DR, Allen RE, Alberts D, Peng YM, Tardelle G, Hutchinson J (1985) A clinical and pharmacokinetic study of isolated limb perfusion with heat and melphalan for melanoma. Cancer 55:2638–2644
9. Wiedemann G, Schem BC, Dahl O, Mella O, Wagner T (1988) Hyperthermie. Grundlagen und Stellenwert einer neuen Therapie modalität in der Onkologie. Dtsch Med Wochenschr 113:787–790

10. Cavaliere R (1987) Perfusion and infusion: indications and techniques. In: Veronesi E, Cascinelli N, Santinami M (eds) Cutaneous melanoma. Status of knowledge and future perspective. Academic, London, pp 577–579
11. Dewey WC, Hopwood LE, Saparto SA et al. (1977) Cellular responses to combinations of hyperthermia and radiation. Radiology 123:463
12. Jönsson P-E, Hafstöm L, Hugander A (1983) Results of regional hyperthermic perfusion for primary and recurrent melanomas of the extremities. In: Schwemmle K, Aigner K (eds) Vascular perfusion in cancer therapy. Springer, Berlin Heidelberg New York, pp 277–282 (Recent results in cancer research, vol 86)
13. Rosin RD, Westbury G (1980) Isolated limb perfusion for malignant melanoma. Practioner 244:1031–1036
14. Lejeune FJ, Deloof T, Ewalenko P et al. (1983) Objective regression of unexcised melanoma in-transit metastases after hyperthermic isolation perfusion of the limbs with melphalan. In: Schwemmle K, Aigner K (eds) Vascular perfusion in cancer therapy. Springer, Berlin Heidelberg New York, pp 268–276 (Recent results in cancer research, vol 86)
15. Vaglini M, Andreola S, Attili A et al. (1985) Hyperthermic antiblastic perfusion in the treatment of cancer of the extremities. Tumori 71:355–359
16. Hahn GM (1979) Potential for therapy of drugs and hyperthermia. Cancer Res 39:2264
17. West KW, Weber TR, Grosfeld JL (1980) Synergistic effect of hyperthermia, papaverine, and chemotherapy in murine neuroblastoma. J Pediatr Surg 15:913–917
18. Krementz ET, Knudson L (1961) The effects of increased oxygen tension on the tumoricidal effect of nitrogen mustard. Surgery 50:266–271

Regional Extremity Perfusion in Patients with Malignant Melanoma

C. Gross, R. Mair, and P. Brücke

I. Chirurgische Klinik, Allgemeines Krankenhaus Linz, Krankenhausstraße 9, 4020 Linz, Austria

Introduction

Malignant melanoma is an unpredictable tumor, especially in its mode and time of metastasis. Although public awareness of this tumor has improved greatly, we are still faced with an alarming number of advanced-stage melanoma.

Since the studies of Clark et al. [1] and Breslow [2], we can distinguish between high- and low-risk melanomas and adapt our therapy accordingly. Wide local excision and lymph node dissection have brought some improvement in treatment. No aggressive regimens of adjuvant therapy, such as systemic chemotherapy, immunotherapy, or a combination of both, have brought any substantial improvement in results.

Creech et al. [3] in 1958 and Cavaliere et al. [4] some years later introduced hyperthemic perfusion with high-dose chemotherapy, exploited the sensitivity of tumor cells to heat and particular drugs. Many studies, that have been done since that time, show encouraging results [5–8], especially in the treatment of local metastases [9]. But because the data of these studies are never comparable, the benefit of this method as adjuvant therapy in stage I high-risk tumors is still under discussion.

We use this kind of treatment in Clark level III, IV, or V tumors of the extremities with invasion greater than 1.5 mm in clinical stage I or II. Stage III tumors are excluded from this therapy, except when psychological factors warrant it.

Since 1977 this mode of treatment has been the therapy of choice in our department, which is still the only one in Austria using this method.

Methods

The tumor is excised and the specimen histologically examined. After verification, that it is a high-risk melanoma, a wide excision is performed and the defect is closed with a split skin graft. After lymph node dissection, perfusion of the extremity is performed. Cannulation of the iliac or axillary vessels is accomplished, and a tourniquet is placed around the root of the limb and held in place by a Steinmannpin. The lines are connected to an extracorporeal circuit consisting of an

R. Jakesz/H Rainer (Eds)
Progress in Regional Cancer Therapy

oxygenator with a heat exchanger and a low flow rotary pump. After preheating the extremity to a tissue temperature of 40°C, 1.2 mg melphalan/kg is administered. After high-temperature perfusion for 1 h, the circuit is washed with plasma protein solution. To control the leakage from regional to systemic circulation, technetium-99-labeled erythrocytes are used. Except in one very obese patient, where we had to stop the perfusion, the leakage never exceeded 10%.

The limitation of this method may be the delay between sampling the blood and receiving the laboratory results. We found that the level in the oxygenator and the central venous pressure give accurate and prompt information concerning the leakage [10]. The mean duration of anesthesia was 3.7 h, including lymph node dissection. A mean 2.7 units of packed red cells were used per patient.

Between 1977 and the beginning of 1987, 43 patients, 18 men and 25 women, were treated in this way. We perfused 7 upper and 36 lower extremities.

Results

We have late information about 35 patients, 10 of whom died. The remaining eight patients were lost to follow-up. Of the 10 patients who died, nine were in stage II at the time of perfusion, some with satellitosis. Six of them died of distal metastases, four of unknown causes. None had local recurrence. Of the eight patients lost to follow-up, three were in stage I, five in stage II. One patient required reperfusion 1 year later because of local recurrence. If we assume that the lost patients also died, we have four deaths among 18 stage I patients, and 14 deaths among 25 stage II patients.

Twenty-five patients were alive at the time of control, 24 of them free of disease an average of 60 months postoperatively (range 6–110 months). One patient (preoperative stage II) required reperfusion 30 months later because of local recurrence. The average recurrence-free interval in stage I patients was 66 months, in stage II 54 months.

Postoperatively, we observed some minor local complications such as lymphatic fistulae and prolonged wound healing, especially in the groin. At the start, we had two neurological lesions requiring prolonged physiotherapy. There were no severe hematological complications.

Discussion

Conventional surgical therapy of high-risk melanoma varies widely. Wide local excision is a commonly accepted procedure. Also, local lymph node dissection should be performed in all cases, even prophylactically in stage I tumors, considering the high incidence of occult metastases.

Hyperthermic perfusion is controversial despite the good results achieved in metastatic cases [5–8, 11–13]. The main reason for these controversies is the lack of prospective randomized studies taking account of different risk factors. However, only Clark level and Breslow depth of invasion are relevant factors. Sex, ulceration, location, and histologic type may have some influence on the prognosis. We are not able to derive any conclusions from our small number of patients, but from our results and the reports in the literature it seems that patients with stage I tumors benefit mostly in terms of avoiding local recurrence and improving 5-year survival rate and disease-free rate. The question of whether there is a real improvement in 10-year survival should be clarified in the ongoing European study.

There is no doubt about the effect of the perfusion in advanced stages of the tumor, especially in local recurrence and satellitosis: our experience is in agreement with the literature [9, 14]. It is possible to control the local disease, but there is probably only little influence on longevity. Nearly all patients die of distant metastases. Nevertheless, hyperthermic perfusion should be the treatment of choice in these advanced stages, thus avoiding mutilation or amputation of an extremity. Repeat perfusions may be necessary to control satellites, but the safety of this procedure and the better quality of life of the patients make the investment in cost and time acceptable.

Conclusion

The results obtained so far indicate that hyperthermic drug perfusion achieves better control of high-risk melanoma than conventional therapy. The effect on long-term survival rates should be clarified in the ongoing prospective European study. The costs of this lengthy treatment do not justify it being withheld from a patient with a high-risk melanoma.

References

1. Clark WH jr, From L, Bernardino EA, Mihim MC (1969) The histogenesis and biologic behavior of primary human malignant melanoma of the skin. Cancer Res 29:705–727
2. Breslow A (1970) Thickness, cross sectional areas and depth of invasion in the prognosis of cutaneous melanoma. Ann Surg 172:902–908
3. Creech O, Krementz ET, Ryan RF (1958) Chemotherapy of cancer: regional perfusion utilizing an extracorporeal circuit. Ann Surg 148:616–632
4. Cavaliere R, Ciocatto EC, Giovanella BC et al. (1967) Selective heat sensitivity of cancer cells: biochemical and clinical studies. Cancer 20:1351–1381
5. Ghussen F, Nagel K, Groth W, Müller JM, Stützer H (1984) A prospective randomized study of regional extremity perfusion in patients with malignant melanoma. Ann Surg 200:764–768
6. Schraffordt Koops H, Oldhoff J, van der Ploeg E, Vermey A, Eibergen R, Beekhuis H (1977) Some aspects of the treatment of primary malignant melanoma of the extremities by isolated regional perfusion. Cancer 39:27–33
7. Martijn H, Schraffordt Koops H, Milton G, Nap M, Oosterhuis W, Shaw H, Oldhoff J (1986) Comparison of two methods of treating primary malignant melanomas Clark IV and V, thickness 1.5 mm and greater, localized on the extremities. Cancer 57:1923–1930
8. Tonak J, Hohenberger W, Weidner F, Goehl H (1983) Hyperthermic perfusion in malignant melanoma, 5-year results. Recent Results Cancer Res 86:229–238
9. Storm K, Morton D (1985) Value of therapeutic hyperthermic limb perfusion in advanced recurrent melanoma of the lower extremity. Am J Surg 150:32–35
10. Necek St, Blauhut B, Bergmann H (1986) Hypertherme Extremitätenperfusion mit Alkeran: Probleme der Anaesthesie und der perioperativen Phase. In: Congress für Anaesthesiologie, Sept 1986 Maudrich, Vienna, p 368

11. Ghussen F, Anderson S, Smalley R (1987) Hyperthermic perfusion with alkeran in patients with melanoma: four year follow up. Proc Annu Meet Am Soc Clin Oncol 6:A829
12. Rege V, Leone L, Soderberg C, Coleman G, Robidoux H, Fijman R, Brown J (1987) Hyperthermic perfusion for stage I malignant melanoma of the extremity. Proc Annu Meet Am Soc Clin Oncol 6:A832
13. Cavaliere R, Di Fillipo F, Aloe L, Carlini S, Piarulli L, Calabro A (1985) Potential of limb perfusion in the treatment of stage 1 high risk limb melanoma patients. In: 3rd European Conference on Clinical Oncology and Cancer Nursing, June 16–20, Stockholm, p 183
14. Nassoor GM, Reinherz RO, Chulengarian JR (1981) Hyperthermia for lower extremity neoplasms. J Foot Surg 20(2):91–92

Preliminary Results of a Double Perfusion Schedule with Melphalan in Measurable Melanoma

B.B.R. Kroon, A.N. van Geel, H.R. Franklin, J.M. Klaase, and C. Benckhuijsen

Department of Surgery, The Netherlands Cancer Institute (Antoni van Leeuwenhoek Huis), Plesmanlaan 121, 1066 CX Amsterdam, The Netherlands

Introduction

Regional isolation perfusion of the limbs is now becoming a standard procedure worldwide. Its advantage is that a high dose of cytostatic drug can be administered to an isolated tumor-bearing region, localizing and enhancing the therapeutic effect without producing the generalized toxicity typical of systemic chemotherapy. The disadvantages of such intrasurgical chemotherapy are that the duration and frequency of drug administration are limited for technical reasons. In other words, the theory of "fractionation and protraction" [7], increasing the difference in tolerance between malignant and normal cells, is difficult to realize.

In order to explore the extent to which multiple perfusions would be feasible, we selected nine patients with locally inoperable melanomas confined to the lower leg, with the intention of treating them with three perfusions of 1 h duration each. The dosage of melphalan chosen was 7.5 mg/liter perfused tissue at each of the three perfusions. Based on schedules used in systemic chemotherapy, an interval of 3 weeks between perfusions was chosen. The perfusions were performed at three different levels: iliac, femoral, and popliteal.

Unfortunately, this treatment schedule proved not to be tolerable. In five patients the intended treatment interval was not realized due to toxicity. Of the remaining four patients who did undergo triple perfusion, however, three achieved complete remission of the inoperable tumor mass. On the basis of this result from the pilot study, we decided to investigate a double perfusion schedule.

Patients and Methods

Only patients with measurable, locally inoperable or recurrent melanomas of the lower leg were selected for double perfusion. For the first perfusion a relatively low dose of melphalan, 6 mg/liter perfused tissue, was administered with the aim of minimizing toxicity, so that an interval of 3 weeks would be possible. For the second perfusion, the dose of melphalan was 9 mg/liter. In general, the first perfusion was administered at the iliac level and the second at the popliteal level.

In order to obtain histological confirmation of response, tumor tissue was left in situ with the intention of removing it 6–12 weeks after the second perfusion. Tattoo

R. Jakesz/H Rainer (Eds)
Progress in Regional Cancer Therapy

marks were made before the perfusion to identify the site of the lesion in case complete remission was obtained.

Upto the time of writing 25 patients (19 women and 6 men, median age 63 years, range 36–76) have been treated according to this schedule. The perfusions were administered at tissue temperatures of 37–38°C ("controlled normothermia") [4] during the whole hour of drug circulation. The indications for perfusion were: neglected primaries (2), local recurrences (3), and satellites or in-transit metastases (20).

Results

The schedule was tolerated well, this being reflected in the toxicity scores. We used the grading system for toxicity developed in our clinics [8]. After the first perfusion, we saw grade I toxicity (no evidence of reaction) in eight patients and grade II (slight erythema and/or slight edema) in 17 patients. After the second perfusion, grade I was seen in two patients, grade II in 14 and grade III (considerable erythema and/or edema with some blistering) in nine.

So far, 22 patients are evaluable for response. For two patients it is still too early, and in one patient two perfusions were performed but the intended interval of 3 weeks was not realized because of wound infection after the first perfusion. Clinical complete remission was achieved in 14 patients, with pathological confirmation in 10 cases. In the remaining four patients, microscopic examination of tissue removed from the tattooed area (where no lesion could be seen or palpated), still revealed melanoma cells. These cases were therefore finally classified as partial remissions (tumor reduction > 50%). Further partial remissions were observed in another three patients, and a "no change" situation was seen in the remaining five.

Of the 10 patients with histologically confirmed complete remission, one developed new tumor growth in the perfused limb (8 months after perfusion); in the others the limb remained disease free (3–21 months). In spite of the success of the local therapy, distant metastases developed in three of the patients, one of whom died 11 months after the perfusion.

Of the four patients with remission which clinically appeared complete but histologically proved to be only partial, two developed recurrence in the limb after 11 and 14 months respectively, one is still disease free (6 months) and one died of distant metastasis (after 9 months), without, however, exhibiting new tumor growth in the perfused limb. For the three other patients with partial remission it is not possible to calculate the duration of the remission because of the administration of supplementary treatment.

Discussion

The clinical remission rate of 64% (14/22) is high. However, in four of these cases, histology revealed that melanoma cells were still present. One problem with this type of response confirmation is that from microscopic examination, it is extremely difficult to assess the melanoma cells' ability to duplicate; i.e., although they may appear vital, they may in fact be dead.

Recently, Baas et al. [1] compared two groups of patients with recurrent melanomas of the leg: 56 who had undergone two perfusions and 37 who had received one perfusion. The interval between the two perfusions in this study was longer than in ours, namely 6 weeks. The cytostatics used were melphalan and actinomycin D. In these patients there was no parameter for assessing response, since no tumor tissue was left in situ. After a 5-year follow-up period there seemed to be no significant difference in local recurrence and survival between the patients treated with one and with two perfusions. However, it is not clear how comparable the two groups really were.

We are of the opinion that the findings of our preliminary report, although not complete in terms of numbers of patients or length of follow-up, are sufficient to advocate consideration of multiple perfusions on the "fractionation and protraction" principle. An option for the future could be the combination of perfusion with repeat infusions (as has recently been reported for osteogenic sarcoma) [5], or with tourniquet infusions [2]. The concept of primary multiple perfusions must also be considered in the efforts to diminish the toxicity of hyperthermic cytostatic perfusions, where it may be advisable to separate treatment modalities. A possibility for instance, would be to start with hyperthermic perfusion without cytostatics, say for 2 h with tissue temperatures of 43°C [6], followed a week later by normothermic perfusion with cytostatics [3]. At this stage of investigation, these experimental perfusions should, as a matter of course, only be administered in situations where measurable, locally inoperable or recurrent disease is left in situ for subsequent objective, clinical, and pathological response evaluation.

References

1. Baas PC, Schraffordt Koops H, Hoekstra HJ, Oosterhuis JW, Van der Weele LT, Oldhoff J (1988) Isolated regional perfusion in the treatment of local recurrence, satellitosis and in-transit metastases of melanomas of the extremities. Reg Cancer Treat 1:33–36
2. Karakousis CP, Kanter PM, Park HC, Sharma SD, Moore R, Ewing JH (1982) Tourniquet infusion versus hyperthermic perfusion. Cancer 49:850–858
3. Kroon BBR, WiebeDink J, Benckhuijsen C et al. (1986) Regional perfusion chemotherapy, sect VIII. 3rd annual report of the Netherlands Cancer Institute, Amsterdam
4. Kroon BBR, Van Geel AN, Benckhuijsen C, Wieberdink J (1987) Normothermic isolation perfusion with melphalan for advanced melanoma of the limbs. Anticancer Res 7:441–442
5. Vaglini M, Bacci G, Baldini M, Belli F, Cascinelli N, Nava M, Picci P, Santinami M, Campanacci M (1987) Limb salvage in osteogenic sarcoma of extremities: a new therapeutic approach associating infusion and hyperthermic antiblastic perfusion. J Extra Corp Technol 19:338–347
6. Van Geel AN, Van der Zeel J, Wieberdink J, Kroon BBR (1985) Isolated hyperthermic perfusion of the extremity (abstract). In: ICRCT 85, Giessen, p 142
7. Wieberdink J (1986) Extracorporeal circulation in regional treatment of cancer. Monograph available on request from the Dutch Society of Extracorporeal Circulation, Langegeer 273, 3075 JJ Rotterdam
8. Wieberdink J, Benckhuijsen C, Braat RP, Van Slooten EA, Olthuis GAA (1982) Dosimetry in isolation perfusion of the limbs by assessment of perfused tissue volume and grading of toxic tissue reactions. Eur J Cancer Clin Oncol 18:905–910

Melphalan in Isolated Limb Perfusion for Malignant Melanoma, Bolus or Divided Dose, Tissue Levels, the pH Effect*

R.N. Scott, R. Blackie, D.J. Kerr, T.E. Wheldon, S.B. Kaye, R.M. MacKie, and A.J. McKay

Department of Vascular Surgery, Gartnavel General Hospital, 1053 Great Western Road, Glasgow G12 OYN, United Kingdom

Isolated limb perfusion (ILP) has now been practised for years [1], but many fundamental issues remain to resolved. This paper summarises three studies we have performed.

Bolus or Divided Dose?

The rationale for ILP depends on enhancing the therapeutic ratio by generating a high concentration of cytotoxic drug within the tumor-bearing limb while sparing the rest of the body. Melphalan (L-phenylalanine mustard, L-PAM) is the drug used most widely in this system. Accurate measurement of this labile drug has become feasible in recent years due to the development of a high-performance liquid chromatography (HPLC) assay [2]. The pharmacokinetics of melphalan in various ILP systems has been described [3–8].

In a phase I study we have increased the dose of melphalan from 1.5 mg/kg to 1.75 mg/kg for iliac ILP with little increase in toxicity. In treating patients according to a protocol for adjuvant perfusion, which involved the administration of 2 mg/kg in divided dose, we observed toxicity which was considered unacceptable for an adjuvant treatment. Uncertain whether this was a simple dose effect or due to the divided dose regime, and because there is no existing data to support either divided dose or single bolus administration, we conducted a study. The aim of the study was to determine whether there is any pharmacokinetic advantage in divided dose or bolus administration of melphalan (1.75 mg/kg) in ILP.

Under balanced general anaesthesia ILP was performed for recurrent or advanced melanoma in 15 patients. The external iliac vessels were cannulated and isolation achieved with an Esmarch bandage tourniquet. The prime consisted of 700 ml packed red cells and 500 ml Ringer's lactate. Melphalan was administered when the calf temperature reached 37.5°C. The oxygenator was supplied with 100% oxygen. The circuit flowed at an average of 370 ml/min for 1 h. Arterial and venous

---

*This work was funded by the Cancer Research Campaign. R.N.S. is in receipt of a travel grant from Lanarkshire Health Board.

R. Jakesz/H Rainer (Eds)
Progress in Regional Cancer Therapy

samples were obtained at 5-min intervals from ports on the oxygenator. The samples were placed on ice immediately and centrifuged as soon as possible. Plasma specimens were frozen for subsequent analysis. A sensitive and specific HPLC assay, based on the method described by Chang et al. [2], was used to measure melphalan concentration. Dansyl proline is added as an internal standard. The lower limit of detection is approximately 0.2 μg/ml and the coefficient of variation is 5.3%.

Figure 1 shows the mean concentration/time curves for the two groups, and Table 1 shows the dose and the areas under the arterial and venous concentration/time curves (AUC_a and AUC_v). There was no significant difference in AUC and no difference in toxicity.

Although this is a small study there is certainly no indication that divided dose administration is associated with any greater AUC than bolus administration of the same dose. Since there was no difference in toxicity, and because melphalan is an unstable drug; we favour the simpler single bolus regime.

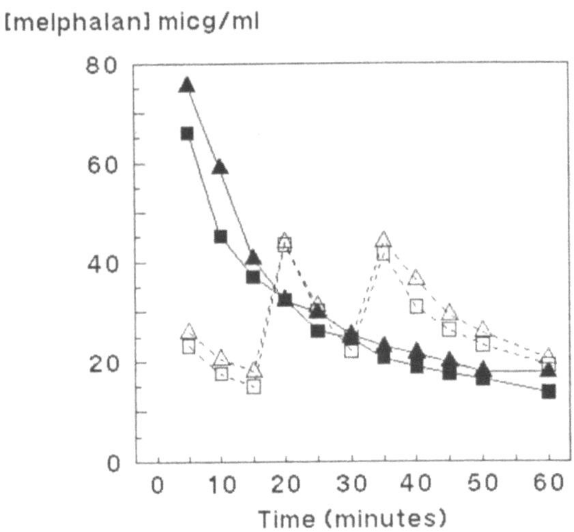

Fig. 1. Concentration/time curves for melphalan (1.75 mg/kg) in ILP. *Filled symbols*, bolus dose; *open symbols*, divided dose; *triangles*, arterial concentration; *squares*, venous concentration

Table 1. Dose and resultant AUC after bolus or divided dose administration of melphalan (1.75 mg/kg)

	Bolus dose ($n = 9$)	Divided dose ($n = 6$)
Dose (mg)	110 (70–165)	110 (84–175)
AUC_a (μg.min/ml)	1649 (1019–4011)	1779 (988–2180)
AUC_v (μg.min/ml)	1570 (990–3056)	1614 (902–2024)

Medians and ranges, Mann–Whitney test.

Tissue Concentrations of Melphalan Achieved by ILP

We have shown previously [6] that ILP achieves high concentrations of melphalan in the plasma of the tumor-bearing limb with low systemic levels during and after ILP. This certainly enhances the therapeutic ratio, but the critical concentrations of cytotoxic drug are those achieved within the viable cells of tumour deposits. The relatively high response rates after ILP with melphalan [9] indicate that effective concentrations can be achieved even in large tumour nodules. Although calculated estimates have been published [7], there have been no reports of direct measurement of tissue concentrations of melphalan achieved by ILP. The aim of this study was to measure the concentration of melphalan achieved by ILP in tumour nodules and in normal tissues, because it cannot be assumed that tumour uptake is simply related to plasma pharmacokinetics.

With ethical committee approval, multiple biopsies were taken from 15 patients with recurrent or advanced melanoma during standard ILP. A total of 55 tissue specimens were taken. The specimens were snap-frozen and stored at −20°C for batch analysis. They were later thawed, weighed and homogenised in a known volume of acidic buffer. Duplicate specimens were then assayed by HPLC as described above.

Table 2 shows the concentrations of melphalan in tumour, fat and skin in the 41 tissue specimens taken at 55 min. Statistical comparisons are made on the basis of paired specimens from each individual patient. The concentration of melphalan in tumour was significantly greater than that in fat, and similar to that in healthy skin. Apparently there was no evidence of preferential accumulation of melphalan in melanoma nodules, but it is encouraging that levels in large necrotic tumour nodules should be as high as in healthy skin. The viable portions of such nodules may yet be shown to selectively accumulate melphalan.

These directly measured tissue concentrations are a little lower than those calculated [7] using an indirect method. We have now established a baseline to determine the effects of physiopharmacological manipulations on tumour concentrations of melphalan in ILP.

pH and Melphalan Cytotoxicity

Physiopharmacological conditions which are unattainable by systemic administration can be achieved and maintained in the tumour-bearing limb during ILP. In

Table 2. Median concentration of melphalan in tumour and normal tissues at 55 min during ILP

Tissue	Melphalan (μg/g)
Tumour ($n = 15$)	3.103
Fat ($n = 14$)	1.15 ($p < 0.01$)[a]
Skin ($n = 12$)	3.54 (n.s.)[a]

[a] Paired Wilcoxon signed rank test.

our standard regime the oxygenator is supplied with 100% oxygen and this produces a profound alkalosis during the hour of perfusion (pH 7.7–8) with no untoward effect. We were interested to determine whether this influenced melphalan cytotoxicity, because the drug hydrolyses to inactive metabolites more slowly in acidic conditions [10].

Multicellular tumour spheroids (MTS) constitute a useful in vitro model for micrometastasis which we have previously used to study thermochemotherapy [11]. MTS are aggregates of tumour cells, growing in liquid suspension culture, which takes a more or less spherical form and which grow by division of cells in the outer rim of the spheroid, which is the part most accessible to nutrients in the culture medium. MTS can be thought of as a system of intermediate complexity between monolayer tissue culture and tumour xenografts.

The aim of this study was to use the B0008 human melanoma MTS model to study the efficacy of melphalan over the pH range relevant to clinical ILP.

In the "agar underlay" static method [12, 13] MTS are formed from monolayers by seeding cells at high density in agar base-coated flasks. The agar prevents cells from adhering to re-form monolayers, and the cells form clumps suspended in the liquid culture medium. Using the B0008 cell line spheroids form in 3–4 days. For experimental therapy, spheroids are pooled, sorted and transferred to thin-walled glass scintillation vials. In studies of pH effect the spheroids are incubated for 1 h at 37°C with and without melphalan (4 μg/ml) at pH 7, 7.4 and 8. The spheroids are then washed with fresh minimum essential medium and 24 spheroids from each experimental group are transferred to individual wells of base-coated multiwell plates. A computerised image analysis system is used to measure the subsequent growth of each individual spheroid. Figure 2 shows an untreated control MTS at 11

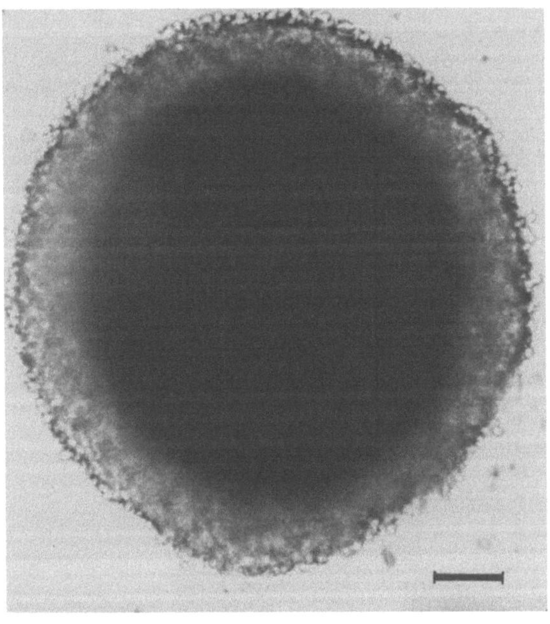

Fig. 2. Untreated control multicellular tumour **spheroid**. *Scale bar*, 100 μm

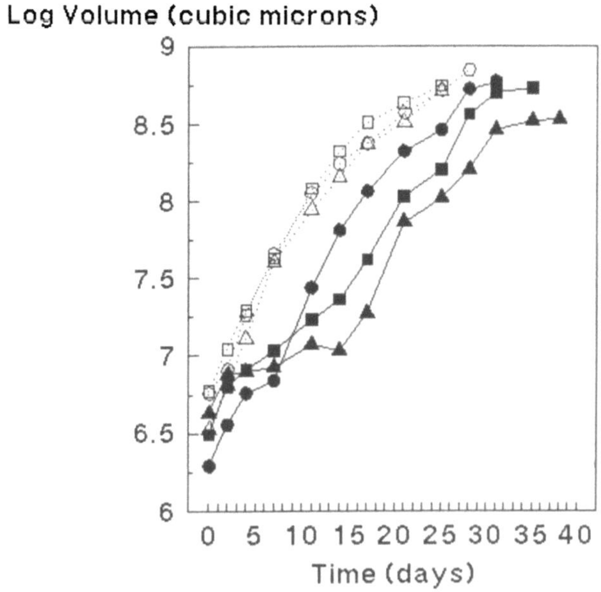

Fig. 3. The influence of pH on melphalan (4 μg/ml) cytotoxicity; growth curves for B0008 human melanoma MTS. *Filled symbols*, melphalan; *open symbols*, controls; *triangles*, pH 7; *squares*, pH 7.4; *circles*, pH 8

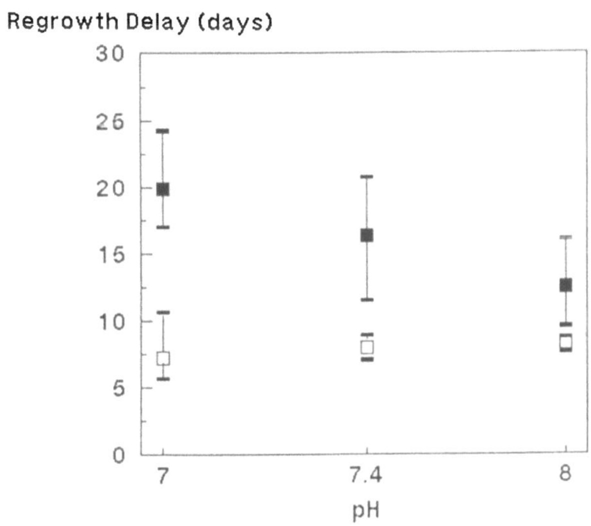

Fig. 4. Regrowth delay of B0008 human melanoma MTS (same experiment as Fig. 3). *Filled squares*, melphalan; *open squares*, controls; *bars*, 95% confidence intervals

days, and Fig. 3 shows the growth curves from a representative experiment. The time taken for MTS to reach 10 times their initial volume is termed the "regrowth delay". In Fig. 4 the median regrowth delays have been plotted against pH (same experiment as Fig. 3). In these experiments altered pH had no effect on the growth of control MTS. There was a significant reduction in melphalan cytotoxicity with increasing pH. The rate of hydrolysis of melphalan was measured at the pH levels employed in these experiments using HPLC, but there was no detectable difference.

These in vitro results suggest that melphalan may be more effective against melanoma cells at normal or acidic pH. The mechanism of this pH effect remains to be discovered. It may involve an effect on the drug itself or on transmembrane carriers [14]. pH is one of a number of critical variables which will determine the optimum regime for clinical ILP.

References

1. Creech OJ, Krementz ET, Ryan RF, Winblad JN (1958) Chemotherapy of cancer: regional perfusion utilising an extracorporeal circuit. Ann Surg 148:616–632
2. Chang SY, Alberts DS, Farquar D, Melnick LR, Walson PD, Salmon SE (1978) Hydrolysis and protein binding of melphalan. J Pharm Sci 67:682–684
3. Hafstrom L, Hugander A, Jonsson P-E, Westling H, Ehrsson H (1984) Blood leakage and melphalan leakage from the perfusion circuit during regional hyperthermic perfusion for malignant melanoma. Cancer Treat Rep 68:867–872
4. Briele HA, Djuric M, Jung DT, Mortell T, Patel MK, Das Gupta TK (1985) Pharmacokinetics of melphalan in clinical isolation perfusion of the extremities. Cancer Res 45:1885–1889
5. Minor DR, Allen RE, Alberts D, Peng Y-M, Tardelli G, Hutchinson J (1985) A clinical and pharmacokinetic study of isolated limb perfusion with heat and melphalan for melanoma. Cancer 55:2638–2644
6. Scott RN, Blackie R, Kerr DJ, Hughes J, Burnside G, MacKie RM, Kaye SB, McKay AJ (1987) Melphalan pharmacokinetics in isolated limb perfusion (ILP) for melanoma (abstract). ICRCT 87, Ulm, p G31
7. Benckhuijsen C, Kroom BBR, van Geel AN, Wieberdink J (1988) Regional perfusion treatment with melphalan for melanoma in a limb: an evaluation of drug kinetics. Eur J Surg Oncol 14:157–163
8. Osterheld HKO, Musch E, von Unruh GE, Loos U, Rauschecker H, Muhlenbruch BJ (1988) A sensitive high-performance liquid chromatographic assay for melphalan and its hydrolysis products in blood and plasma. Cancer Chemother Pharmacol 21:156–162
9. Kroon BBR (1988) Regional isolation perfusion in melanoma of the limbs; accomplishments, unsolved problems, future. Eur J Surg Oncol 14:101–110
10. Furner RL, Brown RK (1980) L-Phenylalanine mustard (L-PAM): the first 25 years. Cancer Treat Rep 64:559–574
11. Scott RN, Wheldon TE, Kaye SB, MacKie RM, McKay AJ (1987) Multicellular tumour spheroids (MTS) as a model for thermochemotherapy with melphalan (abstract). ICRCT 87, Ulm, p A19
12. Yuhas JM, Li AP, Martinez AO, Ladman AJ (1977) A simplified method for production and growth of multicellular tumour spheroids. Cancer Res 37:3639–3643
13. Twentyman PR (1980) Response to chemotherapy of EMT6 spheroids as measured by growth delay and cell survival. Br J Cancer 42:297–304
14. Parsons PG, Carter FB, Morrison L, Regius Mary sr (1981) Mechanism of melphalan resistance developed in vitro in human melanoma cells. Cancer Res 41:1524–1534

Isolation Perfusion of Malignant Soft Tissue Tumors

W. Hohenberger, J. Göhl, and C. Kessler

Chirurgische Universitätsklinik, Maximiliansplatz, 8520 Erlangen, FRG

Introduction

There is no doubt that surgical excision is the first-choice treatment for soft tissue sarcomas. In the limbs, however, resection of the tumor with the requisite margins of clearance (4 cm in the longitudinal and transverse planes and 2 cm in the vertical plane) [7] is often hindered by the proximity of nerves and vessels.

In these situations amputation represents the only chance of adequate clearance, but is often refused by the patients. Furthermore, many patients with soft tissue sarcomas are transferred with a history of evidently inadequate primary treatment and an increased risk of local recurrence. Thus, some therapy adjuvant to surgery is often mandatory for potential curability. Isolation perfusion with or without hyperthermia offers this option at low risk and with high theoretical efficacy.

Patients and Method

From 1976 to 1987, 32 patients with soft tissue sarcomas of the limbs were treated by hyperthermic isolation perfusion, in addition to local excision of the primary tumor if present, at the Department of Surgery of the University of Erlangen. Elective lymph node dissection was performed in those patients judged to be at high risk of developing lymph node metastases (rhabdomyosarcomas, synovial sarcomas and malignant fibrous histiocytomas). The mean age of these patients (13 males, 19 females) was 46.4 years. The leg was involved in 28 cases and the arm in four. The median follow-up of all patients was 73 months, with a minimum of 18 months, and that of the patients alive at the time of writing was 87 months.

The indications for isolation perfusion were:

- Curative excision but limited margin of clearance ($n = 19$, including five patients with macroscopic residual tumor after previous operation)
- Noncurative excision (R1: no residual tumor seen macroscopically, but tumor found to reach margin of specimen on histological examination),
- recurrence limited to limb ($n = 12$) and limited margin of clearance in solitary tumors

R. Jakesz/H Rainer (Eds)
Progress in Regional Cancer Therapy

Malignant fibrous histiocytoma ($n = 11$) was the most frequent tumor type.

There were seven synovial sarcomas, six liposarcomas, five rhabdomyosarcomas, one fibrosarcoma, one extraskeletal chondrosarcoma, and one unclassified malignant sarcoma.

Tumor staging (UICC 1978) was as follows:

IA	2	IIIA	4
IB	2	IIIB	5
IIA	7	IIIC	—
IIB	5	IVA	5
		IVB	1

Hyperthermic isolation perfusion was performed for 1 h at a maximal tissue temperature between 40°C and 42°C with the same technique as for melanomas [8]. The combination of drugs usually used was melphalan (1.2 mg/kg body weight for legs, 0.5 mg/kg body weight for arms) with actinomycin D (1 mg and 0.5 mg respectively). In one patient, 250 mg cisplatin was used for leg perfusion.

Eight patients received additional systemic chemotherapy and 10 had local radiotherapy, including four patients receiving both.

Results

There were no postoperative complications. Local recurrences occurred in six (19%) of the 32 patients:

G3	5/13	T1	3/14
G2	1/14	T2	3/12
G1	0/5	T3	0/6

Local relapse was diagnosed between 5 and 85 months (median 43 months) after isolation perfusion. However, none of the six patients with previous noncurative excision (R1) developed any local recurrence. Twenty-three patients were still alive at the time of writing. The remaining nine died from distant metastases, with additional local recurrence in three cases. Median survival of all patients was 73 months.

Discussion

Local recurrence is an important problem in the treatment of soft tissue sarcomas and is significantly correlated to survival. Tumor-specific factors and adequacy of primary treatment also influence the rate of cure.

The basic prerequisite for local surgical control of the primary is adequate margins of clearance, namely 4 cm in the transverse planes and 2 cm in depth. These margins often cannot be achieved because of the presence of structures essential for acceptable function. Thus, adjuvant therapy may be mandatory.

A high but localized tumor killing effect may be achieved by any modality focusing high doses in a limited area, so that systemic toxicity is insignificant. Such modalities are radiotherapy and selective chemotherapy via the intra-arterial route or by isolation perfusion. The isolation perfusion technique has been successfully used for soft tissue sarcomas in many centers [1, 2, 4–6]. In our experience, isolation perfusion alone was effective for local tumor control even in noncurative excisions (R1), with no local recurrence in six patients.

However, as yet unsettled aspects of the use of isolation perfusion in melanomas (e.g., effect of neoadjuvant perfusion, role of hyperthermia, reduction of local recurrences in the case of a limited margin of clearance by perfusion vs external radiotherapy; see Hohenberger, this volume), are also matters for future studies in soft tissue sarcomas.

References

1. Braat RP, Wieberdink J, van Slooten E, Olthuis G (1983) Regional perfusion with Adriamycin in soft tissue sarcomas. In: Schwemmle K, Aigner K (eds) Vascular perfusion in cancer therapy. Springer, Berlin Heidelberg New York, pp 260–263 (Recent results cancer research, vol 86)
2. DiFilippo F, Calabro AM, Cavallari A, Carlini S, Buttini GL, Moscarelli F, Cavaliere F, Piarulle L, Cavalliere R (1988) The role of hyperthermic perfusion as a first step in the treatment of soft tissue sarcomas of the extremities. World J Surg 12:332–339
3. UICC (1978) TNM classification of malignant tumours, 3rd edn. Springer, Berlin Heidelberg New York
4. Krementz ET, Carter RD, Sutherland CM, Hutton I (1977) Chemotherapy of sarcomas of the limbs of regional perfusion. Ann Surg 185:555
5. Lejeune FJ, Lienard D, Ewalenke P (1988) Hyperthermic isolation perfusion of the limbs with cytostatics after surgical excision of sarcomas. World J Surg 12:345–348
6. Stehlin JS, Giovanelli BC, Gutierrez AE, Delpolyi PD, Greef PJ (1984) 15 years' experience with hyperthermic perfusion for treatment of soft tissue sarcoma and malignant melanoma of the extremities. Front Radiat Ther Oncol 18:177
7. Tonak J (1986) Maligne Weichteiltumoren. In: Gall FP, Hermanek P, Tonak J (eds) Chirurgische Onkologie. Springer, Berlin Heidelberg New York, pp 643–671
8. Tonak J, Hohenberger W, Weidner F, Göhl J (1983) Hyperthermic perfusion in malignant melanoma: 5-year results. In: Schwemmle K, Aigner K (eds) Vascular perfusion in cancer therapy. Springer, Berlin Heidelberg New York, pp 229–238 (Recent results cancer research, vol 86)

The Effect of Topical Adriamycin in Superficial Bladder Tumors: A 5-Year Follow-up

K. Burk, W. Schultze-Seemann, and G. Rodeck

Abteilung für medizinische Onkologie, Farmitalia Carlo Erba GmbH, Merzhäuserstraße 112, 7800 Freiburg, FRG

Patients and Methods

Two hundred and forty patients with superficial bladder carcinoma were treated in the Department of Urology of Marburg University between 1979 and 1984. Patients with primary tumors had transurethral resection (TUR) alone, whereas patients with at least two recurrences in their prior history received doxorubicin (Adriamycin, Farmitalia; ADM) as recurrence prophylaxis in addition to TUR. In the case of further recurrence without muscle invasion, local treatment with ADM was repeated for patients in the ADM group and was offered to patients in the TUR alone group. The results presented in the following refer to patients who received either TUR plus ADM or repeated TUR alone, without a topical recurrence prophylaxis.

Although the patients were not randomized, the two groups are well balanced with regard to stage, grade, age, and sex. The proportion of Ta tumors was 72% in the TUR alone grop and 74% in the TUR + ADM group, and high-grade tumors constituted 43% and 47% respectively (Table 1). One hundred and fourteen patients had repeated TUR alone till tumor progression and 126 patients had additional recurrence prophylaxis with ADM, repeatedly if necessary. The median follow-up was 42 months (range 3–72 months) for the TUR group and 47 months (9–72 months) for the ADM group.

Four and three patients respectively were lost to follow-up, 20 and 11 patients respectively died during the observation period. Half of the deaths in the TUR group were due to tumor progression, whereas in the ADM group only one patient died of tumor progression (Table 2).

Results

In the group with primary tumors (TUR only), the mean recurrence-free interval for Ta tumors was 29.5 months and for T1 tumors only 13.5 months. In the group receiving recurrence prophylaxis with ADM the mean recurrence-free interval for Ta tumors was increased from 14.2 to 28.9 months which is comparable to the group with primary tumors. The enhancement of the mean recurrence-free interval for T1 tumors from 7.4 months up to 20.6 months is even more striking (Table 3).

R. Jakesz/H. Rainer (Eds.)
Progress in Regional Cancer Therapy

Table 1. Material

	TUR $n = 114$	TUR + ADM $n = 126$
Tumor extent		
Tis	—	1
Ta	82	93
T1	32	32
Grade		
G0	9	7
G1	56	60
G2	34	43
G3	15	16
Previous recurrences	None	$\geqslant 2$
Median age in years (range)	68(52–96)	67(47–82)

Table 2. Recurrence-free interval and recurrence rate

	TUR $n = 114$	TUR + ADM $n = 126$	
		Before ADM	After ADM
Mean recurrence-free interval (months)			
Ta	29.4	14.2	28.9
T1	13.5	7.4	20.6
Recurrence rate (1%)			
Ta	3.4	7.01	3.45
T1	7.4	13.40	4.85

Looking at tumor progression, defined as invasion of the muscular layer, we found that 9.8% of patients with Ta tumors in the TUR group suffered from tumor progression, compared with only 1% in the ADM group. The proportions of T1 tumors with muscle-invasive recurrences – 31% vs 0%—were significantly different ($p < 0.005$).

The progression rate obviously influences the rate of deaths due to tumor. In the TUR group 6% of the patients with Ta tumors and 15.6% of those with T1 tumors died due to tumor progression. In contrast, only 1 of 93 patients with Ta tumors in the ADM group died because of tumor progression.

Discussion

According to the literature about 10% of patients with Ta tumors and about 30% of those who have T1 tumors suffer from muscle-invasive recurrences when treated by TUR alone. More than half of the patients suffering from progression die due to the

Table 3. Follow-up and results

	TUR $n = 114$		TUR + ADM $n = 126$
Median Follow-up in months (range)	42 (3–72)		47 (9–72)
Lost to Follow-up	4		3
Tumor Progression			
Ta	8/82		1/93
T1	10/32	$p < 0.005$	0/32
Tis	—		0/1
Tumor mortality			
Ta	5/82		1/93
T1	5/32	$p = 0.005$	0/32
Tis	—		0/1
Total mortality			
Ta	17/82		9/93
T1	10/32	$p < 0.025$	0/32
Tis	—		0/1

tumor. In our study three of the patients who developed muscle-invasive recurrences had G2 tumors, all the others had G3 tumors.

In our study, of 126 patients with recurrent superficial bladder cancer who had adjuvant local treatment with ADM only one displayed tumor progression. This patient had received only four instillations when the treatment was stopped because of chemocystitis. Progression in this case occurred 13 months after the termination of adjuvant ADM therapy with a T2-3 G3 tumor. The patient refused the suggested cystectomy but received irradiation to the bladder and the local lymph nodes. This patient died due to her tumor 18 months after radiotherapy.

All other patients in the ADM group with recurrence of their superficial bladder tumors received repeated local adjuvant therapy with ADM (up to four courses).

This clearly indicates that repeated adjuvant local treatment with ADM is able to prevent tumor recurrence. The number of patients observed is too small to state that tumor progression will be prevented in all cases. Nevertheless it is evident that the high-risk group with high-grade recurrent superficial bladder carcinoma will have significantly less tumor invasion into the muscular layer, provided they receive repeated adjuvant local treatment.

We showed that the recurrence-free interval for patients with recurrent Ta tumors could be improved to 28 months which is similar to that in patients with primary Ta tumors. For patients with recurrent T1 tumors the recurrence-free interval could be raised to 20.6 months, 1.5 times higher than in primary T1 tumors treated by TUR alone. The recurrence rate exhibits the same development.

We presume that local adjuvant chemotherapy does not prevent recurrence, but prolongs the recurrence-free interval and so reduces the progression rate. Our results also demonstrate that patients in a high-risk group (recurrent Ta, G2, G3, and T1 tumors) will benefit more from local adjuvant chemotherapy.

Conclusions

1. Patients with recurrent Ta, G2, and G3 tumors, as well as patients with T1 tumors, belong to a high-risk group.
2. Patients in this high-risk group will benefit most from adjuvant local treatment with ADM.
3. Adjuvant local chemotherapy with ADM prolongs the recurrence-free interval of patients with recurrent Ta tumors of all grades.

Topical Instillation of Mitomycin C in the Treatment of Superficial Bladder Tumors: Long-Term Observation

H. Leyh

Urologische Klinik und Poliklinik der TU München, Klinikum rechts der Isar, Ismaningerstraße 22, 8000 München 80, FRG

Patients and Methods

This study was set up to help answer two questions:

- Does temporary topical chemotherapy with mitomycin C (MMC) substantially reduce the recurrence rate of bladder tumors in the long term?
- For what kind of superficial bladder tumors is topical instillation therapy best suited?

The course of disease in 85 patients with recurrent superficial transitional cell carcinoma of the bladder was analyzed. Following transurethral resection (TUR), patients were treated by intermittent intravesical MMC chemotherapy for 1 year.

Tumor recurrence and progression were compared with the course of disease in a retrospective group of 350 patients with similar staging and grading who had been treated by TUR only. The minimum postoperative observation time in both groups was 5 years.

As shown in Table 1, when MMC was first administered, tumor staging and grading were pTis G3 in two patients, pTaG1 in nine, pTa G2 in 54, pT1 G2 in 17, and pT1 G3 in three. Seven patients had unifocal, 78 patients multifocal tumor recurrences.

A dose of 20 mg MMC was given once a week for 12 weeks after TUR and once a month for the subsequent 9 months. Urinary cytology and cystoscopy as follow-up examinations were carried out in 3-month intervals. When recurrent bladder tumor growth without tumor progression was found, the initial therapeutic regimen was restarted.

Results

In 47% of patients treated with MMC, tumor recurrence was found during observation period. In half of these cases tumor recurred during the year of MMC therapy, in 83% during the first 2 years. Yet, compared with controls, patients with MMC therapy showed a distinct lower recurrence rate (Fig. 1). While in the MMC group 76% of patients were without tumor recurrence after 1 year and 61% after 2

R. Jakesz/H Rainer (Eds)
Progress in Regional Cancer Therapy

Table 1. Tumor staging and grading before initiation of MMC therapy ($n = 85$)

	pTis	pTa	pT1	
G1	—	9	—	9
G2	—	54	17	71
G3	2	—	3	5
	2	63	20	85

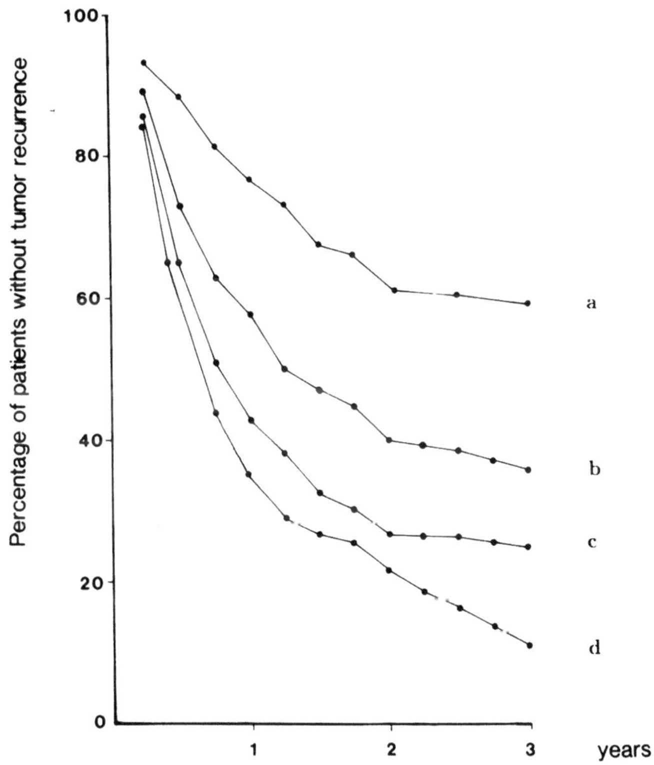

Fig. 1. Recurrence rate after transurethral resection with or without topical instillation of mitomycin C. *a*, after tumor recurrence (TUR + MMC); *b*, after primary disease (TUR); *c*, after one to three tumor recurrences (TUR); *d*, after 4–25 tumor recurrences (TUR)

years, only 40% of patients in the retrospective group were free of tumor recurrence after 1 year and only 25% after 2 years.

Intravesical MMC therapy reduced the annual individual recurrence rate from 0.95 to 0.28, i.e., to 29% of the rate before topical treatment. The best results were found in G1 tumors, pTa tumors, and unifocal tumors (Fig. 2).

Among MMC-treated patients with tumor recurrence, 50% revealed no change in tumor staging and grading and 17% showed improvement in staging or grading.

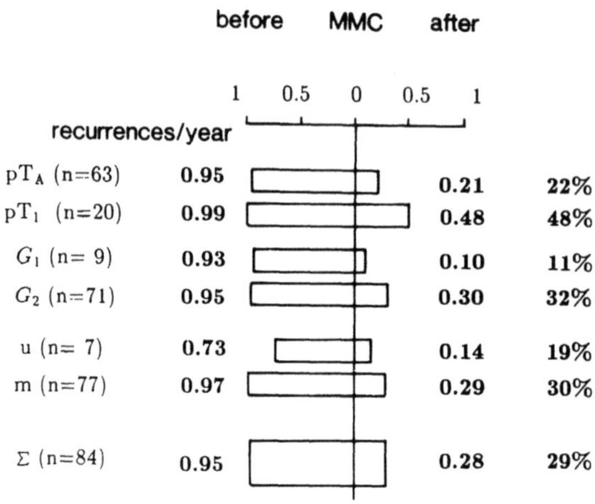

Fig. 2. Recurrence rate during equal periods of time before and after initiation of MMC chemotherapy (average 69 months; $n = 84$). *U*, unifocal; *m*, multifocal

Table 2. Tumor recurrence during or after MMC therapy

	n	%
Tumor recurrence	40	47
With regression in T or G	7	8
Without progression in T or G	20	24
With progression in T or G	13	15

Table 3. Rate of tumor progression after TUR alone and TUR + MMC

	Tumor progression (%) TUR	TUR + MMC
Muscle infiltration after:		
Ta tumor	16	6
T1 tumor	33	25
Total	23	11
G3 tumor after:		
G1 tumor	16	0
G2 tumor	24	13
Total	21	11

Fifteen percent of all patients treated with MMC showed progress in staging or grading during or after topical chemotherapy, on average $1\frac{1}{2}$ years after initiation of treatment (Table 2). Most of these cases were then in a stage of disease no longer curable by TUR.

During the observation time 11% of patients had tumor progression from pTa or pT1 to an invasive stage, and likewise 11% went from G1 or G2 to G3. In the retrospective group the corresponding values were 23% for muscle infiltration and 21% for progression to a G3 tumor. In both groups higher risk was found in patients with pT1 or G2 tumors compared to pTa respectively G1 tumors (Table 3).

Conclusion

Temporary MMC therapy reduces the recurrence rate of superficial bladder tumors significantly for a period of at least 5 years and lengthens the disease-free interval. Our study revealed intravesical MMC to be most effective in G1, pTa, and unifocal tumors.

The fact that nearly half the tumor recurrences developed in the 2nd year after initiation of instillation therapy casts doubt on the practice of terminating topical chemotherapy after a period of 12 months. Although the tumor progression rate under MMC therapy is lower than in patients treated only by TUR, close attention should be paid to the cases with fast progression of disease.

Taking into account cost and side effects of treatment (15%–30%), topical chemotherapy should be recommended only for superficial bladder tumors involving a high risk of recurrence and progression, such as recurrent or multifocal G2 tumors, superficial tumors with concomitant carcinoma in situ, or primary carcinoma in situ.

Mitomycin and Hyaluronidase in the Prevention of Recurrent Bladder Tumor

U. Maier and G. Baumgartner

Urologische Universitätsklinik Wien, Alser Straße 4, 1090 Wien, Austria

Methods

Numerous studies have shown mitomycin to have a significant effect on the recurrence rate of bladder tumors [1–5]. We report here on three clinical trials of mitomycin in the treatment of bladder cancer: (1) a randomized study of mitomycin vs control; (2) a long-term study of mitomycin; (3) a randomized study of mitomycin vs mitomycin + hyaluronidase. In all three trials 20 mg mitomycin was given after transurethral resection (TUR) of bladder tumor stage Ta to T2 of all grades of malignancy over a period of 2 years; in the first 6 months at intervals of 2 weeks and thereafter every 4 weeks. Endoscopic follow-ups, combined with bladder washing cytology, were scheduled at intervals of 3 months in the first 2 years and then half-yearly. Intravenous pyelography and sonography were carried out once a year in the first 2 years and then every 18 months.

Randomized Study: Mitomycin Vs Control ($n = 62$)

In the first study [6] the groups were statistically well comparable in terms of age, sex, number of primary and recurrent tumors, and follow-up time (Table 1) as well as staging and grading of the tumors. The recurrence rate (Table 2) was significantly lower in the mitomycin group (21.9%) than in the control group (56.7%). Mapping of normal looking bladder epithelium was carried out with every endoscopic control. Surprisingly, the rate of dysplasia was nearly twice as high in the mitomycin group as in the control group, despite the lower recurrence rate (Table 2).

Long-Term Study: Mitomycin ($n = 157$)

The results of the long-term study with mitomycin confirmed the findings of the previous randomized trial, with a recurrence rate of 25.5%. Side effects such as cystitis and exanthema were observed in 7.6% of patients.

R. Jakesz/H Rainer (Eds.)
Progress in Regional Cancer Therapy

Table 1. Randomized study: mitomycin vs control. (Patient characteristics)

	Mitomycin $n = 32$	Control $n = 30$
Age in years (mean)	63.1	66.4
Males/females	22/10	19/11
Primary tumor	23	22
Recurrent tumor	9	8
Observation time in months (mean)	24.2	25.1

Table 2. Randomized study: mitomycin vs control. (Recurrences and dysplasia)

	Mitomycin $n = 32$	Control $n = 30$
Recurrences	7/32 (21.9%)	17/30 (56.7%)
Mean disease-free interval (months)	13	10
Dysplasia	43.8%	23.3%

Randomized Study: Mitomycin vs Mitomycin + Hyaluronidase ($n = 56$)

Hyaluronidase splits hyaluronic acid. As a result, the intercellular substance is loosened and tissue transport is accelerated. In 1982 Baumgartner [7] noted a dramatic improvement of clinical symptoms in a patient with myeloma after paravenous injection of cytostatics and consecutive local treatment with hyaluronidase. This prompted a series of investigations designed to show whether or not hyaluronidase had any effects on the growth of neoplasms or the action of cytostatics [8–11]. Most of these investigations indicated a beneficial effect of hyaluronidase. In the light of these reports, it appeared logical to make use of this treatment concept in the prevention of recurrent bladder cancer and set up a randomized clinical trial.

Fifty-six patients who had undergone histologically verified radical TUR for bladder cancer were treated [12]. After randomization, 28 patients received mitomycin and the remaining 28 were given mitomycin + hyaluronidase 200 000 U. The treatment groups were statistically well comparable (Table 3). The distribution of stage and grade showed good correlation between the groups (Table 4). During the observation time, nine of the 28 patients (32.1%) receiving mitomycin alone developed recurrent tumors after periods of 6–24 months. Four of the regrowths had the same stage and grade as the primary tumor, while three were downstaged and two were upstaged in terms of malignancy rather than infiltration depth. Of these nine patients, four had primary tumors before their entry into the trial, while five had recurrent tumors. Of the 28 patients with additional hyaluronidase, two (7.1%) developed recurrences after 6 and 20 months; both were downstaged and downgraded. One of these patients had a primary tumor when entering the trial, the

Table 3. Randomized study: mitomycin vs mitomycin + hyaluronidase, patient characteristics

	Mitomycin $n = 28$	Mitomycin + hyaluronidase $n = 28$
Age in years (mean)	62.8	67.3
Males/females	17/11	18/10
Primary tumor	15	16
Recurrent tumor	13	12
Observation time in months (mean)	21.1	20.2

Table 4. Randomized study: mitomycin vs mitomycin + hyaluronidase. Stage and grade

	Mitomycin $n = 28$			Mitomycin + hyaluronidase $n = 28$		
	G1	G2	G3	G1	G2	G3
Ta	8	2	—	9	1	—
T1	7	7	—	5	8	—
T2	—	3	1	—	1	4

other had his second recurrence. Hyaluronidase thus significantly ($p < 0.05$) improved the well-known effect of mitomycin in preventing tumor regrowth.

In the group treated with mitomycin alone, five patients (17%) who altogether received 788 instillations developed side effects. These consisted in skin rashes and cystitis. Patients receiving additional hyaluronidase showed similar side effects at a rate of 14%.

The data presented establish a significant additive effect of hyaluronidase ($p < 0.05$) in the prevention of recurrent bladder tumors, but afford no definitive conclusions concerning such things as the optimal time to begin treatment, cycle interval, duration, dosage, and choice of cytostatic. With the treatment and follow-up schedule reported, however, it is clear that supplementary hyaluronidase enhanced the action of the cytostatic chosen. As hyaluronidase did not increase the rate of side effects, it appears to have a place as an adjuvant to cytostatic chemotherapy for further reducing the rate of recurrences in patients with bladder cancer. The possibility of reducing the hyaluronidase dose without any loss of protective effect, as well as the use of supplementary hyaluronidase in the systemic treatment of metastatic urothelial cancers, remains to be studied.

Conclusions

1. Mitomycin reduces the recurrence rate of bladder tumors after TUR significantly ($p < 0.01$), with a low rate of side effects.
2. The addition to hyaluronidase (200 000 U) further reduces the recurrence rate significantly ($p < 0.05$) without increasing the rate of side effects.

References

1. Huland H, Otto U (1983) Mitomycin instillation to prevent recurrence of superficial bladder carcinoma. Urology 9:84–86
2. Maier U, Kautzky W (1983) Intravesical mitomycin instillation therapy after transurethral resection of bladder tumor. In: Proceedings, 13th International Congress of Chemotherapy, Vienna, 28 Aug–2 Sept
3. Bauer HW (1984) Mitomycin C – Ergebnisse bei Harnblasentumoren. Tumordiagn Ther 5:1–34
4. Huland H, Brachmann W, Hubmann R, Kaufmann J, Knipper W, Lantzius-Beninga F, Klöppel G (1986) Rezidivprophylaxe oberflächlicher Harnblasenkarzinome. Ergebnisse einer multizentrischen Hamburger Studie. Verhandlungsberichte der Deutschen Giesellschaft für Urologie, Würzburg, 23–28 Sept
5. Maier U (1987) Erfahrungen mit Mitomycin C in der topischen Rezidivprophylaxe von Blasentumoren. Proceedings, 10th International Symposium, Ludwig-Boltzmann-Institut zur Erforschung der Infektionen und Geschwülste des Harntraktes, Vienna, 19–21 Feb 1987
6. Maier U, Holzner JH (1985) Stellenwert der Urotheldysplasien in makroskopisch normaler Schleimhaut bei Patienten mit Blasentumoren. Ergebnisse einer randomisierten Studie mit und ohne intravesicale Mitomycin C Rezidivprophylaxe. Onkologie 8:232–240
7. Baumgartner G (1987) Hyaluronidase in der Therapie maligner Erkrankungen. Wien Klin Wochenschrift [Suppl 174]
8. Baumgartner G, Baumgartner M, Alth G, Beck A, Hentschel E, Klaushofer E, Klein D, Neumann H, Stierer M (1985) Hyaluronidase as supplement to cytostatic chemotherapy. A pilot study. J Exp Clin Cancer Res 4:279–291
9. Baumgartner G, Horaczek A (1987) Hyaluronidase combined with cytostatic chemotherapy in glioblastomas. In: Sack H, Bamberg M (eds) Abstracts symposium on therapy of primary brain tumors, Essen, 26–28 March. Strahlenklinik des Westdeutschen Tumorzentrums, Essen, p 43
10. Baumgartner G, Horaczek A, Grunert P, Kitz K, Wunsch M (1987) Hyaluronidase als Zusatz zur zytostatischen Chemotherapie bei Glioblastomen. Onkologie 10:100–103.
11. Baumgartner G, Neumann H (1987) Die Hyaluronidase in der zytostatischen Therapie von HNO-Tumoren. Laryngol Rhinol Otol (Stuttg) 66:195–199
12. Maier U, Baumgartner G (1989) Metaphylactic effect of mitomycin C with and without hyaluronidase after transurethral resection of bladder cancer. Randomized trial. J Urol 141:528–530

How Effective Is Topical Interferon-α 2b for Preventing Recurrence of Superficial Bladder Cancer

R. Hasun, W. Höltl, W. Albrecht, and M. Marberger

Abteilung für Urologie, Krankenanstalt Rudolfstiftung, Juchgasse 25, 1030 Wien, Austria

Introduction

The close association between bladder cancer and modulation of the immune system has been known for many years. Reactivity to surface antigens, such as the ABO blood group antigens and the T group antigens, is often lost with the development of bladder cancer. These findings, together with the accessibility of the bladder mucosa to direct, topical treatment, have permitted and justified an immunotherapeutic approach to bladder cancer.

Experimental and clinical data showed the efficacy of interferon in preventing recurrent superficial bladder cancer [1, 2]. We introduced a randomized phase III trial of high-dose interferon vs low-dose interferon vs ethoglucid. Interferon-α2b was produced by the bacterium *E. coli*.

Material and Methods

A total of 42 patients with primary multifocal urothelial tumors pTa and pT1, G1–2, recurrent unifocal or multifocal urothelial tumors pTa and pT1, G1 or Tis were included. Other inclusion criteria were complete resection of the transitional cell carcinoma, Karnofsky status of more than 50%, and adequate renal, hepatic, and bone marrow function.

Every patient had complete removal of all superficial tumor tissue by transurethral resection (TUR) followed by multiple random biopsies at the end of TUR. None had undergone previous local chemotherapy or immunotherapy. Therapy started within 36 h after TUR. Thirty-two patients were available for response. Eight patients were lost due to noncompliance, and two died from unrelated causes.

The median follow-up period was 26 months overall, with 26.3 months in the low-dose group, 27 months in the high-dose group, and 21.9 months in the ethoglucid group.

R. Jakesz/H Rainer (Eds)
Progress in Regional Cancer Therapy

Results

The results were assessed in terms of the recurrence rate, which is the quotient of the number of recurrences and the patient months of follow-up multiplied by 100.

The overall median recurrence rate was 4.6. In the low-dose group the figure was 5.8, in the high-dose group, 3.7. In the ethoglucid group we found a recurrence rate of 4.5. In none of the three groups was any systemic toxicity observed. No local toxicity was found in either of the interferon groups. In the ethoglucid group three patients dropped out of the study because of severe chemocystitis.

Conclusion

Topical treatment of superficial bladder cancer with interferon-α is effective. In our study the best results were achieved in the high-dose interferon group. We found that intravesical interferon-α has no toxic side effects.

Further trials with higher numbers of patients should identify those patients who can benefit from topical interferon treatment and ascertain the optimal interferon concentrations and therapy intervals. Perhaps combination of interferon with another cytotoxic or immunomodulatory drug will improve its efficacy.

References

1. Torti FM et al. (1984) Superficial bladder cancer is responsive to Alpha-2b-Interferon administered intravesically. Proc ASCO:C-628
2. Borden EC et al. (1984) L Antiproliferative activities of interferons against human bladder carcinoma cell lines in vitro. J Urol 132:800

Neo-adjuvant Intra-arterial Chemotherapy for Treatment of Locally Advanced Bladder Cancer: Therapeutic Protocol and Preliminary Report

M. Bonsignori, F. Sturba, A. Paccapelo, R. Bencivenga, L. Zepponi, M. Polito, G. Muzzonigro, D. Minardi, L. Graziani, R. Montironi, and L. Possati

Oncology Department, Regional Hospital Torette, 60020 Ancona, Italy

Introduction

Locally advanced bladder cancer (T3ab-T4a NO-1-2 MO) is not always amenable to radical surgery, and the search for the best treatment continues. The 5-year survival rate is generally 12%–20% for T3 tumors [1, 2] and 5% for T4 tumors [3, 4]. New (preoperative) neo-adjuvant therapy protocols intends to produce better results in such bladder tumors have recently been described [5–8]. The biologic rationale for this kind of treatment is that the drugs achieve a very high concentration in the neoplasm, more than with systemic administration, and toxicity, in contrast is slight. Cisplatin + 4-epidoxorubicin has been shown to be one of the more active combinations [8, 9].

Patients and Methods

We are carrying out a nonrandomized pilot study to establish the efficacy of neo-adjuvant local intra-arterial chemotherapy in enabling radical surgery of T3ab-T4a NO-1-2 MO G1-2-2 bladder cancer. The patients are followed up to a new manifestation of the pathology.

The neo-adjuvant chemotherapy protocol is as follows:

Cisplatin (CDDP): 25 mg/day for 6 days, each dose diluted in 100 ml physiologic saline and infused using a pump over a period of 4 h bilaterally into the hypogastric arteries.

4-Epidoxorubicin (4-EPI): 25 mg/day for 6 days, dilution and infusion as for CDDP, administration commencing immediately after completion of CDDP infusion. Total dosage: 150 mg CDDP, 150 mg 4-EPI.

The chemotherapy is administered via two catheters with their tips in the hypogastric arteries downstream from the gluteal arteries, catheter access is via the percutaneous transfemoral route. If it is possible to catheterize only one of the hypogastric arteries, we advance the catheter to the cancer site in the bladder and reduce the total dose by one third.

Surgery is performed 3 weeks after the end of chemotherapy. The criteria for evaluation are:

R. Jakesz/H Rainer (Eds.)
Progress in Regional Cancer Therapy

1. Efficacy of neo-adjuvant chemotherapy
   - in vitro biologic assessment of mitotic index
   - histologic assessment after chemotherapy of change in grade, if any, and percentage necrosis of neoplastic tissue
   - clinical assessment during operation
2. Side effects of neo-adjuvant chemotherapy
   - systemic and local toxicity, assessed using the UICC criteria
   - local accidents of regional arterial access
3. Disease-free interval before local recurrences and distant metastases
4. Survival

We began the study in February 1986 and have, upto the time of writing, treated 12 patients with an average of 60 years (range 50–70): three patients with stage T3a, eight with stage T3b, and one with stage T4. It was possible to insert the catheters bilaterally in 10 cases; in the remaining two cases one catheter was placed as described above.

Preliminary Results

Seven patients had total cystectomy and the remaining five underwent partial cystectomy. All of them had a radical operation and we observed marked reduction of neoplastic volume, easy isolation from adjacent tissues, and minor bleeding. The histologic control showed substantial deep necrosis of the tumor mass (average 67.4%). The biologic assessment revealed in all cases either no in vitro growth or early depletion of cell populations.

Metastases. One patient (PT3b G2) treated with monolateral chemotherapy and subsequent total cystectomy had a pelvic recurrence 2 months after the treatment and died of renal failure and cardiac crisis. One patient (PT3b M2 G2) who was treated with chemotherapy for only 3 days because of skin necrosis and subsequently underwent cystectomy had a vaginal metastasis after 5 months. One patient (PT3a G1–2) had metastases after 18 months.

Survival. Eight patients are still alive after follow-up of 6–29 months; three of them received radical cystectomy, the other five partial cystectomy. Four patients have died: one after 9 months (PT3b G2), one after 4 months (PT3b N2 G2), one after 18 months (PT3a G1–2), one after 10 months. In the last case death was unconnected with the bladder cancer.

Toxicity and Local Side Effects. Only 1 patient discontinued the chemotherapy because of a severe local side effect (gluteal skin necrosis). Many patients had psychological problems (insomnia, erethism) related to staying in bed throughout the period of treatment. The systemic toxicity and local side effects were graded as follows: grade 1 = mild; grade 2 = moderate; grade 3 = severe; grade 4 = very severe.

Systemic Toxicity. Nausea and vomiting: grade 1 ($n = 5$); hematologic: grade 1 ($n = 1$), grade 2 ($n = 1$), grade 3 ($n = 1$): Renal: grade 2 ($n = 1$); cardiac: none; hepatic: grade 1 ($n = 3$); alopecia: grade 1 ($n = 7$).

Local Side Effects. Gluteal erythema: grade 1 ($n = 5$); gluteal perineal skin necrosis: grade 3 ($n = 1$); grade 4 ($n = 1$).

Conclusions

From our preliminary experience we can state the following:

—Locoregional neo-adjuvant chemotherapy reduces the tumor volume and leads to demarcation between cancer and adjacent tissues; this permits more radical surgery.
—Postoperative histologic evaluation reveals substantial deep necrosis of the tumor mass (average 67.4%).
—In vitro biologic assessment shows in all cases no growth or early depletion of cell populations.
—The treatment is generally well tolerated.
—The side effects and toxicity are so far moderate and always temporary. Only one patient discontinued the chemotherapy, because of a gluteal perineal skin necrosis and this patient recovered in 15 days.

References

1. Resnick MI, O'Connor VJJ (1973) Segmental resection for carcinoma of the bladder: review of 102 patients. J Urol 109:1007
2. Utz DC et al. (1973) A clinicopathologic evaluation of partial cystectomy for carcinoma of the urinary bladder. Cancer 32:10075
3. Miller LS (1977) Bladder cancer: superiority of preoperative irradiation and cystectomy in clinical stages B2 and C. Cancer 39:973
4. Goffinet DR, Schneider MJ et al. (1975) Bladder cancer: results of radiation therapy in 384 patients. Radiology 117:149
5. Grigoletto E et al. (1982) Intra-arterial cisplatinum in head and neck cancer. Preliminary results. Chemioterapia 1:204
6. Madajewicz S et al. (1981) Plasma, spinal fluid and organ distribution of cisplatinum (DDP) following intravenous (IV) and intracarotid (IC) infusion. Proc Am Assoc Cancer Res Am Soc Clin Oncol 22:176 (abstr 697)
7. Calvo D et al. (1980) Phase I–II trial of percutaneous intraarterial cis-diammine-dichloro platinum (II) for regional confined malignancy. Cancer 45:1278
8. Smith PH (1981) Chemotherapy of bladder cancer: a review. Cancer Treat Rep 65:165 [Suppl. 1]
9. Soloway MS, Ikard M, Ford K (1981) Cis-diamminodichloroplatinum (II) in locally advanced and metastatic urothelial cancer. Cancer 47:476

RADIOTHERAPY

Reconstructive Microsurgery and Radiotherapy in Advanced Tumors of the Head and Neck

H. Kärcher and K.-H. Kärcher

Abteilung für Kiefer- und Gesichtschirurgie, Universitäts-Zahn-Klinik,
Auenbruggerplatz 12, 8010 Graz, Austria

Introduction

The possibilities for reconstruction have increased substantially with the development of microsurgery. Microvascular free tissue transplantation is now an established procedure in head and neck surgery. Nearly every specific tissue defect can be repaired with appropriate donor tissue. Radiation therapy is very often combined with surgery of head and neck tumors. The different treatment modalities – pre- or postoperative irradiation – also influence the reconstructive procedures. Especially when a microvascular transfer is planned, the status of the recipient vessels is of utmost importance. Irradiated vessels show thickening of all parts of the vessel wall and fibrosis of the surrounding tissue. Therefore exact preoperative planning is necessary before any free flap transplantation. One has to distinguish between primary reconstruction and secondary reconstruction of the defect after tumor resection: in both cases the vessels can be irradiated beforehand but the situation is not the same.

The vessel damage after preoperative irradiation is, of course, not as bad as after combined surgery and postoperative irradiation. That means that secondary reconstructions after postoperative irradiation are among the most difficult reconstructive procedures of all: in particular, bone defects of the mandible require vital revascularized bone grafts because of the bad transplantation bed. The classical indication is still reconstruction of osteoradionecrosis of the mandible.

Primary reconstructions after composite resections of tumors of the head and neck have increased during the past 10 years and have brought changes in surgeon's attitudes. One must not remove only the tumor, because modern reconstructive techniques permit preservation of the quality of life to a certain degree independently of curative or palliative intent.

Previously, when no reconstruction was performed, the radiotherapist had to treat badly oxygenated tissues. The development of musculocutaneous, fasciocutaneous, or musculoperitoneal flaps and free jejunal grafts has transformed the treatment and the functional results [1, 4]. The most important single advance in the treatment of head and neck cancer is the fact that aggressive radiotherapy can now be given to a healthy, well-oxygenated area without danger to the transplanted tissue.

R. Jakesz/H Rainer (Eds)
Progress in Regional Cancer Therapy

Primary Reconstruction and Postoperative Radiotherapy

In eight cases of advanced tumors of the head and neck a composite resection was performed simultaneously with reconstruction of the defect using a "free flap" and postoperative irradiation.

The latissimus dorsi musculocutaneous flap was the flap of choice for defects of the tongue and the floor of the mouth (Fig. 1). But the latissimus dorsi was also used for external tumors of the face, because of its long vascular pedicle.

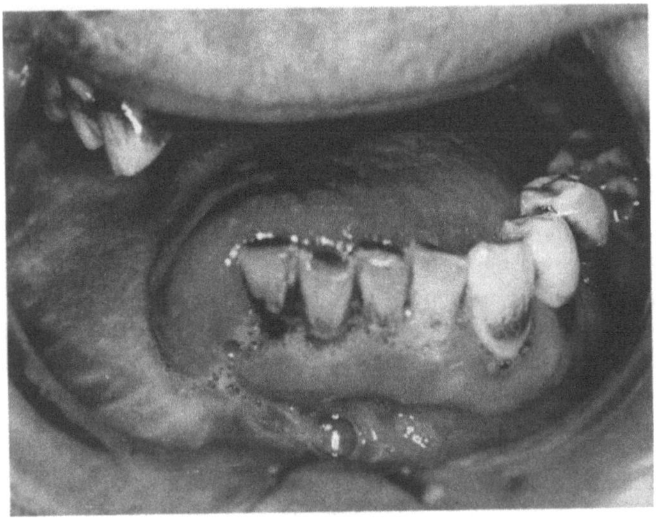

Fig. 1. Free latissimus dorsi flap after irradiation (70 Gy) of a T4 tongue cancer

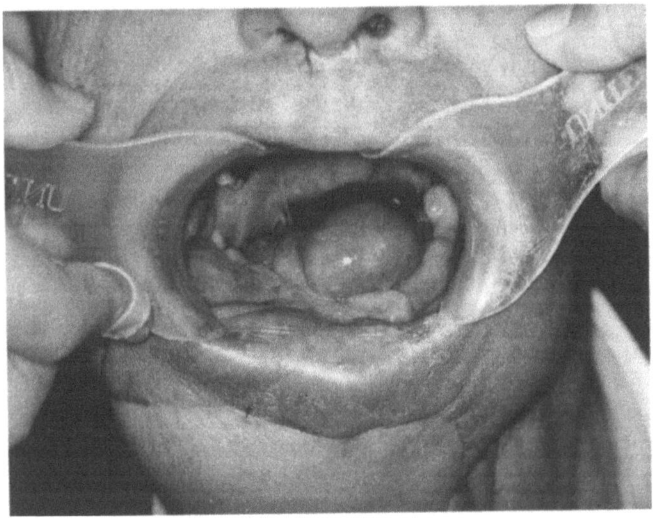

Fig. 2. Free peritoneal groin flap and osteomusculocutaneous groin flap after irradiation (60 Gy) of a T4 cancer of the floor of the mouth

In carcinomas of the floor of the mouth we also used the myoperitoneal groin flap [3]. This flap can be combined with an osteomusculocutaneous groin flap [5] on one pedicle (Fig. 2).

Secondary Reconstruction After Surgery and Radiotherapy

Especially bone defects have to be reconstructed after ablative surgery. We favored the vascularized iliac bone graft, because of its long pedicle and the large bone (Fig. 3). If possible we performed the anastomoses at the opposite side from the neck dissection, because of the lesser degree of vessel damage.

In cases of osteoradionecrosis the defects were successfully reconstructed (Figs. 4, 5). The bone grafts were revascularized and stayed viable as shown by technetium scans during the first week after operation. Large bone defects after composite resection and radiotherapy need vital bone reconstruction because of the poor

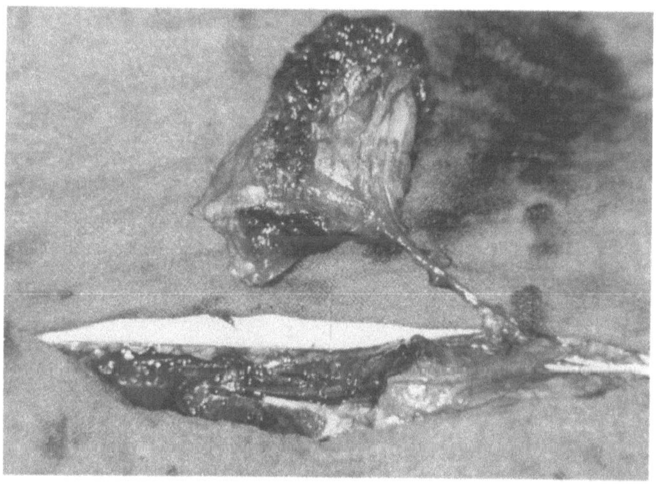

Fig. 3. Pedicled iliac bone graft

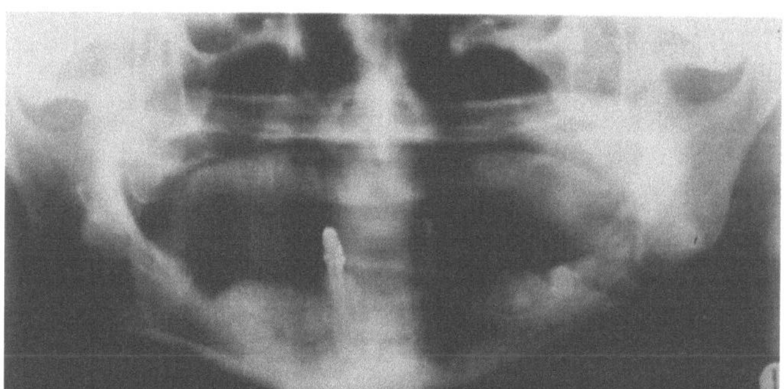

Fig. 4. Osteoradionecrosis of the mandible

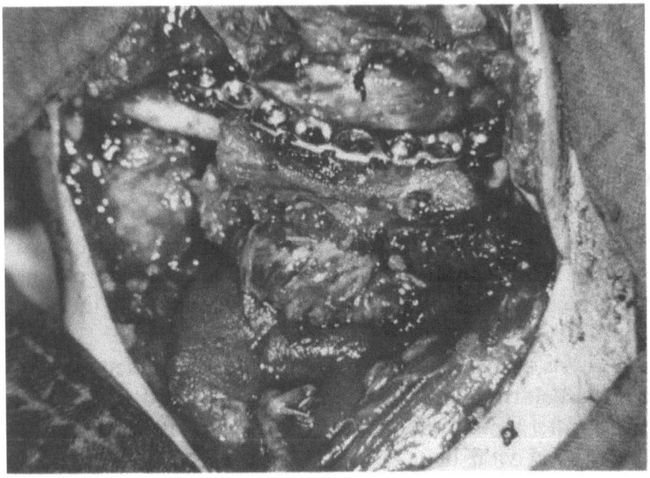

Fig. 5. Microvascular iliac bone reconstruction

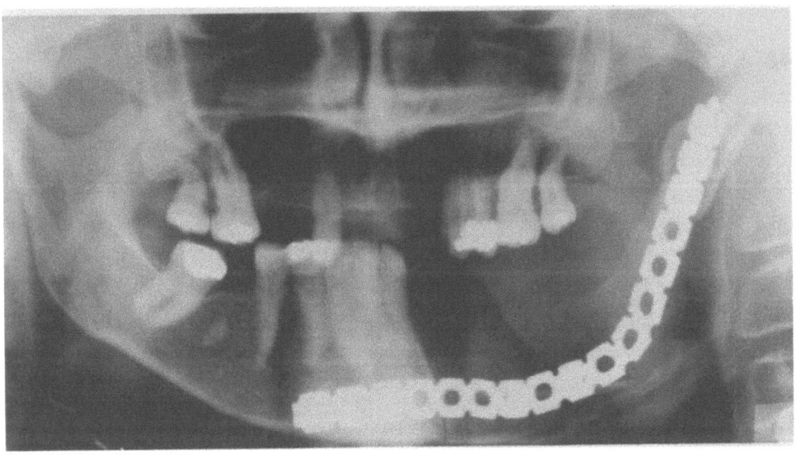

Fig. 6. Successful secondary bone reconstruction of the mandible with a revascularized iliac bone graft

transplantation bed. Even under the worst conditions these revascularized transplants succeeded (Fig. 6).

In one case an iliac bone flap was lost due to venous thrombosis, because the recipient vessels were of poor quality and a vein graft was used for venous drainage of the flap.

Discussion

Composite defects after ablative surgery of carcinomas of the head and neck can be reconstructed by means of free vascularized tissue transfer. A good functional result and a well-vascularized target region for postoperative radiotherapy can be achieved with free microvascular flaps. It is possible to reconstruct every different tissue defect using specific donor sites, such as the iliac bone for the mandible or the jejunum or peritoneum for oropharyngeal defects. In no case was the primary microvascular reconstruction adversely affected by postoperative irradiation. Animal experiments afforded similarly good results [2].

Quite different problems arise in secondary reconstructions in irradiated areas, where the failure rate is certainly higher than in primary reconstructions. This is due not so much to radiofibrosis as to the surgical difficulty in finding recipient vessels. Therefore one should perform the anastomosis under the best tissue conditions possible, even if vein grafts are necessary. Preoperative irradiation of up to 30 Gy does no harm to the recipient vessels. From the point of view of reconstruction, therefore, preoperative irradiation up to 30 Gy and postoperative dose completion up to 70 Gy is to be recommended. The reaction of transplanted tissue is limited and the functional results remain acceptable.

References

1. Daniel RK, Taylor GI (1973) Distant transfer of an island flap by microvascular anastomoses. Plast Reconstr Surg 52:111
2. Kärcher H, Kleinert R (1986) The regeneration in vascularized and free nerve grafts – a comparative study in rats. J Maxillofac Surg 14:341
3. Kärcher H, Hellbom B, Radner H (1989) The osteomusculocutaneous musculoperitoneal groin flap in head and neck reconstruction. J Reconstr Microsurg 5(1):31–35
4. McCraw JB, Dibell DG, Carraway JH (1977) Clinical definition of independent myocutaneous vascular territories. Plast Reconstr Surg 60:341
5. Taylor GI, Townsend P, Corlett R (1979) Superiority of the deep circumflex iliac vessels as the supply for free groin flaps. Clinical work. Plast Reconstr Surg 64:745

Palliation of Nonresectable Esophageal Cancer by Iridium-192 Intraluminal Afterloading

P. Kohek, B. Pakisch, F.-M. Smolle-Jüttner, P. Rehak, G. Stückelschweiger, and G. Friehs

Department für Thoraxchirurgie, Universitäts-Klinik für Chirurgie, Auenbruggerplatz 15, 8036 Graz, Austria

Introduction

Patients with malignant esophageal obstructions pose a difficult therapeutic problem. Advanced stage of the disease, reduced nutritional status caused by mechanical irradiation of the esophagus, and poor cardiopulmonary condition rule out major therapeutic interventions (resection, bypass) in most cases. A variety of palliative measures are in use to eliminate dysphagia and improve the quality of life (bouginage, endoprosthesis, gastrostomy, high-dose teletherapy, chemotherapy, laser, and brachytherapy) [1, 2, 3, 5, 10, 17].

In recent years fiberendoscopic Nd-Yag laser debulking of malignant obstructions of the esophagus has been shown to be of value. This method frequently provides prompt and effective symptomatic improvement, but rapid regrowth necessitates frequent endoscopic procedures with decreased efficacy over time [2]. Palliation by external irradiation alone is limited by the presence of radiosensitive structures (mediastinum, spine). Periesophageal tumor masses often show insufficient response or quick relapse, resulting in recurrence of esophageal stenosis [5, 10].

High-dose-rate (HDR) irridium-192 intraluminal afterloading therapy has shown favorable results in stenoses of the esophagus. The only limitation of this method might be the narrow range of the effective dose in certain cases [10, 11, 16, 18].

Specifically to overcome these problems, a combined modality treatment (CMT) consisting of combined bouginage-laser treatment (CBLT), HDR intraluminal ^{192}Ir afterloading, and high-voltage external irradiation was developed in order to prolong the palliative effect (oral intake of all kinds of properly chewed food).

Patients and Methods

CBLT was performed for initial recanalization in patients with high-grade stenoses (St3, St4). After dilation using the Gilliard-Savary Dilator Set (Wilson Cook Medical Inc., Winston-Salem, USA), retrograde Nd-Yag laser coagulation (Medilas, MBB AT, Munich, FRG) was performed until a lumen permitting the insertion of

R. Jakesz/H. Rainer (Eds.)
Progress in Regional Cancer Therapy

the afterloading applicator was achieved [11]. For intraluminal brachytherapy (afterloading) we used remote HDR ^{192}Ir afterloading systems (Selectron and Micro-Selectron, Nucleotron Inc., Leersum, The Netherlands). Both are HDR devices with ^{192}Ir sources. The activity of the sources ranges between 2 and 5 Ci for the Selectron and between 5 and 10 Ci for the Micro-Selectron.

Afterloading

After pretherapeutic computed tomography and endoscopic determination of the proximal and distal tumor margins, a special applicator (PVC catheters: Selectron 8 mm outer diameter, Micro-Selectron 2 and 5 mm outer diameter) is passed over a previously inserted guide wire or directly through the channel of the fiberendoscope to the estimated position of the tumor in the esophagus. For final radiological localization an inner tube with metal marker pellets (Selectron) or a metal wire (Micro-Selectron) as a radiopaque marker was inserted into the applicator. Those nonradioactive markers ("dummy sources") permit very accurate positioning of the device under X-ray control. After definitive positioning of the applicator, the dummy was replaced by a flexible tubing system connected to a radiation "safe". CBLT and afterloading were performed under anticholinergic/sedative premedication and topical anesthesia.

During afterloading the staff had to leave the room and the patients were monitored via an intercom system. The transfer of the iridium sources down a flexible tubing system into their precalculated position inside the applicator tube was controlled by a microprocessor. The advantage of HDR ^{192}Ir brachytherapy is the short application time of the high-dose irradiation to the region of interest. The duration of intraluminal irradiation varied, depending on the activity of the sources and the extent of the tumor, between 10 and 25 min with the Selectron and between 2 and 5 min with the Micro-Selectron. A dose of 6 Gy was administered to the point of reference within a radius of 10 mm from the surface of the source. If any problems occurred during afterloading, the procedure could be interrupted at any time by automatic withdrawal of the sources within 5 s. Each patient underwent two afterloading sessions within a period of 1 week.

External Irradiation

In order to prolong the palliative effect, high-voltage external teletherapy was administered (25 MeV Linear Accelerator, General Electric Inc., Milwoukee, USA). The total dose ranged between 50 and 66 Gy (2 Gy per day, 5 times a week)

Patients

Since May 1987, 28 patients (23 males, 5 females; age 42–84 years, mean 66.25 years) with malignant esophageal obstruction have undergone HDR ^{192}Ir intraluminal afterloading therapy. Functional (8/28) or anatomical (20/28) inoperability was present in all cases (Table 1). High clinical (UICC) tumor stage, severe dysphagia, or

Table 1. Esophageal carcinoma: histology, grading and site

Site		Histology	
		Squamous cell carcinoma ($n = 22$)	Adenocarcinoma ($n = 6$)
Cervical	4	G1 3	G1 1
Upper third	9	G2 7	G2 2
Middle third	5	G3 8	G3 2
Distal third	10	Gx 4	Gx 1

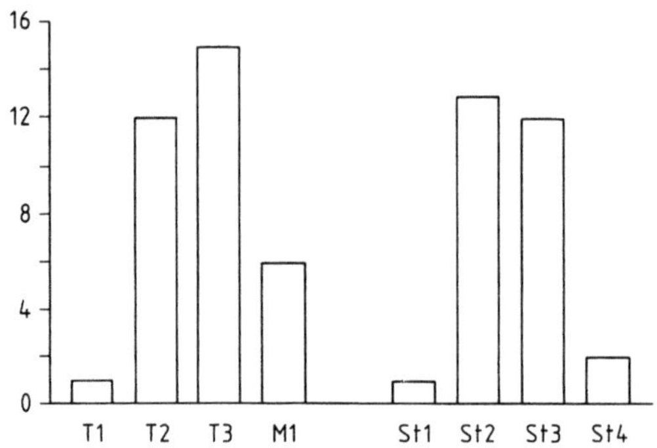

Fig. 1. Clinical tumor stage (UICC) and initial degree of stenosis. *St1*, 50% stenosis; *St2*, passable for endoscope (9.5 mm); *St3*, passable for guidewire (0.6 mm); *St4*, total stenosis

aphagia were documented in a high proportion of these patients (Fig. 1). In 14 cases CBLT was necessary to enable insertion of the afterloading tube into the esophagus straddling the tumor.

Results

Fourteen of the 28 patients (50%) were able to complete the CMT. A marked improvement of dysphagia was documented in this group. The palliative effect lasted for between 3 and 18 months (mean 285 days) (Table 2). In five patients external irradiation was limited (18–36 Gy) for functional reasons. Four of this group died within 1–5 months after onset of therapy. At the time of writing, the fifth patient is alive with a follow-up of 9 months and has moderate dysphagia. In nine patients (32.14%) intraluminal afterloading was the sole therapy, because of distant metastasis (6), death during therapy (1), or refusal of further therapy (2). Five of these nine patients showed progression of the disease and died within 1–3 months. One of the nine is still alive with local expansion of the tumor.

In 16 of the 28 patients (57.14%) oral nutrition was possible until their death or up to the time of writing. The mean duration of the palliative effect was 170 days (Table 3). The mean survival time after 18 months follow-up is 205.5 days (Fig. 2). Seventeen patients are still alive. The only serious therapy-related complication was a fatal esophagotracheal fistula in one case.

Table 2. Dysphagia score before and after CMT

Before CMT (n = 14)		After CMT (n = 14)	
D0	—	D0	5
D1	3	D1	5
D2	5	D2	3
D3	5	D3	1
D4	1	D4	—

D0, none; D1, minimal; D2, moderate; D3, severe; D4, aphagia.

Table 3. Dysphagia score before and after therapy (all patients)

Before (n = 28)		After (n = 23[a])	
D0	—	D0	6
D1	4	D1	8
D2	6	D2	7
D3	14	D3	2
D4	4	D4	—

D0, none; D1, minimal; D2, moderate; D3, severe; D4, aphagia.
[a]Two patients were lost to follow-up, three patients died during therapy.

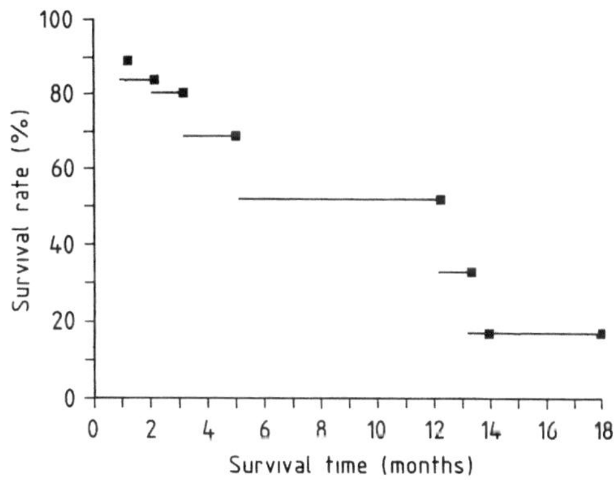

Fig. 2. The survival rate after 18 months is 20% ($n = 28$)

Discussion

Compared to other methods, CMT seems to have a synergistic effect on the duration of the palliation. Though bouginage is a simple, fast, and safe method of relieving obstruction, the duration of the palliative effect is short (3–45 days) [2]. CBLT alone achieves palliation lasting between 1 and 7 weeks and offers quick reopening of tumor stenoses. Rapid regrowth necessitates frequent endoscopic procedures with decreased efficacy over time [11, 14, 18]. The long-term results of endoprosthesis (mean 4.9 months) and gastrostomy (mean 6.3 months) were better than those of CBL in our patients, but the incidence of fatal complications was high (Fig. 3) [4, 16, 19].

The combined modality treatment (CMT) consisting of CBLT afterloading and high-voltage external teletherapy seems to be valid as a first-stage palliation of nonresectable esophageal cancer. To what extent long-term remission could be achieved by means of this treatment schedule remains to be ascertained.

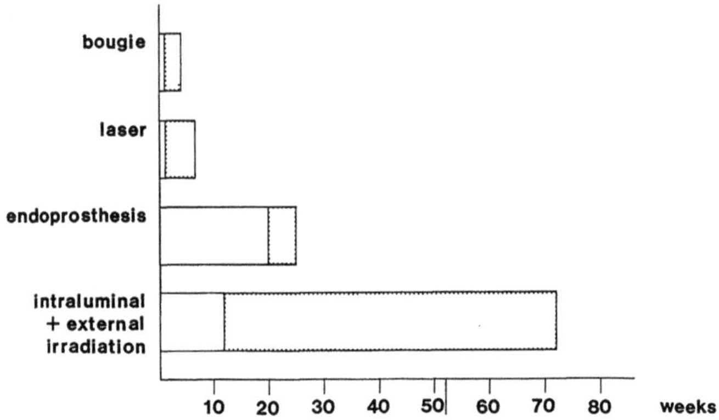

Fig. 3. Duration of palliation achieved by various methods in a total of 184 patients from 1982 to 1988. *Stippled area*, range of palliative effect

Summary

Since May 1987, 28 patients with nonresectable malignant esophageal stenoses have been treated by combined bouginage-laser treatment, ^{192}Ir afterloading and high-voltage external irradiation (combined modality treatment, CMT). Twenty-two squamous cell carcinomas and six adenocarcinomas of the esophagus were histologically verified. High clinical tumor stages and functional or anatomical inoperability were present in all cases. After CMT the mean duration of satisfactory palliative effect (oral intake of all kinds of properly chewed food) was 170 days, median survival time was 205.5 days, and the survival rate after 18 months is 17.6%.

References

1. Advani SH, Saikia TK, Swarood S, Ramakrishnan G, Nair CN, Dinshaw KA, Sharma S, Vyas JJ (1985) Chemotherapy in esophageal cancer. Cancer 56:1502–1506
2. Aste H, Munzzi F, Martines H, Pugliese V (1985) Esophageal dilation in malignant dysphagia. Cancer 56:2713–2715
3. Beatty JD, De Boer G, Ridder WD (1979) Carcinoma of the esophagus. Pretreatment, assessment, correlation of radiation treatment parameters with survival, and identification and management of radiation treatment failure. Cancer 43:2254–2267
4. Boyce EHW (1982) Medical management of esophageal obstruction and esophageal pulmonary fistula. Cancer 50:2597–2600
5. Caspers RJL, Welvaart K, Verkers RJ, Hermans J, Leer JWH (1988) the effect of radiotherapy on dysphagia and survival in patients with esophageal cancer. Radiother Oncol 12:15–23
6. Chavy AL, Rougier M, Pie de Loup C, Kac J, Laplanche AC, Elias DM, Ducreux MP, Zummer-Rubinstein K, Zimmermann PA, Charbit MA, Crespon BM (1986) Esophageal prothesis for neoplastic stenosis. A prognostic study of 77 cases. Cancer 57:1426–1431
7. Fischer SA, Brady LW (1987) Carcinoma of the esophagus. In: Perez CA, Brady LW (eds) Principles and practice of radiation oncology. Lippincott, Philadelphia
8. Hishikawa J (1983) Radiation treatment of esophageal carcinoma using a high-dose-rate remote afterloader. Radiat Med 1:237–244

9. Hishikawa J, Kamikonya N, Tanaka S, Miura T (1987) Radiation of esophageal carcinoma. Role of high-dose-rate intracavitary irradiation. Radiother Oncol 9:13–20
10. Jobson JJ, van Andel JG, Eijkenboom WMH, van Houten H, Müd HJ, Obertop H, van Pütten WLJ (1986) Carcinoma of the esophagus: treatment results. Radiother Oncol 5:101–108
11. Jüttner FM, Kohek P, Pinter H, Friehs G (1988) Palliation of esophageal carcinoma in cardiopulmonary high-risk patients. In: Siewert JR, Hölscher AH (eds). Diseases of the esophagus. Springer, Berlin Heidelberg New York, pp 722–724
12. Karlin DA, Fischer RS, Krevsky B (1987) Prolonged survival and effective palliation in patients with squamous cell carcinoma of the esophagus following endoscopic laser therapy. Cancer 59:1969–1972
13. Kies MS, Rosen ST, Tsang TK, Shetty R, Schneider PA, Wallemark CB, Shileds TW (1987) Cisplatin and 5-fluorouracil in the primary management of squamous esophageal cancer. Cancer 60:2156–2160
14. Kutzner J (1986) Strahlentherapie des Oesophagus-Carcinoms. Strah-lentherapie 1:13–16
15. Mathus-Vliegen EMH, Tytgat GNJ (1986) Laser photocoagulation in the palliative treatment of upper digestive tract tumors. Cancer 57:396–399
16. Ries G, Bader M, Hagenmüller F, Kneschaurek P, Dittler HJ (1988) Das High-Dose-Rate Iridium-192-Afterloading-Verfahren in der Behandlung inoperabler Tumoren des oberen Digestivtraktes. In: Hammer J, Kärcher KH (eds) Fortschritte in der interstitiellen und intracavitären Strahlentherapie. Zucker-schwerdt, pp 60–66
17. Rosenberg JC, Lichter AS, Roth JA, Kelsen DP (1985) Cancer of the esophagus. In: de Vita VT, Hellmannen S, Rosenberg SA (eds) Principles and practice of radiation oncology, 2nd edn. Lippincott, Philadelphia, pp 621–657
18. Rowland CG (1984) Treatment of carcinoma of the esophagus with a new Selectron applicator. In: Mould RF (ed) Brachytherapy. Proceedings of 3rd International Selectron Users Meeting, Innsbruck, pp 248–250. R.F. Mould, Westminster Hospital, London
19. Valbuena J (1984) Endoscopic palliative treatment of esophageal and cardial cancer: a new antireflux prosthesis. A study of 40 cases. Cancer 53:993–998
20. Van Andel TG, Dees J, Eijkenboom WMM, van Houten H, Jobsen JJ, Mud HJ, Obertop H, van Putten WLJ, Von Blanvenstein M, Leftinck-Schattenkerk M, de Jong PC, Knegt P, Splinter TAW, Verweis I (1986) Therapy of esophageal carcinoma. Acta Radiol Oncol 25:115–120

Interstitial Radiotherapy with Iridium 192 in the Treatment of Early Breast Cancer

G. Reiner, W. Seitz, A.P. Schmid, R. Jakesz, R. Kolb, M. Sperlich, A. Reiner and J. Spona

1. Chirurgische Universitätsklinik, Alser Straße 4, 1090 Wien, Austria

Introduction

Reports on conservative surgery of small breast carcinoma have accumulated over recent years, and the results seem to be very promising [4, 9, 12–14]. The necessity of postoperative radiation therapy after conservative breast surgery was clearly demonstrated by the 5-year results of the NSABP trial B06 [7] and earlier by the Milan group [17] and by Hayward [8] and Atkins et al. [1]. B. Fisher et al. [7] have reported a local recurrence rate of 7.7% after segmental mastectomy and axillary dissection followed by irradiation of the breast vs 30% without radiotherapy. The aim of our study was to further reduce the local recurrence rate by adding interstitial radiotherapy with iridium-192 implants at the site of the primary lesion to the percutaneous irradiation of the breast.

Material and Methods

The study was initiated in March 1983 at the First Department of Surgery and the Department of Radiotherapy of the University of Vienna. So far, 165 consecutive patients with operable breast cancer (T1–2 up to 4 cm diameter, N0–1) have entered the trial. The criteria for exclusion were tumor diameter of more than 4 cm, central tumor location, clinical or mammographic evidence of multicentricity, and involvement of more than seven axillary lymph nodes. Of the 165 patients, 156 had invasive breast cancer, six had microinvasive tumors, and three had ductal carcinoma in situ. A total of 113 patients were microscopically free of tumor spread to the axillary lymph nodes; 86 of those had tumors staged as T1, 27 staged as T2. Forty-seven patients had metastatic spread to the axillary nodes, with a T1 tumor in 28 cases and a T2 tumor in 19 cases. Five patients did not undergo axillary nodal dissection. Histologic tumor grading could be performed in 127 cases according to Bloom and Richardson [2]. Thirty-two patients had G1 tumors, 57 tumors were G2, and 38 tumors were undifferentiated (G3). In all but 33 cases estrogen and progesterone receptor content was determined by the dextran-coated charcoal method [15]. Some 55% were estrogen receptor positive and 40% were progesterone

R. Jakesz/H Rainer (Eds)
Progress in Regional Cancer Therapy

receptor positive. The patients' age ranged from 31 to 79 years with a mean of 55 years. Fifty-three patients were premenopausal and 112 postmenopausal.

Surgical Procedure

Breast conservation was achieved by performing 148 quadrantectomies and 17 tumorectomies, all margins being histologically free of tumor. Axillary lymph node dissection was obligatory and done either en bloc or through a separate incision. It extended up to the apex of the axilla, leaving the minor pectoral muscle intact.

Whenever the diagnosis of carcinoma was impossible on frozen section, axillary dissection was performed as a second step after definitive diagnosis based on the paraffin-embedded material. Five patients refused this second operation.

Radiation Therapy

Irradiation of the breast was an integral part of the treatment. A total dose of 45–50 Gy (1.8 Gy daily) was delivered percutaneously to the operated breast by a 6-MeV Linac apparatus. In addition, the area of the primary breast lesion itself was boosted with 15–25 Gy given interstitially by a ^{192}Ir implant, when two-thirds of the percutaneous dose had been delivered. 139 patients received the ^{192}Ir implant via a manual afterloading system as a low dose rate procedure lasting approximately 30 h. Since March 1987, 26 patients have had the ^{192}Ir administered using an automated afterloading system as a high dose rate procedure, delivering 10–15 Gy interstitially during a 10 to 20-min period only. In these cases percutaneous irradiation of the breast required 50 Gy.

Adjuvant Treatment

Postoperative adjuvant treatment was given to 73 patients. They were mostly high-risk cases with positive axillary lymph nodes, estrogen receptor-negative tumors, progesterone receptor-negative tumors, or G3 tumors. Thirty-eight patients entered studies on adjuvant treatment and were randomized into various treatment regimens (Table 1).

Thirty-six patients received chemotherapy (one cycle AV-CMF or six cycles CMF). AV-CMF was administered prior to radiation therapy. When six cycles of CMF was the treatment of choice, two cycles were given before and four after radiotherapy. Thirty-five patients received 20–30 mg tamoxifen daily for at least 2 years, and two patients had chemohormonotherapy with one cycle AV-CMF + 30 mg tamoxifen daily.

Statistical Methods

The relevant data of all patients were recorded and stored in an automated data system continuously updated according to the information drawn from follow-up

Table 1. Adjuvant treatment and prognostic factors in 165 patients with conservative surgery of breast cancer

	n	No adjuvant treatment	Adjuvant chemo-therapy	Adjuvant hormono-therapy	Adjuvant chemohormono-therapy
T1	118	74 (9)	22 (12)	20 (4)	2 (2)
T2	47	18 (1)	14 (6)	15 (4)	0
N0	113	77 (8)	15 (9)	21	0
N+	47	12 (2)	21 (9)	12 (8)	2 (2)
Nx	5	3	0	2	0
G1	32	18	4 (2)	10 (2)	0
G2	57	28 (1)	13 (6)	15 (5)	1 (1)
G3	38	21 (5)	13 (7)	4	0
Gx	38	25 (4)	6 (3)	6 (1)	1 (1)
ER−	60	32 (7)	23 (17)	4	1 (1)
ER+	72	35 (2)	8	29 (8)	0
ERx	33	25 (1)	5 (1)	2	1 (1)
PgR−	80	40 (9)	28 (17)	12 (1)	0
PgR+	52	25 (1)	4	22 (7)	1 (1)
PgRx	33	27	4 (1)	1	1 (1)

Data in parentheses are numbers of randomized patients.

examination. Life table analysis was performed by the actuarial Kaplan–Meier method [11] using the programs of the BMDP statistics package.

Results

The median follow-up period in our study is 2.5 years. We observed recurrence of disease in 16 patients (10%). One of these patients presented with axillary recurrence alone. Three patients had a local recurrence in the operated breast with simultaneous generalization. Twelve patients developed distant metastases without any sign of locoregional recurrence. Eight patients died from metastatic disease (seven with distant metastases only, one with additional local recurrence). Two patients died free of recurrence for reasons unrelated to cancer. Two other patients died with unknown status of disease.

The overall survival of all patients after 2.5 years of follow-up was 97% (Fig. 1). The influence of prognostic factors such as lymph node involvement, tumor differentiation, steroid hormone receptor status and tumor diameter on overall survival was separately analyzed and proved to be insignificant for each subgroup. Recurrence of disease occurred more frequently in patients with T2 tumors, in receptor-negative patients, and in patients with positive axillary lymph nodes or undifferentiated tumors (Table 2).

Overall, the interstitial radiotherapy with ^{192}Ir was well tolerated by the patients and the cosmetic result was judged good to excellent in 84%. The main side effects of

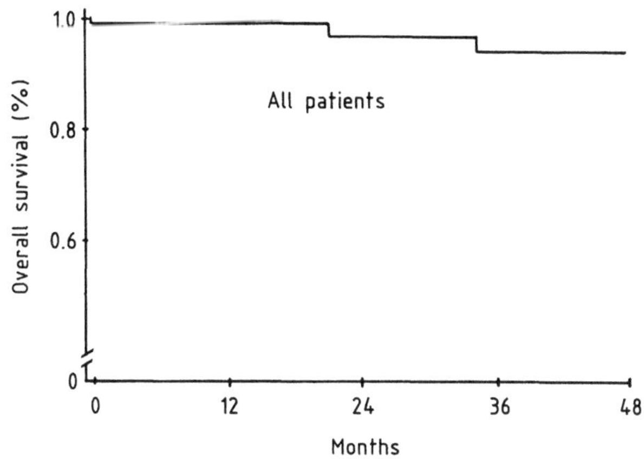

Fig. 1. Overall survival of 165 patients after conservative surgery of breast cancer and interstitial irradiation with Iridium-192. Median follow-up 2.5 years

Table 2. Recurrences and prognostic factors after 2.5 years of follow-up in 165 patients with conservative surgery of breast cancer and interstitial irradiation with ^{192}Ir

	n	Local recurrence	Distant metastases	Local and distant recurrence	Total	(%)
T1	118	1	7	1	9	(8)
T2	47	0	5	2	7	(15)
N0	113	1	3	3	7	(6)
N+	47	0	8	0	8	(17)
Nx	5	0	1	0	1	
G1	32	0	2	0	2	(6)
G2	57	0	2	2	4	(7)
G3	38	0	4	1	5	(13)
Gx	38	1	4	0	5	(13)
ER −	60	1	6	2	9	(15)
ER +	72	0	3	1	4	(6)
ERx	33	0	3	0	3	(9)
PgR −	80	0	9	3	12	(15)
PgR +	52	0	1	0	1	(2)
PgRx	33	1	2	0	3	(9)

ER, estrogen receptor; PgR, progesterone receptor.

the procedure were edema of the irradiated breast due to damage to skin and lymphatics, and parenchymal induration. 20 patients developed tumors in the treated breast where recurrence could not be ruled out. These tumors thus had to be removed, but all turned out to be benign lesions on histologic examination (necrosis of fatty tissue, inflammatory granulomas, etc.).

Discussion

The addition of interstitial irradiation with ^{192}Ir to the basic external radiation therapy of breast tissue after conservative surgery for primary breast cancer has yielded, after 2.5 years of follow-up, a slightly lower rate of local treatment failure than percutaneous irradiation alone [7]. So far, we have observed local recurrences in 2.4% of patients. Similar results were obtained by other groups with comparable treatment regimens [3, 5, 6, 16] and also, for instance, by boosting the tumor bed with 10–15 Gy using a ^{60}Co unit.

Our results clearly show the significant influence of the prognostic factors on the incidence of early recurrence of disease. Patients with axillary lymph node involvement or with large undifferentiated, or steroid hormone receptor-negative tumors suffered more frequently from recurrent disease than others. Also, analysis of the disease-free survival shows that lymph node involvement and lack of steroid receptors are significant predictors of early recurrence, whereas tumor diameter and histologic tumor grading did not reach significance in this regard.

Surprisingly, none of the patients with local recurrence had had positive axillary nodes at the time of initial operation. The one patient with axillary recurrence alone had obviously had an incomplete initial axillary dissection.

Overall survival was not significantly influenced by the prognostic factors defined earlier. This finding might be explained by the fact that most patients at high risk for early recurrence were subjected to adjuvant cytotoxic chemotherapy or treatment with tamoxifen. On the other hand, overall survival of patients receiving adjuvant therapy was not significantly different from that of patients without systemic treatment. These results underline the effect of adjuvant treatment on the prognosis of high-risk patients that we could show in a previous study [10], and suggest that adjuvant treatment possibly reduces the rate of local recurrence.

Since our follow-up period of 2.5 years is still short compared to those in other published studies, our good results have to be considered as preliminary. Interstitial irradiation with ^{192}Ir may possibly prove simply to prolong the disease-free interval with no impact on overall survival.

References

1. Atkins H, Hayward JL, Klugman DJ et al. (1972) Treatment of early breast cancer: a report after ten years of clinical trial. Br Med J 2:423–429
2. Bloom HJG, Richardson WW (1957) Histological grading and prognosis in breast cancer. Br J Cancer 11:359–377
3. Bulman AS, Zeitman A, Phillips RH, Ellis H (1987) Interim results of treatment of breast cancer with breast conservation for all patients. Surgery 101:395–399
4. Calle R, Pilleron JP, Schlienger P, Vilcoq JR (1978) Conservative management of operable breast cancer: ten years experience at the Foundation Curie. Cancer 42: 2045–2053
5. Calle R, Vilcoq JR, Zafrani B, Vielh P, Fourquet A (1986) Local control and survival of breast cancer treated by limited surgery followed by irradiation. Int J Radiat Oncol Biol Phys 12:873–878
6. Clark RM, Wilkinson RH, Mahoney LJ, Reid JG, MacDonald WD (1982) Breast cancer: a 21 year experience with conservative surgery and radiation. Int J Radiat Oncol Biol Phys 8:967–975

Intracavitary High-Dose-Rate Afterloading Irradiation in the Treatment of Cancer of the Esophagus and Gastroesophageal Junction

K. Koch, J. Frohwein, W. Bergemann, F. Gramlich, P. Semler, and M. Zschiederich

Abteilung für Strahlentherapie, Universitätsklinikum Rudolf Virchow, Augustenburger Platz 1, 1000 Berlin, FRG

Esophageal cancer often has troublesome consequences such as stenosis, dysphagia, weight loss, and pain. As a result, patients are often in poor general condition. Although the prognosis remains poor, therapy with immediate effect is needed. For this reason we developed a new combination technique consisting of laser therapy, endoluminal afterloading, and external irradiation.

Patients with a narrow stenosis or a larger endoluminal tumor first underwent laser therapy. The Nd:YAG laser not only coagulates, but can also vaporize tissue when applied for a longer time. The immediate effect of laser vaporization enlarges the esophagus at once, but satisfactory long-term results are obtained only in exceptional cases.

Afterloading irradiation reaches not only the tumor in the lumen but also the esophageal wall and nearby surroundings. Long stenoses are easier to treat by this means. Endoluminal irradiation, a modern afterloading technique, is a two-step procedure. First, an applicator is inserted in the esophagus. After the hospital staff have left the room, the source is removed from its radiation-proof container and placed in the applicator by remote control. This procedure avoids the exposure of hospital personnel while allowing the use of a highly radioactive source (iridium-192, maximum activity 740 GBq) for short exposure periods. The rapid fall-off in radiation dose (Fig. 1) permits the use of high single doses. The dose of 15 Gy for nearly all of our endoluminal applications is calculated at a distance of 5 mm from the axis of the source. More than half the patients recieved 3–4 applications at 2-week intervals.

Because of tumor growth and lymph node metastases and endo-esophageal treatment alone therapy is not sufficient. Adequate combination therapy must include external irradiation. The characteristic isodose curves of internal and external irradiation allow very high doses in combination. Thus, we had tumor doses up to 80–100 Gy with doses of 40–60 Gy at the lymph nodes while protecting the parenchyma of the lung. The internal and external therapy were carried out simultaneously.

A total of 139 patients with esophageal and cardiac cancer were evaluated. Of the 96 male and 43 female subjects with a mean age of 68 years (range 37–89 years), 12 had carcinoma in the upper third of the esophagus, 47 in the middle third, 42 in the lower third, and 38 in the cardia. Some 70% had squamous cell carcinoma, 30%

R. Jakesz/H. Rainer (Eds.)
Progress in Regional Cancer Therapy

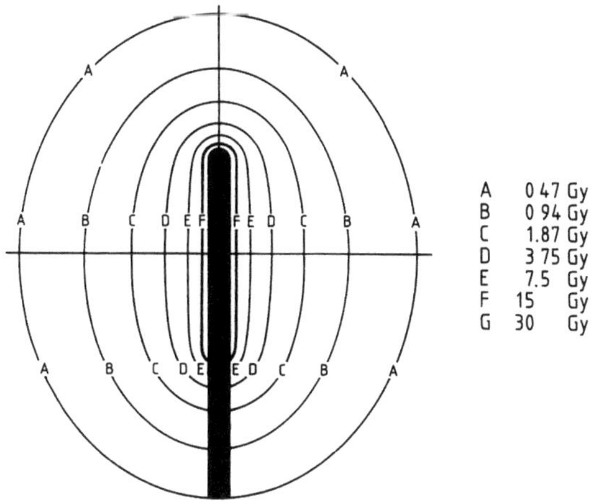

Fig. 1. Isodose curves for ^{192}Ir afterloading irradiation. Activity 740 GBq, treatment time 77 s

adenocarcinoma. Many of them suffered from advanced disease: 7% had a T1 tumor, 58% a T2 tumor, and 35% a T3 tumor; 24% had lymph node metastasis and 14% distant metastasis at the time of diagnosis.

A total of 488 afterloading applications were performed in 139 patients (mean 3.5, range 1–11). Thirty-four patients received laser therapy (76 applications) and 90 patients had external irradiation with a mean dose of 50 Gy (range 4–100 Gy). The overall response rate was 58%, with no significant difference between squamous cell carcinomas (59%) and adenocarcinomas (57%).

Survival (Fig. 2) data are unsatisfactory. The overall mean duration of survival is 10 months (range 1–49 months), with 9 (1–49) months for squamous cell carcinoma and 11 (1–48) months for adenocarcinoma.

Twelve patients, all from the squamous cell carcinoma group, developed fistulae. The mean interval before the fistula was 9 months (range 1–18 months). There was no significant correlation with dosage, but all had extensive local tumors.

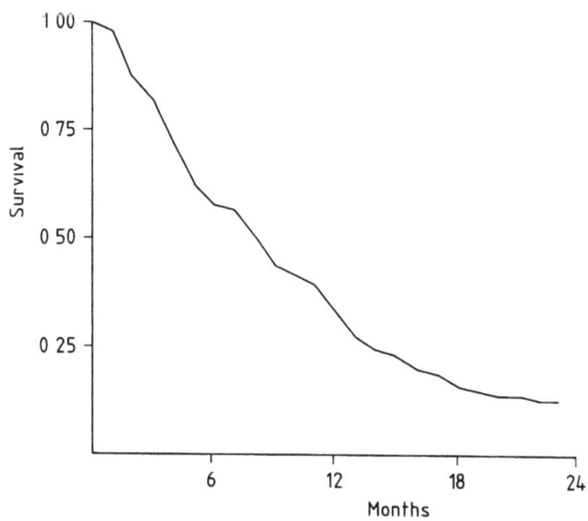

Fig. 2. Survival after endoluminal irradiation of patients with carcinoma of esophagus and gastroesophageal junction

Endoluminal laser and afterloading therapy should be employed within the framework of the overall treatment concept for carcinoma of the upper gastrointestinal tract.

Summary

We treated 139 patients with carcinoma of the upper gastrointestinal tract with endoluminal afterloading irradiation by remote control. In this way it is possible to use a highly radioactive ^{192}Ir source, for example 20 C = 740 GBq, for only a few minutes. More than half the patients received three to four doses of 15 Gy at 5 mm from the source axis at intervals of 2 weeks. Thirty-four patients first had laser therapy for immediate tumor reduction, 90 patients underwent combined treatment with external irradiation. The response rate was 58% and the mean survival time was 10 months.

External Radiotherapy for Local and Regional Control of Lung Cancer

H.D. Kogelnik

Institut für Radiotherapie und Radio-Onkologie, Landeskrankenanstalten Salzburg, Müllner Hauptstraße 48, 5020 Salzburg, Austria

Introduction

Surgery and radiotherapy are the only means of achieving permanent local and regional tumor control in patients with lung cancer. All resectable carcinomas should be treated surgically. Although the ultimate incidence of distant metastases is very high, freedom from locoregional cancer is the prerequisite for long-term survival and cure of the disease. Currently, the overall 5-year survival rate of patients with bronchogenic carcinoma is about 10%.

The incidence of ipsilateral hilar node metastases from the different lobes ranges from 60% to 77% [21]. Even in early (operable) cases, mediastinal adenopathy is found in 40%–50% of surgical specimens [2]. With the aid of CT scans for patient selection, about 15%–20% are operated on, with a resectability rate higher than 90% [8].

In unresectable advanced stage III non-small cell lung cancer, not only is the ultimate rate of distant metastases for all histologies 75–80% [8], but also the ultimate intrathoracic failure rate ranges from 70%–80% [17]. However, there is clear evidence that increased locoregional tumor control leads to improved survival rates [8, 14, 18]. In patients with small cell bronchogenic carcinoma, who mostly present with widely disseminated disease, higher intrathoracic tumor control rates also lead to increased long-term survival [1, 13, 16, 20]. Overall, local failure is a major cause of death, accounting for approximately 10% of all patients with lung cancer [24].

Three groups of factors affect the response to irradiation and survival:

1. Patient characteristics (e.g., initial performance status, weight loss in past 6 month, age)
2. Tumor characteristics (e.g., clinical stage, size of lesion, histologic type)
3. Technical parameters relating to delivery of irradiation (e.g., quality assurance programs, tumor dose, tumor volume treated)

In addition, tumor response to irradiation itself also has prognostic significance [8]. Quality assurance programs are of particular importance, because both tumor response and survival decrease if radiotherapy is not performed under optimal conditions [14].

R. Jakesz/H. Rainer (Eds.)
Progress in Regional Cancer Therapy

Non-Small Cell Lung Cancer

Non-small cell lung cancer accounts for approximately 80% of all malignant lung tumors. Less than 20% of such cases are operable. Whether definitive or palliative irradiation is used depends on a variety of factors, including the results of cardiopulmonary function tests.

Postoperative Irradiation

Postoperative radiotherapy is not indicated in pT1, T2, N0 patients with no residual disease. However, irradiation is most beneficial for N0 patients with residual disease [23]: With radiation doses of 5000 cGy in 5 weeks, followed by a boost of 500–1000 cGy, there was only one local failure (4%) among 22 patients with residual disease (9 gross, 13 microscopic). The 5-year actuarial survival rate of this group is 70%. Of all 115 patients receiving postoperative irradiation, only 11% failed intrathoracically, although 77 patients had stage III disease. Distant metastatic relapse occurred in 4% of N0, 28% of N1, and 60% of N2 patients.

From these data, and also from the results of a randomized study of completely resected stage II and stage III epidermoid cancer of the lung [12] it is evident that a striking and significant reduction of intrathoracic recurrences is achieved by postoperative irradiation. However, despite the beneficial effect on the quality of life, there is no statistically significant increase in survival rates in N1 and N2 patients, largely because of the high incidence of distant metastases (especially in N2 patients). On the other hand, several reports in the literature suggest that postoperative radiation therapy does increase survival for these patients [6, 10, 11]. Currently most centers recommend postoperative irradiation for patients with hilar and mediastinal nodal metastases as well as for T3 tumors.

Preoperative Irradiation

With the information from CT scans available, preoperative radiotherapy might well be a realistic approach for a selected group of patients with "marginally resectable" lung cancer. In a study by Sherman et al. [22], complete resectability was achieved in 83% of such patients, who were operated on within 2 weeks after radiotherapy. Tumor doses of 3000 cGy in 2 weeks were used for most of the patients. The 5-year survival rate for those with resectable tumors was 27%. The authors concluded that in selected patients with marginally resectable to unresectable lung cancer (without demonstrated distant disease), preoperative irradiation improves survival to a level comparable to that in patients with less advanced lesions treated with surgery alone.

Definitive Radiation Therapy

The requirements for definitive radiotherapy in non-small cell lung cancer are:

1. Curative surgery not possible (medically inoperable or unresectable cancer)
2. Disease localized to the chest

Table 1. Definitive radiotherapy in unresectable non-small cell carcinoma of the lung ($n = 378$) [14]

Dose	Intrathoracic recurrences	Two-year survival (overall)
4000 cGy	52% [a]	10%–11%
5000 cGy	41%	19%
6000 cGy	30% [a]	

[a] f = 0.006.

3. Good performance status (Karnofsky)
4. Adequate cardiopulmonary function

Five-year survival rates of up to 10% are obtained [7, 14, 19].

From studies by the Radiation Therapy Oncology Group it is evident that increasing radiation doses not only decrease intrathoracic recurrences but also increase survival rates (Table 1) [14, 19]. With precision radiotherapy and the use of CT scans for treatment planning, tumor doses of up to 7000 cGy may be given using a shrinking-field technique. Patients in whom intrathoracic tumor control is achieved within 6 or 12 months exhibit a statistically significant improvement in survival [19].

In most advanced stage III cases, a marked improvement in quality of life was demonstrated by continuing relief of signs and symptoms of pain, hemoptysis, and pleural effusion in 50%, 50%, and 62% respectively of patients who received 3000 cGy in 2 weeks [3]. In stage III patients with less extensive tumors, who received a tumor dose of 6000 cGy (split-course irradiation) there was continuing relief in 60%, 100%, and 75% respectively.

Current results of chemotherapy in non-small cell bronchogenic carcinoma are not encouraging [8]. Results of trials on chemotherapy are usually reported in terms of response, which is not the same as tumor control. A short-lived "partial response" or "stable disease" are of no ultimate value. Moreover, initial chemotherapy may lead to an accelerated regeneration of clonogenic tumor cells. Thus, not only will the more effective treatment form (surgery, radiotherapy) be delayed, but also the biological tumor situation will become worse.

Small Cell Lung Cancer

In contrast to non-small cell bronchogenic carcinoma, chemotherapy is very valuable in small cell lung cancer. The combination of radiotherapy (5000–6000 cGy tumor dose) and multidrug chemotherapy has increased both locoregional tumor control and survival compared with chemotherapy alone (Tables 2 and 3). Also, there is evidence that intrathoracic tumor control is associated with improved survival up to 5 years [5]. All patients who fail in the chest (with or without distant metastases) die within 36 months. Long-term survival is observed only in patients, who do not develop chest relapses or distant metastases.

Table 2. Small cell carcinoma of the lung: loco-regional recurrence after chemotherapy alone (CT) vs chemotherapy plus radiotherapy (CT + RT)

Reference	CT	CT + RT
Salazar et al. [20]	82%	28%
Mira et al. [13]	55%[a]	24%[a]
Perez et al. [16]	52%	36%
Arriagada et al. [1]	—	20%

[a] Extensive disease.

Table 3. Small cell lung cancer (limited disease): survival after chemotherapy alone (CT) vs chemotherapy plus radiotherapy (CT + RT)

	Two-year survival		Three-year survival	
Reference	CT	CT + RT	CT	CT + RT
Bunn and Ihde [4]	7%	17%	—	—
Perez et al. [15, 16]	23%	40%	5%	20%
Arriagada et al. [1]	—	35%	—	28%
Glatstein [9]	11%	32%	—	—

All patients with limited disease who achieve complete remission intrathoracically after initial chemotherapy, or after subsequent radiotherapy, should also receive elective brain irradiation (3600 cGy in 18 fractions over $3\frac{1}{2}$ weeks). In this way the incidence of brain metastases, which would be in excess of 50% in long-term survivors without elective brain irradiation, is reduced to below 5% [8].

Apical (Superior Sulcus) Lung Carcinoma

Superior sulcus tumors are treated either by preoperative irradiation (when operable) or by definitive radiotherapy. Preoperatively, tumor doses ranging from 3000 cGy in 2 weeks to 4500 cGy in 5 weeks are given, followed by en bloc resection 4–6 weeks later. Using definitive irradiation, about 6500 cGy are administered in 6–7 weeks. With either form of therapy, 5-year survival rates in the range of 15%–30% are obtained [8].

Superior Vena Cava Syndrome

Because 10%–20% of patients with a superior vena cava syndrome survive longer than 2 years, aggressive treatment is indicated when the disease is still localized. In these situations, tumor doses between 6000 and 7000 cGy may be given (with higher fractions initially). Overall, good improvement of symptoms is achieved in about

70% of patients. Radiotherapy is usually the initial treatment of choice; in small cell carcinoma, however, patients with less severe symptoms are initially treated by chemotherapy.

Complications of Therapy

Depending on dose, volume of tumor and normal tissues within the radiation field, size of fraction, radiation energy, age, preexisting diseases, additive chemotherapy, availability of CT planning, etc., various moderate to severe complications may occur after definitive radiotherapy. Pneumonitis, pulmonary fibrosis, esophagitis, esophageal stenosis, pericarditis, subcutaneous fibrosis, and costochondritis are among the more common side effects, and should be anticipated in a reasonably low proportion of patients treated aggressively.

Treatment Planning

Computed tomography is an essential prerequisite for radiotherapy treatment planning in about 50% of all patients with lung cancer (i.e., for those who receive definitive radiotherapy). With the help of CT it has been shown that previously about 30% of all treatment plans were inadequate. With precision radiotherapy (including the use of CT scans and three-dimensional planning), significant improvements in uncomplicated intrathoracic tumor control rates (and possibly in survival) may be expected, because higher tumor doses can be applied with sparing of larger volumes of normal tissues.

Outlook

Because the ultimate rates of locoregional and especially of distant failure in lung cancer are still very high, there is a continuing necessity for further improvements in locoregional therapy, and a crucial need for effective systemic chemotherapy. Progress in radio-oncology is expected in the fields of intraoperative radiotherapy, altered fractionation schedules, radiosensitizers and radioprotectors, hyperthermia and radiotherapy, radio-immunotherapy, heavy particles, and precision radiotherapy (including three-dimensional planning).

References

1. Arriagada R, Le Chevalier T, Ruffié P et al. (1987) Optimizing combinations of alternating radiotherapy and chemotherapy in limited small cell lung cancer. In: Kärcher KH, Kogelnik HD, Szepesi T (eds) Progress in radio-oncology III. International Club for Radio-Oncology, Vienna, pp 226–230
2. Baird JA (1965) The pathways of lymphatic spread of carcinoma of the lung. Br J Surg 52:868
3. Barkley HT (1980) Lung. In: Fletcher GH (ed) Textbook of radiotherapy, 3rd edn. Lea and Febiger, Philadelphia, pp 664–688

4. Bunn PA, Ihde DC (1981) Small cell bronchogenic carcinoma: a review of therapeutic results. In: Livingston RB (ed) Lung cancer. Nijhoff, The Hague, pp 169–308
5. Bunn PA et al. (1985) Paper at Fourth world conference on lung cancer, Toronto, 25–30 Aug
6. Choi NCH, Grillo HC, Gardiello M et al. (1980) Basis for new strategies in postoperative radiotherapy of bronchogenic carcinoma. Int J Radiat Oncol Biol Phys 6:31–35
7. Coy P, Kennelly GM (1980) The role of curative radiotherapy in the treatment of lung cancer. Cancer 45:698–702
8. Emami B, Perez CA (1987) Carcinoma of the lung. In: Perez CA, Brady LW (eds) Principles and practice of radiation oncology. Lippincott, Philadelphia, pp 650–683
9. Glatstein E, Ihde D, Bunn P et al. (1985) Radiotherapy in management of limited small cell lung carcinoma: a randomized prospective study. Cancer Treat Symp 2:97–100
10. Green N, Kurohara SS, George FW III et al. (1975) Postresection irradiation for primary lung cancer. Radiology 116:405–407
11. Kirsh MM, Rotman H, Argenta L et al. (1976) Carcinoma of the lung: results of treatment over ten years. Ann Thorac Surg 21:371–377
12. Lung Cancer Study Group (1986) Effects of postoperative mediastinal radiation on completely resected stage II and stage III epidermoid cancer of the lung. N Engl J Med 315:1377–1381
13. Mira JG, Livingston RB, Moore TN et al. (1982) Influence of chest radiotherapy in frequency and patterns of chest relapse in disseminated small cell lung carcinoma. A Southwest Oncology Group Study. Cancer 50:1266–1272
14. Perez CA, Stanley K, Grundy G et al. (1982) Impact of irradiation technique and tumor extent in tumor control and survival of patients with unresectable non-oat cell carcinoma of the lung. Report by the Radiation Therapy Oncology Group. Cancer 50:1091–1099
15. Perez CA, Einhorn L, Oldham RK et al. (1983) Preliminary report of a randomised trial of radiotherapy to the thorax in limited small cell carcinoma of the lung treated with multiagent chemotherapy. Proc Am Soc Clin Oncol 2:190
16. Perez CA, Einhorn L, Oldham RK et al. (1984) Randomized trial of radiotherapy to the thorax in limited small cell carcinoma of the lung treated with multiagent chemotherapy and elective brain irradiation: a preliminary report. J Clin Oncol 2:1200–1208
17. Perez CA, Bauer M, Birch R (1985) Impact of tumor control on survival in carcinoma of the lung (Abstract). In: Third Rome International Symposium: The challenge of local tumor control and its impact on survival. Rome, May 12–17, pp I–V
18. Perez CA (1985) Non-small cell carcinoma of the lung: dose-time parameters. Cancer Treat Symp 2:131–142
19. Perez CA, Bauer M, Edelstein S et al. (1986) Impact of tumor control on survival in carcinoma of the lung treated with irradiation. Int J Radiat Oncol Biol Phys 12:539–547
20. Salazar OM, Creech RH, Rubin P et al. (1980) Half-body and local chest irradiation as consolidation following response to standard induction chemotherapy for disseminated small cell lung cancer: an Eastern Cooperative Group pilot report. Int J Radiat Oncol Biol Phys 6:1093–1102
21. Seydel HG, Chait A, Gmelich JT (1975) Cancer of the lung. Wiley, New York
22. Sherman DM, Neptune W, Weichselbaum R et al. (1978) An aggressive approach to marginally resectable lung cancer. Cancer 41:2040–2045
23. Slater JD, Ellerbroek NA, Barkley HT et al. (1988) Radiation therapy following resection of bronchogenic carcinoma (Abstract). Int J Radiat Oncol Biol Phys 15 [Suppl 1]:118
24. Suit HD (1969) Introduction: statement of the problem pertaining to the effect of dose fractionation and total treatment time on response of tissue to x-irradiation. In: Time and dose relationships in radiation biology as applied to radiotherapy. Brookhaven National Laboratory, Associated Universities, Brookhaven, pp VII–X

Clinical Experience with a Multifrequency Hyperthermia System and Chemotherapy in the Treatment of Superficial Metastases*

G. Cruciani, V. Salerno, E. Crippa, M. Morelli, G. Gnani, and M. Marangolo

Department of Medical Oncology, SMC Hospital, 48100 Ravenna, Italy

Introduction

In cancer therapy, hyperthermia as sole treatment modality yields only a moderate rate of objective responses, in the order of < 20% (mostly partial responses). On the other hand, chemotherapy or radiotherapy alone rarely achieves cure, especially in bulky solid tumors, due to cellular resistance and to poor vascular supply, which causes hypoxia and reduced drug access [9].

From clinical trials it appears to be advantageous, in terms of complete response, to add hyperthermia to radiotherapy [3], but the control of bulky neoplastic disease by local modalities is often difficult, and in sites like head and neck the incidence of locoregional recurrence is reported to be as high as 60%, while distant metastases develop in more than 10% of cases [1]. This justifies the introduction of effective chemotherapy as part of the definitive treatment in patients with locally advanced disease.

Furthermore, many experimental studies support the combination of hyperthermia and drugs, because at least for some drugs there is an increased cell killing proportionally to the temperature rise and in some cases even resistant cell lines can be rendered susceptible to combined chemotherapy by means of hyperthermia [6]. Two randomized trials have demonstrated a significant advantage when local hyperthermia is added to chemotherapy in head and neck cancer [2] and in vulvovaginal cancer [8].

The aim of this study is to evaluate the role of local hyperthermia in combination with systemic chemotherapy in patients with superficial metastases.

Patients and Methods

Twenty patients with superficial metastases from epithelial neoplasms were treated with combination chemotherapy plus local hyperthermia as shown in Table 1 [5]. Seventeen of the 20 patients had been previously treated with chemotherapy (14

*Supported by the Regione Emilia Romagna and the Istituto Oncologico Romagnolo.

R. Jakesz/H. Rainer (Eds.)
Progress in Regional Cancer Therapy

Table 1. Protocol for combination chemotherapy plus local hyperthermia

Agent	Dosage	Day(s)
Cisplatin	20 mg/m^2	1, 2, 3, 4, 5
Bleomycin	10 mg/m^2	8, 12
Methotrexate	100 mg/m^2	15
Folinic acid	100 mg/m^2	16
Hyperthermia	30 min, 43°C	1, 5, 8, 12, 15

patients) or radiotherapy. The majority had metastases from epidermoid cancer. The histology was adenocarcinoma according to undifferentiated carcinoma in two, and melanoma in one. The site of the primary cancer was prevalently the head and neck. A further four patients were treated according to a second protocol—weekly epirubicin 20 mg/m^2 combined with local hyperthermia 60 min at 43°C. Three of these four patients had locoregional relapse from breast carcinoma, previously treated except in one case. One patient had a relapse of liposarcoma, already treated with surgery and radiation therapy.

The median age of all patients was 65 years (range 55–83). Performance status (ECOG) was 0 in six patients, 1 in 11 patients, 2 in three patients, 3 in three patients and 4 in one patient.

The drugs were always infused in 15 min, overlapping the last 5–10 min of the local hyperthermia.

Hyperthermia

All patients were treated with a radiative hyperthermia system working at 144 and 432 MHz, designed in Italy by ENEA-SMA [4]. Applicators of different shapes and sizes were available in order to optimize the thermo-electromagnetic coupling between antennas and tumors. The applicators were filled with de-ionized water, acting as both dielectric and cooling fluid. The thermometry was carried out with multisensor thermocouple probes connected to a 15-channel computerized clinical thermometer. During the treatment the temperature was measured in at least five locations within the tumor, at different depths and distances from the cutaneous center of the hyperthermic field.

A hyperthermic treatment was defined as optimal when at least in one session it was possible to maintain a minimum tumor temperature of 42.5–43°C for 30 min.

Response and Toxicity

In the case of patients with more than one lesion, response was assessed separately for neoplastic lesions within and outside the hyperthermia field. Complete response (CR) was defined as the absence of evidence of disease. Partial response (PR) was defined as a reduction of at least 50% in the sum of the products of the perpendicular diameters of measurable lesions. Stable disease (SD) was defined as a regression of less than 50% of measurable lesions. Progressive disease (PD) was defined as an increase greater than 25% in any measurable lesion or the appearance of new lesions. Duration of response was defined, as the period between the beginning of the treatment and the time of PD. The evaluation of response was made at the end of the combined treatment. Toxicity from chemotherapy was evaluated according to Miller et al. [10]. Cutaneous toxicity of hyperthermic treatment was defined in terms of cutaneous burns (0 = absent, 1 = blisters, 2 = necrosis $< 10\,cm^2$, 3 = necrosis $> 10\,cm^2$).

Results

The local response to the first protocol was 65% (eight PR and five CR). Median duration of response was 5 months (range 2–22 + months). Local response was similar in all histologic types. Four CR were achieved in patients pretreated with radiotherapy or chemoradiotherapy, while another CR was obtained in one patient not pretreated (Table 2).

Among 8 patients with more than one evaluable site of metastasis, no objective response was achieved outside the hyperthermia field, while a 50% rate of objective response (two PR and two CR) was noted in the lesions treated with hyperthermia. It was not possible to attain good hyperthermia in all patients. No CR was obtained in patients suboptimally treated (Table 3). Toxicity was generally due to the systemic treatment, and only two cutaneous burns were noted (Table 4).

Of the four patients treated with the second protocol (weekly epirubicin plus hyperthermia), three responded to the combined treatment (two PR and one CR). The durations of response were 5, 8, and 10 months. One patient, with a bulky relapse on the chest wall, had PD after combined treatment. This patient had been

Table 2. Local response according to previous treatment

Previous treatment	*n*	CR	PR	SD	PD
Chemotherapy	4	—	1	3	—
Radiotherapy	11	3	5	3	—
Chemoradiotherapy	2	1	1	—	—
No treatment	3	1	1	1	—

Table 3. Hyperthermic treatment and local response

Hyperthermia	*n*	CR	PR	SD	Percentage response
Optimal	14	5	5	4	71.04
Suboptimal	6	—	3	3	50.0

Table 4. Toxicity after combined treatment

Grade	Vomiting	Hematological	Mucositis	Cutaneous burns
1	5	—	1	—
2	5	4	3	2
3	3	2	—	—
4	—	—	—	—

heavily pretreated with chemoradiotherapy. The 2 PR were rendered CR, by surgery in one case and radiotherapy in the other.

The toxicity of this protocol was mild, always of grade 1, except for alopecia.

Discussion and Conclusion

The high rate of objective remissions obtained in pretreated patients gives a confirmation of the thermal enhancement observed with different drugs in vitro. Noteworthy is the high response rate in patients previously treated with radiation therapy (8/11). The observation of a response in the hyperthermia field while other metastatic lesions were progressing prompts a search for the mechanism by which hyperthermia overcomes drug resistance. Plasma membrane components are relevant as markers of drug resistance and as targets for thermotherapy [7].

In some cases patients in PR after combined thermochemotherapy were rendered disease free by subsequent radiotherapy or surgery. Toxicity was generally mild and never of grade 4. Cutaneous toxicity from local hyperthermia was also mild.

In conclusion, thermochemotherapy can be safely applied as palliative therapy in patients with superficial relapses, even in preirradiated areas.

A new concept for consideration is the application of thermochemotherapy, possibly with the best chemotherapy regimen for a given neoplastic disease, as neoadjuvant treatment in patients with bulky locoregional disease before definitive surgery and/or radiotherapy.

The same approach could be applied to deeper tumors, if in future the technical limitations on deep heating can be overcome.

References

1. Al-Sarraf M (1988) Chemotherapy concepts. Head and neck cancer. Semin Oncol 15: 70–85
2. Arcangeli G, Cividalli A, Lovisolo G, Mauro F, Creton G, Nervi C, Pavin G (1980) Effectiveness of local hyperthermia in association with radiotherapy or chemotherapy: comparison of multi-modality treatments on multiple neck node metastases. In: Arcangeli G, Mauro F (eds) Proceedings of the first meeting of the European Group of Hyperthermia in radiation Oncology. Masson, Milano, pp 257–265
3. Arcangeli G, Overgaard J, Gonzalez Gonzalez D, Shrivastava PN (1988) Hyperthermia trials. Int J Radiat Oncol Biol Phys 14:S93–S109

4. Borrani A, Calamai G, Lachi L, Lovisolo GA, Marsiglia G, Mauro F (1988) MHS experience and improvements after one year of activity (meeting abstract). 5th International Symposium on Hyperthermic Oncology, Aug 29–Sept 3, 1988, Kyoto
5. Cruciani G, Molinari AL, Marangolo M, Morelli M, Gnani G, Mazzotti A, Mauro F (1987) Applicability of local hyperthermia as adjuvant to systemic chemotherapy. Tumori 73:629–633
6. Dahl O (1988) Interaction of hyperthermia and chemotherapy. Recent Results Cancer Res 107:157–169
7. Greco C (1988) Drug resistance and hyperthermia (meeting abstract). In: 5th international symposium on hyperthermic oncology, Aug 29–Sept 3 1988, Kyoto
8. Kohno I, Kaneshige E, Fujiwara K, Sekiba K (1984) Thermochemotherapy (TC) for gynecologic malignancies. In: Overgaard J (ed) Hyperthermic oncology, vol I. Taylor and Francis, London, pp 753–756
9. Maher EJ (1987) Problems in cancer treatment. In: Field SB, Franconi C (eds) Physics and technology of hyperthermia. Nijhoff, Dordrecht, pp 3–18 (Applied sciences, vol 127)
10. Miller AB, Hoogstraten B, Staquet M, Winkler A (1981) Reporting results of cancer treatment. Cancer 47:207–214

Recent Clinical Experience with an Annular Phased Array Hyperthermia System in the Treatment of Advanced Recurrences in the Pelvis

P. Steindorfer, R. Germann, A. Berger, G. Wolf, H.J. Mischinger, S. Uranus, P. Rehak, K. Arian-Schad, and M. Klimpfinger

Chirurgische Abteilung, Medizinische Hochschule, Auenbruggerplatz 1, 8030 Graz, Austria

Introduction

The sometimes disappointing results in the treatment of advanced disease of gastrointestinal tumors, especially pelvic recurrences of rectal cancer patients, have prompted studies of different local treatment modalities to enhance the effect of local tumor control. One of the main concerns of surgeon and radio-oncologist is to prevent the very damaging pelvic recurrence, but if the tumor does relapse one should seek an effective method of local tumor control.

Deep regional hyperthermia (HT) has therefore come more and more into the domain of oncologists. The biological principles of HT in the treatment of different malignancies in vitro and in vivo have been presented by many authors [1, 3, 4, 6, 7, 16, 17]. So-called moderate HT, between 41.5 and 45 °C, has a lot of different effects on the growth of tumor cells in vitro and in vivo, depending on duration and temperature level of heat exposure [8, 9, 16]. The enhanced cell-killing effect obtained by using HT as one part of combined treatment modalities, e.g., with radiotherapy (RTX) and/or chemotherapy (CTX), has been proven in several experimental and clinical trials [3, 4, 6, 7, 10, 11, 14, 15, 17, 18]. These biological and clinical investigations provided the rationale for initiating a clinical study of the use of HT in patients with advanced pelvic recurrences of colorectal cancer.

Technical Equipment

In the clinical practice of HT many different devices are available and in use, but only a few have the facility to monitor the temperature within the tumor continuously during the HT procedure. We are using the BSD 1000 hyperthermia System (BSD Medical Corp., Salt Lake City, Utah) Which is an annular phased array system (APAS) of 16 microwave antennas (applicators) guided by computer. Thermistor probes inserted within the tumor area monitor the temperature continuously during the treatment [2]. To achieve better coupling to the surface of the patient's body, the antennas are connected to water boluses filled with de-ionized water. A radio-frequency generator produces the energy and sends it to the applicators. This system is widely used for clinical deep regional HT [13, 16, 19]. The average frequency we

R. Jakesz/H Rainer (Eds)
Progress in Regional Cancer Therapy

used during the HT procedure ranged between 60 and 70 MHz, the average energy being about 1000 W.

Design of the Study

Only pretreated patients with advanced recurrences in the pelvis after surgery, RTX, and/or CTX were entered in the study. All patients had a rectal cancer recurrence – we did not want to mix tumor types because of differences in biological reaction to different treatment modalities. This study was also designed as a pilot study, so we selected two different patient groups:

Group A: Patients irradiated previously with a residual RTX dose of at least 20 Gy, which is inadequate in such large tumors. All had undergone previous radical or palliative surgery, and a few of them had also received CTX, mainly systemic 5-fluorouracil (5-FU).

Group B: Patients with a residual dose lower than 20 Gy, a few of them with previous CTX. All of them had undergone surgery, as in group A.

Before starting the therapy, all patients were subjected to the following investigations: CT scan, ECG, blood cell count, renal function test, X-ray of the lungs, and ultrasound of the liver. The Karnofsky performance status of the patients was more than 50%. Distant metastases were excluded before starting therapy. Tumor volume was estimated from CT scans of the pelvic region.

The treatment plan in group A was a sequential combination of regional HT (RHT) with high-voltage RTX in once-daily fractions of 2 Gy. RHT was given twice a week for at least 40 min at a temperature of about 42°C within the tumor area.

The treatment protocol of group B was quite different regarding the systemic therapy. We combined the RHT with 5-FU, the cytotoxic drug used most commonly in colorectal cancer. RHT was given twice a week as in group A, but during each HT treatment the patient received 1000 mg 5-FU intravenously. We started the infusion about 1 h before the HT procedure and continued during the whole treatment. On the days without HT the patients received 750 mg 5-FU orally. During the whole RHT procedure the patients were supervised by intensive care nurses and physicians. Blood pressure, heart rate, core temperature, and the patient's subjective sensations were monitored continuously.

After the end of the course of treatment another CT scan was done to look for necrosis and reduction of tumor volume. It is very difficult, however, to evaluate the response in nonmeasurable disease like recurrences in the pelvic area. Thus we decided to perform second- or third-look operations after finishing HT.

Results

When we started using the APAS in HT treatment in 1983, we emphasized CT as a means for ascertaining remission. We have since done second-look operations in seven patients and now have to view the results more critically. We cannot evaluate the remission rates in our series objectively except by means of surgery and histopathology. Even CT in combination with serological markers (carcino-embryonic antigen, alkaline phosphatase) and needle biopsies is not able to produce any objective remission criteria, because of the difficulties in discriminating between necrotic tissue and viable tumor. To evaluate our response, we used the guidelines of the UICC for nonsuperficial tumors.

Analyzing our collected data and relating them to the remission rates, we found a significant correlation of the median energy used over all the treatments (Fig. 1) but not for the average temperature profiles (Fig. 2). We reached the desired temperature in nearly 80% of the treated cases (Fig. 3) but the temperature changes from treatment to treatment due to the different setup techniques. Very precise treatment planning is therefore not possible at this moment. We did not use the mapping

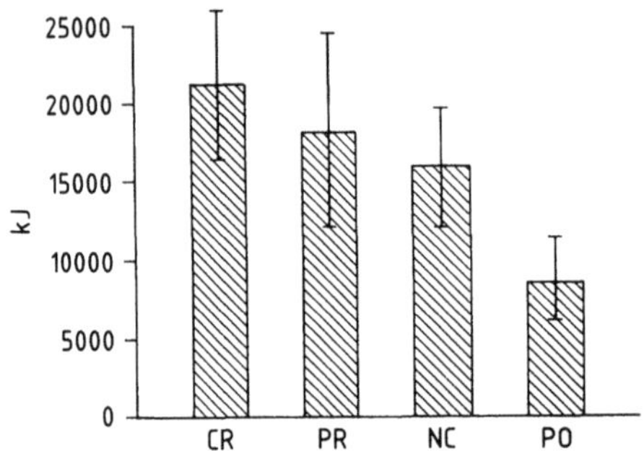

Fig. 1. Average energy used in HT treatments. *CR*, complete remission; *PR*, partial remission; *NC*, no change; *PD*, progressive disease

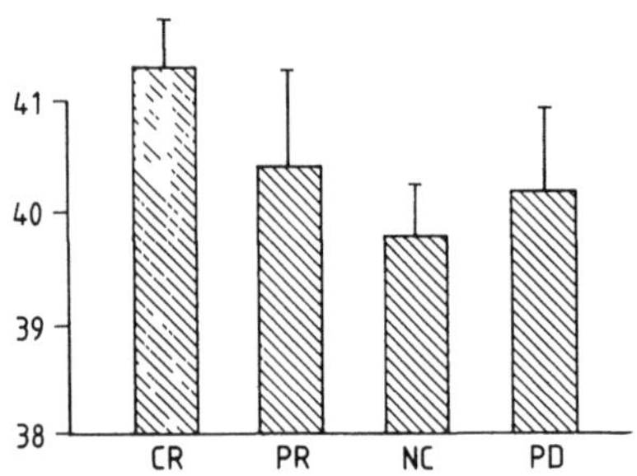

Fig. 2. Average temperature achieved in HT treatments

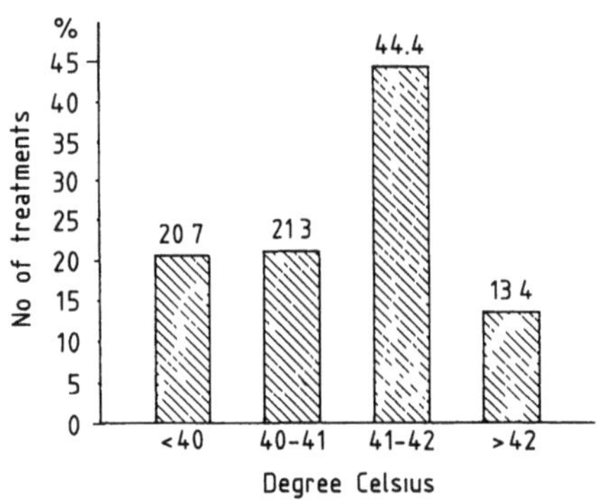

Fig. 3. Temperature distribution in HT treatments

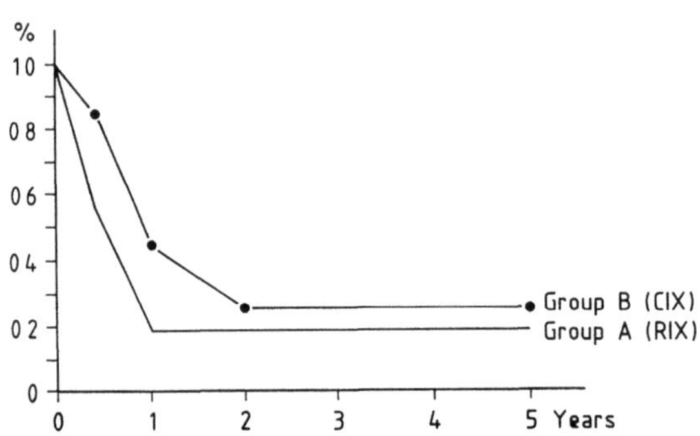

Fig. 4. Actuarial survival rate

Table 1. Remission rates

	CR	PR	NC	PD
Group A HT + RTX (20–32 Gy)	0	6	4	3
Group B HT + CTX (1000 mg/750 mg 5-FU)	1 (7)[a]	8	4	3

CR, complete remission; PR, partial remission; NC, no change; PD, progressive disease.
[a] Seven patients are in CR after surgery, but if only the HT treatment is taken into consideration there was only one case of CR, because a few viable tumor cells were found within the resected material on histological investigation.

procedure described by Gibbs [5], because of the very prototypical nature of the HT device.

Groups A and B did not differ significantly in survival, which may be explained by the very advanced and heavily pretreated cases we entered in the study (Fig. 4). After second-look operation in seven cases of group B, we performed histopathological investigation of the resected specimen. The tumor was embedded in paraffin after fixation with formaldehyde, then stained with hematoxylin and eosin. Within the investigated sections the tumor was mainly necrotic or necrobiotic, but we also found intact tumor formations.

The question as to whether the tumor cells have any viability or are thermoresistant clones cannot be answered yet.

Conclusions

In our feasibility study of the clinical use of HT in very advanced pelvic recurrences we could show that HT is effective in combined therapy with RTX and/or CTX. The assessment of response is very difficult, and still only possible by objective histological investigation. The treatment planning is at the moment very prototypical and one cannot correlate the setup to any objective response of the tumors being treated. Nevertheless, in certain carefully selected cases deep regional HT is effective, and more detailed prospective randomized trials are necessary to obtain more and better information on how to use deep HT in clinical oncology.

References

1. Bichel P, Overgaard J, Nielsen OS (1979) Synergistic cell cycle kinetic effect of low doses of hyperthermia and radiation on tumor cells. Eur J Cancer 15:1191
2. Bowman RR (1976) A probe for measuring temperature in radio frequency-heated material. IEEE Trans Microwave Theory Tech 24:43
3. Dahl O (1983) Hyperthermic potentiation of doxorubicin in a transplantable neurogenic rat tumor (BT4A) in BDIX rats. Int J Radiat Oncol Biol Phys 9:203
4. Dahl O, Mella O (1983) Effect of timing and sequence of hyperthermia and cyclosphosphamide on a neurogenic rat tumor BT4a in vivo. Cancer 52:983–998

5. Gibbs FA (1983) Thermal mapping in experimental cancer treatment with hyperthermia: description and use of a semiautomatic system. Int J Radiat Oncol Biol Phys 9:217
6. Hahn GM, Strande DP (1976) Cytotoxic effects of hyperthermia and adriamycin on Chinese hamster cells. JNCI 57:1063
7. Hahn GM, Braun J, Har-Kedar I (1975) Thermochemotherapy: synergism between hyperthermia (42–43°) and adriamycin (or bleomycin) in mammalian cell inactivation. Proc Natl Acad Sci USA 72:937
8. Jorritsma JBM, Kampinga HH, Scaf AHJ, Konings AWT (1985) Strand break repair, DNA polymerase activity and heat radiosensitization in thermotolerant cells. Int J Hyperthermia 1:131–147
9. Li GC, Petersen NS, Mitchel HK (1982) Induced thermal tolerance and heat shock protein synthesis in Chinese hamster ovary cells. Int J Radiat Oncol Biol Phys 8:63
10. Marmor JB (1969) Interactions of hyperthermia and chemotherapy in animals. Cancer Res 39:2269
11. Mella A (1985) Combined hyperthermia and cis-diamminedichloroplatinum in BDIX rats with transplanted BT4A tumors. Int J Hyperthermia 1:171–185
12. Muller WU, Li GC, Goldstein LS (1985) Heat does not induce synthesis of heat shock proteins or thermotolerance in the earliest stage of mouse embryo development. Int J Hyperthermia 1(1):97–103
13. Oleson JR, Sim DA, Conrad J, Fletcher AM, Gross EJ (1986) Results of a phase I regional hyperthermia device evaluation: microwave annular array versus radiofrequency induction coil. Int J Hyperthermia 2(4):327–336
14. Overgaard J (1976) Combined adriamycin and hyperthermia treatment of a murine mammary carcinoma in vivo. Cancer Res 36:3077
15. Overgaard (1978) The effect of local hyperthermia alone, and in combination with radiation, on solid tumors. In: Streffer C et al. (eds) Cancer therapy by hyperthermia and radiation. Urban and Schwarzenberg, Munich, p 49
16. Short GJ, Turner PF (1980) Physical hyperthermia and cancer therapy. IEEE Proc 68 (1):133
17. Steindorfer P (1985) Hyperthermie und Chemotherapie solider Tumore (Experimentelle Doppelblindstudie an transplantierten 5123-Morris-Hepatomen). Acta Chir Austriaca [Suppl] 63
18. Steindorfer P, Germann R, Klimpfinger M (1988) Experience with an annular phased array hyperthermia system in the treatment of advanced recurrences of the pelvis. In: Issels RD, Wilmann SW (eds) Application of hyperthermia in the treatment of cancer. Springer, Berlin Heidelberg New York, pp 226–235 (Recent results in cancer research, vol 107)
19. Turner PF (1984) Hyperthermia and inhomogeneous tissue effects using an annular phased array. IEEE Trans Microwave Theory Tech 32(8):874
20. Van der Zee J, van Putten WLJ, van den Berg AP, van Thoon GC et al. (1986) Retrospective analysis of the response of tumours in patients treated with a combination of radiotherapy and hyperthermia. Int J Hyperthermia 2(4):337–350

The Viennese Interstitial System KHS 9/W 18: Homogeneous Hyperthermia with Simultaneous Radiation in Deep-seated Tumors with Integrated Heat Protection of Normal Tissue

L. Handl-Zeller, K. Schreier, K.H. Kärcher, M. Budihna, and H. Lesnicar

Universitätsklinik für Radiotherapie und Radiologie, Alser Straße 4, 1090 Wien, Austria

Introduction

The sequence of application must be carefully considered if heat and irradiation are to be combined effectively.

As early as 1978 Sapareto et al. [8], Dewey et al. [1], and Li and Kal [6] had clearly demonstrated in vitro that the maximum interaction between heat and radiation in terms of cell killing occurs when the two are given simultaneously. They found that as much as a six-fold increase in survival could occur when the two treatments were separated by as little as 5–10 min.

Small changes in the sequential timing of heat and radiation may therefore cause large variations in survival, even when the time period between exposure to heat and radiation is brief.

Overgaard [7] studied the influence of sequence and interval between the two modalities on local tumor control and normal tissue damage in a C3H mouse mammary carcinoma transplanted into the feet of C3D2F1 mice in order to optimize the therapeutic effect of a combined hyperthermia radiation treatment. An increased thermal enhancement ratio (TER) was observed after simultaneous treatment. TER values ranged from 1.2 at 41°C to about 5 at 34.5°C after 1 h of heating, but in all simultaneous treatment schedules the TER values were similar in tumor and normal tissue, so that no improvement in therapeutic gain was obtained. Overgaard concluded that if hyperthermia was to play a useful therapeutic role, the combined treatment had to result in an improved therapeutic effect in terms of increased tumor response and/or decreased damage to normal tissue. Similar conclusions were reached by Hill and Denekamp [5] and Field [2]. If selective tumor heating cannot be obtained, simultaneous heat-radiation treatment therefore appears to be of doubtful value, because the thermal enhancement may be of similar magnitude in both tumor and normal tissue.

Clinical Implications

Despite differences in proliferation kinetics and environmental conditions, the almost identical TER values found in tumor and skin after simultaneous treatment,

R. Jakesz/H Rainer (Eds.)
Progress in Regional Cancer Therapy
© Springer-Verlag Berlin·Heidelberg 1990

make it reasonable to assume that direct radiosensitization and reduced accumulation of sublethal damage are mainly responsible for hyperthermic sensitization [7].

In the event of selective or partly selective tumor heating being obtained, the optimal therapeutic effect of hyperthermia and radiation will be achieved when the radiosensitizing effect of heat is utilised simultaneously. The joint application of heat and radiation involve only minor difficulties when treating mice in a waterbath, but the adaption of this protocol to human cancer treatment is considerably more difficult [8]. For this reason, few clinical trials in which heat and radiation are given simultaneously have been proposed. The development of a two-zone needle for use in conjunction with the interstitial hyperthermia unit KHS 9/W 18 has provided the answer to the problem.

Methods

Implants for radiotherapy can also be employed as interstitial sources of heat. The micro heat exchangers used consist of metal needles or plastic tubes 1.6–2.0 mm in diameter and with a wall thickness of 0.1 mm [3, 4]. There are two practical ways of heating a tumor:

1. The simple **through flow method**, where warm water flows from the unit into the implant on one side and out on the other (superficial tumors)
2. The **counter flow method**, where warm water flows into the implant and out on the same side.

For deep seated tumors the counter flow needles can be made of metal or consist of plastic tubes which are closed at the end.

The heat transfer to the tissue is exclusively dependent on thermal conduction. A water flow rate of at least 2 ml s^{-1} through each needle is necessary to procure the turbulent conditions which are important if heat transfer is to be maximal. Theoretical temperature distributions calculated by J.W. Hand and S. Clegg and the values shown in our own experiments [9] reveal an energy transfer in the micro heat exchangers of the order of 200–400 mW cm^{-1}°C. The capacity for heating muscle tissue is about 0.5 mW cm^{-1}°C. This means that the water-heated implants of 1.6–2.0 mm diameter provide a high energy reserve and can function as sources of heat at constant temperature in tissue in which a high degree of homogeneity temperature distribution can be expected.

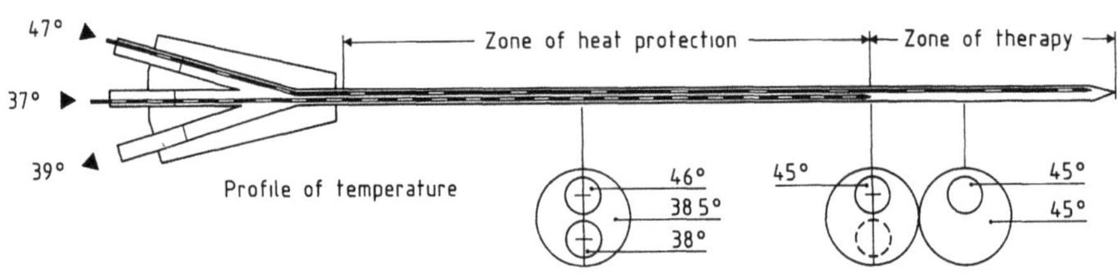

Fig. 1. Schematic presentation of the two-zone needle

The Two-Zone Needle

The lengths of the warm water and the cold water supply in the implant correspond to the warming zone and to the radiation zone of the needle respectively. The uncooled area of the needle allows space for the radioactive source.

Results

Whereas with through flow and counter flow as normally used the heating area is limited to two dimensions, the two-zone needle provides radiation and hyperthermia simultaneously in order to confine this to three-dimensional radiation and heat.

References

1. Dewey WC, Hopwood LE, Sapareto SA, Gerweck LE (1977) Cellular responses to combinations of hyperthermia and radiation. Radiology 123:463–474
2. Field SB (1980) Cancer therapy by hyperthermia, drugs and radiation. In: The third international symposium, Fort Collins CO, June 22–26, 1980. p 83 (abstr)
3. Handl-Zeller L, Kärcher KH, Schreier K, Handl O (1986) Optimierung interstitieller Hyperthermiesysteme. Strahlentherapie 163:460–463
4. Handl-Zeller L, Kärcher KH (1987) Hyperthermie als adjuvante Behandlung bei der Radiatio. In: Neugebauer H (ed) Medizinisches Jahrbuch. Müller, Wien, pp 111–117, 211
5. Hill SA, Denekamp J (1980) In: The third international symposium on cancer therapy by hyperthermia, drugs and radiation. Fort Collins CO, June 22–26, 1980. p 91 (abstr)
6. Li GC, Kal HB (1977) Effect of hyperthermia on the radiation response of two mammalian cell lines. Eur J Cancer 13:65–69
7. Overgaard J (1980) Simultaneous and sequential hyperthermia and radiation treatment of an experimental tumor and its surrounding normal tissue in vivo. Int J Radiat Oncol Biol Phys 6:1507–1517
8. Sapareto SA, Hopwood LE, Dewey WC (1978) Combined effects of X-irradiation and hyperthermia on CHO cells for various temperatures and orders of application. Radiat Res 73:221–223
9. Schreier K, Budihna M, Lesnicar H, Handl-Zeller L, Hand JW, Prior MV, Clegg ST (in press) Preliminary studies of interstitial hyperthermia using hot water. Int J Hyperthermia

Thermoradiotherapy of Superficial and Half Deep-seated Tumors: Thermal Profiles and Tumor Response*

H.J. Feldmann, M. Molls, S. Adler, and H. Sack**

Abteilung für Radiotherapie, Westdeutsches Tumorzentrum, Hufelandstraße 55, 4300 Essen, FRG

Introduction

About one third of all cancer patients die as a result of locoregional failure. To improve local control hyperthermia is being increasingly used in clinical tumor therapy [1, 2, 4, 7]. It has been demonstrated that hyperthermia in combination with irradiation increases the response rate. Our aim was to evaluate heating equipment, tumor response and toxicity in different anatomical regions of superficial tumors and of these located 3 to 7 cm beneath the surface (half deep-seated).

Materials and Methods

Fifty two patients (22 female, 30 male) with a total of 63 tumors were treated with a combination of radiotherapy and local hyperthermia. The patient characteristics are given in Table 1. The patients had locally advanced head and neck cancer, locoregional disease of malignant melanoma, presacral recurrences of rectal carcinoma, lymph node metastases of breast cancer, locally advanced or metastatic soft tissue sarcoma, and tumors of other origins (Table 1). In eight patients hyperthermia was performed as an adjuvant therapy after macroscopically radical resection of the tumors. Previous irradiation limited the actual radiation dose, and therefore radiotherapy was combined with hyperthermia. Up to now 700 single hyperthermia sessions have been performed; most treatments were superficial. Two heating devices were used: a 27-MHz diathermic generator (HMS 200, HMS Elektronik, Leverkusen, FRG) and a microwave generator (BSD-1000; BSD Medical Corporation, Salt Lake City, USA) with four radiative contact applicators, the MA 150 (450 MHz), the MA 120 (680 MHz), the MA 200 (80–180 MHz), and the MA 201 (80–180 MHz). The applicators have an attached variable bolus for coupling of heat and control of surface temperature. Two patients with large presacral recurrences of rectal cancer were treated with the annular phased array of

*This clinical study was supported by the German Cancer Foundation.
**The authors wish to acknowledge the valuable technical assistance of Mrs. H. Ophey.

R. Jakesz/H Rainer (Eds)
Progress in Regional Cancer Therapy

Table 1. Patient characteristics

Number of patients: 52		Age (years): 11–81 (mean 54)
Number of tumors: 63		Sex (M/F): 30/22
Histology	—	Site(s)
Squamous cell cancer	27	N3 lymph nodes/head and neck primaries
Melanoma	16	Paravertebral/chest wall/lymph nodes
Rectal cancer	6	Sacral/presacral
Breast cancer	6	Sternal/chest wall
Soft tissue sarcoma	4	Lower leg/foot/chest wall
Askin tumor	2	Paravertebral
Renal cancer	1	Sacral/presacral
Plasmocytoma	1	Chest wall
Tumor volume (0.5–377 cm^3; mean 94 cm^3)		
0–99 cm^3	64%	
100–199 cm^3	17%	
200–377 cm^3	19%	

the BSD-1000 apparatus using a partial array activation. In this arrangement power was delivered to the two adjacent quadrants which were closest to the tumor and which surrounded the target volume best.

Heat was delivered within about 20 min after irradiation twice or four times per week, and the goal was to maintain the temperature of the tumor center at 42.5 °C for 30–60 min. Bowman probes or copper constantan thermocouples were introduced into the tumor along blind-ended 16-G Teflon catheters (Deseret Inc., USA), which had been inserted under local anesthesia. One or two catheters were inserted into the tumor center and left in situ for the total duration of the treatment series.

Radiation was given using photon or electron beams of adequate energies. Conventional fractionation was preferred. In 57% of the tumors the actual radiation dose was kept between 0 and 49 Gy due to previous irradiation or palliative intention of the treatment. In the remaining 43% of the tumors radical irradiation could be performed with doses from 50 to 72 Gy.

Tumor response was classified according to the WHO criteria: complete response (CR) was defined as the disappearance of tumor, partial response (PR) as a reduction in total tumor volume of greater than 50%, and no change (NC) as a reduction of less than 50% or as an increase of 25% or less in tumor dimension.

Tumor volume was calculated as the volume of a regular ellipsoid $= (\pi/6) \cdot abc$, where a, b, and c are the orthogonal diameters.

Results

In 51% of the tumors temperatures of 42–48 °C were reached in the tumor centers. Thermal doses were calculated as minutes equivalent at 42.5 °C in the tumor center using a standard formula [5]. The total heat doses of fractionated hyperthermia treatments were determined by summarizing the heat doses of single treatments. In

Table 2. Response according to histology

Histology	CR	PR	NED	NC
Squamous cell cancer	13/26	6/26	1/26	6/26
Melanoma	4/16	8/16	3/16	1/16
Breast cancer	5/6	0/6	1/6	0/6
Rectal cancer	0/6	1/6	0/6	5/6
Soft tissue sarcoma	1/4	2/4	1/4	0/4
Others	0/4	1/4	2/4	1/4

Sixty-two of 63 tumors were evaluable. CR, complete remission; PR, partial remission; NED, no evidence of disease (after adjuvant radiotherapy plus hyperthermia); NC, no change.

60% of the tumors total heat doses higher than 100 minutes equivalent were obtained, in 13% heat doses between 50 and 100 min, and in 27% heat doses of only up to 49 min could be achieved. The impression that the tumors became easier to heat with an increasing number of treatments was not received.

Patient follow-up ranged from 3 to 24 months with a mean of 6 months. The response rates in terms of no evidence of disease (NED), CR, PR, and NC for all tumors treated are given in Table 2. The response was determined 3 months after the end of the treatment. NED was seen in 13%, CR in 38%, PR in 28%, and NC in 21% of the tumors. A very low response rate was seen in patients with presacral recurrences of rectal cancer: In five of six the status was NC. The tumors had infiltrated from the presacral region into the sacrum. In the other histologies the rate of CR–PR ranged between 50 and 83%.

In a subgroup of patients ($n = 8$) with locally advanced head and neck cancer radical irradiation (dose: 60–70 Gy) was combined with hyperthermia. Five patients suffered from locally advanced (T3, T4) primary tumors (tongue, floor of mouth) with N3 lymph node metastases (TNM–UICC); two patients had only N3 lymph node metastases, and one patient had a large primary tumor (T3; UICC TNM classification). Capacitive heating technique was used for the primaries, microwave heating equipment for the N3 lymph nodes. All five patients with advanced primaries and N3 nodes showed CR, which was also observed in those two patients presenting only with N3 nodes. In one patient with a large tumor of the floor of the mouth a partial remission was observed. In this case the follow-up has been too short to evaluate the final outcome.

In eight patients we performed adjuvant therapy after macroscopically radical resection of the tumor. In seven of these eight, with a follow-up from 3 to 18 months, there was no evidence of disease. Only one patient died due to distant metastases.

Local control of irradiated and heated tumors does not appear to be influenced by tumor size. Complete and partial response rates were approximately 80% despite different tumor volume groupings (Table 3). In 75% to 80% of the responding tumors (CR + PR), radiation doses from 40 to 72 Gy were given, with no differences between the various groups being seen.

The analysis of treatment parameters indicates that total radiation dose correlates with clinical response: CR and PR occur more frequently in the group with higher radiation doses. In the 40–72 Gy range an 89% tumor control rate

Table 3. Response according to tumor volume, total heat dose, and total radiation dose

	Tumor volume (cm³)[a]		
	< 100	100–109	≥ 200
CR	12/27 (45%)	2/7 (29%)	3/8 (38%)
PR	9/27 (33%)	4/7 (57%)	4/8 (50%)
NC	6/27 (22%)	1/7 (14%)	1/8 (12%)

	Total heat dose (min eq 4.25°C)[b]	
	< 100	≥ 100
CR	5/14 (36%)	9/21 (43%)
PR	4/14 (28%)	8/21 (38%)
NC	5/14 (36%)	4/21 (19%)

	Total radiation dose (Gy)[c]	
	18–39	40–72
CR	5/16 (31%)	18/37 (49%)
PR	2/16 (13%)	15/37 (40%)
NC	9/16 (56%)	4/37 (11%)

[a] Forty-two tumors evaluable, eight microscopically residual tumors, 13 tumors not evaluable.
[b] Thirty-five tumors evaluable, eight microscopically residual tumors, 20 tumors not evaluable (total heat dose could not be determined during the whole treatment).
[c] Fifty-three tumors evaluable, eight microscopically residual tumors, two patients without radiation.

(CR + PR) was observed, vs 44% in the 0–39 Gy range. Nonetheless the difference was not statistically significant.

Considering thermal treatment parameters we analyzed the influence on tumor regression of the total heat dose given to the tumor center (min eq 42.5 °C). A 67% tumor control (CR + PR) was achieved in the 0–99 min range extending longer as opposed to 81% control in tumors with heat doses higher than 100 min (range 100–863 min). Thus, although a trend could be observed, there was no clear correlation between response at 3 months and total heat dose. Acute treatment complications in the hyperthermia field occurred in about 10% of the tumors. They included local infection ($n = 3$), thermal blister ($n = 2$), and perineal hematoma ($n = 1$). Acute side effects of irradiated and heated regions were not enhanced in patients with large cervical lymph node metastases of head and neck cancer when compared with only irradiated contralateral neck regions in the same patient. Severe side effects occurred in less than 5% of cases. They comprised ulceration ($n = 2$) and osteoradionecrosis ($n = 1$). Cutaneous ulcerations of up to a few centimeters in diameter were seen in skin uninvolved by tumor, and probably arose from local overheating.

Discussion and Conclusion

Appropriate heating (total heat doses higher than 100 min eq 42.5 °C) could be performed in 60% of the tumors. There was no positive correlation between response and heat dose, although a trend favoring higher heat doses was noticed. Such a correlation has been described by Arcangeli et al. and Storm et al. [1, 6]. Other authors [3, 8] showed that tumor response correlates best with a minimum total heat dose. The controversial results in the literature can be explained by the fact that other important biologic parameters such as thermotolerance and radiosensitization also greatly affect the clinical outcome.

Tumor volume showed an important influence on clinical outcome. The response rate decreased with increasing volume. This relationship is well known in tumors which are only irradiated. Several authors [1, 3] have found the same trend for the combination of radiotherapy and hyperthermia, but the difference in the response rates of small and large lesions was comparatively small in the combined treatment. We found no association between tumor volume and incidence of complete or partial response. The influence of the radiation dose on the response of different tumor volume groupings can be neglected because of the nearly identical radiation dose distribution. Especially our experience in the treatment of malignant melanoma shows that a relatively good response can also be achieved in large tumors by comparison with the response rates in small tumors. Bulky tumors with poor vascularization may be easier to heat.

The magnitude of the radiation dose is clearly of extreme importance in the response of neoplastic lesions. Complete and partial responses were more frequent after high radiation doses. Our results are in agreement with those obtained by other investigators [1, 7, 8].

With regard to tumor response our preliminary results demonstrate the advantage of adding hyperthermia to conventionally fractionated palliative irradiation in patients with previously irradiated tumors in different anatomical regions. We believe that the total response rate (CR + PR) of 66% can be ascribed to the combination of radiotherapy and hyperthermia, because the majority of patients had been previously irradiated and presented with large tumors, so that the response to radiotherapy alone would have been poor. Our initial experience of adding hyperthermia to radical irradiation of previously unirradiated advanced tumors of the head and neck justifies to moving hyperthermia into the front line with curative irradiation.

References

1. Arcangeli G, Arcangeli G, Guerra A, Lovisolo G, Cividalli A, Marino C, Mauro F (1985) Tumour response to heat and radiation: prognostic variables in the treatment of neck node metastases from head and neck cancer. Int J Hyperthermia 1:207–217
2. Molls M, Feldmann HJ, Bamberg M, Sack H (1988) Hyperthermie als Radiosensibilisator. Tumordiagn Ther 9:S41–48
3. Oleson JR, Sim DA, Manning MR (1984) Analysis of prognostic variables in hyperthermia treatment of 161 patients. Int J Radiat Oncol Biol Phys 10:2231–2239
4. Overgaard J (1987) Hyperthermia as an adjuvant to radiotherapy. Review of the

randomized multicenter studies of the European Society for Hyperthermic Oncology. Strahlenther Onkol 163:7–13
5. Sapareto SA, Dewey WC (1984) Thermal dose determination in cancer therapy. Int J Radiat Oncol Biol Phys 6:1507–1517
6. Storm F, Roe D, Drury B (1987) The magnetrode study group: analysis of thermal dose response to heat. In: Abstracts of 35th annual meeting of Radiation Research Society, Feb 21–26, p 16
7. Valdagni R, Amichetti M, Pani G (1988) Radical radiation alone versus radical radiation plus microwave hyperthermia for N_3 (TNM–UICC) neck nodes: a prospective randomized clinical trial. Int J Radiat Oncol Biol Phys 15:13–24
8. Van der Zee J, van Dutten LJ, van den Berg AP, van Rhoon GC, Wike-Hooley JL, Broekmeyer-Reurink MP, Reinhold HS (1986) Retrospective analysis of the response of tumours in patients treated with a combination of radiotherapy and hyperthermia. Int J Hyperthermia 2:337–349

Comparison of Leakage Measurement Using ^{99m}Tc-Labeled Red Blood Cells and Peripheral Melphalan Determination in Hyperthermic Isolation Perfusion of the Extremities*

H. Foth, H. Rauschecker[1], C. Willenbrock[1], H.C. Michaelis, F. Horst[1], E. Voth[2], E. Musch[3], U. Loos[3], and G.F. Kahl

Institut für Pharmakologie und Toxikologie, Universität Göttingen, Robert-Koch-Straße 40, 3400 Göttingen, FRG

Introduction

The effectiveness of the therapy of malignant melanoma is thought to be improved by in addition hyperthermic isolation perfusion with the alkylating agent melphalan to wide excision [3, 7, 10, 12]. The advantages offered by this technique are the limitation of hyperthermia to the tumor-bearing extremities and the establishment of high concentrations of the cytostatic in the perfusion circuit. Judged on the basis of tissue weight the dosage of melphalan which can be administered during isolation perfusion exceeds manyfold the dosages tolerated during multiple oral dosing [1, 2, 5, 13]. Despite attempts to isolate the extremity completely by surgical techniques, leakage of perfusate containing high amounts of cytostatics into the systemic circulation cannot be prevented completely [6, 8]. In this study an attempt is made to determine whether or not the concentrations of melphalan in the systemic circulation correlate quantitatively with the leakage of ^{99m}Tc-labeled erythrocytes. If such a correlation exists, then Tc leakage could indicate the amount of drug reaching the systemic circulation. This information may influence intraoperative decisions.

Methods

Three male and five female patients aged 29 to 67 years were included in the study. Their body weight ranged from 50 to 85 kg. They were suffering from histologically typed high-risk melanoma of the lower extremities with a vertical tumor size equal to or larger than 1.5 mm.

---

*This study was supported by the Deutsche Krebshilfe/Dr. Mildred Scheel Stiftung.

[1] Abteilung für Allgemeinchirurgie, Zentrum Chirurgie, Universitätsklinikum, Robert-Koch-Straße 40, 3400 Göttingen, FRG

[2] Abteilung Nuklearmedizin, Zéntrum Radiologie, Universitätsklinikum, Robert-Koch-Straße 40, 3400 Göttingen, FRG

[3] Abteilung für Innere Medizin, Universitätsklinik, Sigmund-Freud-Straße 25, 5300 Bonn, FRG

R. Jakesz/H Rainer (Eds)
Progress in Regional Cancer Therapy

Hyperthermic isolation perfusion was carried out using an artificial perfusion circuit composed of a Ben V Bentley oxygenator and a roller pump. A semisynthetic medium prepared from concentrated human erythrocytes, human albumin, and saline supplemented with $NaHCO_3$, hematocrit $15 \pm 3\%$, was used. The extremity was perfused via the external iliac artery and vein at a mean pressure of 104 ± 7 mmHg. It was additionally isolated by a tight tourniquet. The mean flow rate during perfusion was 418 ± 75 ml/min. After heating to a subcutaneous temperature of 38°C, melphalan (Alkeran) and ^{99m}Tc-labeled erythrocytes (0.5 mCi) were administered as bolus injections. The melphalan dosage was 10 mg/l limb volume as determined by water displacement. Hyperthermic perfusion was performed for 1 h. Prior to disconnection the melphalan-containing perfusate was washed out and the tubings were primed with drug-free medium.

Samples from the perfusion circuit and peripheral venous blood were drawn at appropriate time points and were immediately stored on ice. ^{99m}Tc-derived radioactivity was counted in a well-type Beckman scintillation counter, and the results were corrected for spontaneous radioactive decomposition. Plasma was prepared by centrifugation and frozen at −20 °C until analysis. Melphalan was extracted from plasma according to [14]. Analysis was performed by HPLC on a Hypersil-phenyl column with 25% acetonitrile in 0.01 *M* phosphate buffer (pH 3.0) as the mobile phase; fluorescence was determined at 270 nm/350 nm. Elution was performed isocratically at a flow rate of 2.0 ml/min. The pharmacokinetic parameters were derived by least squares regression analysis of the terminal phase of the concentration-time curve. Areas under the concentration-time curves (AUC) were determined by the trapezoidal method and extrapolated to infinity. Clearance values were estimated by dose/AUC. The total volume of perfusate after connection was derived from the initial volumes of distribution (V_D) of Tc divided by the extrapolated concentration of radioactivity at zero time (C_0). Alternatively, the volume of perfusate was estimated by the hematocrit method according to Lejeune [8]. The mean value obtained in another series of perfusions ($n = 14$) was used for this purpose. The plasma flow rate was calculated from the volume of perfusate × Tc leakage (%/min) corrected for individual plasma fractions. The drug leakage to be expected was obtained by plasma flow rate × average melphalan concentration in the perfusate, which was estimated according to the basic relationships during multiple dosing with fluctuating concentrations (AUC/τ). All data shown are either individual values or arithmetic means ± S.E.

Results

The pharmacokinetic parameters of melphalan elimination from the perfusion circuit are shown in Table 1. During hyperthermic perfusion the elimination half-life of melphalan in the perfusion medium (32 ± 3 min) was threefold shorter than the reported values during systemic elimination [1, 4, 5]. In control experiments in which no limb was inserted into the circuit the apparent half-lives were 102 and 103 min (data not shown). The decrease of melphalan concentrations during blank perfusion is considered to be caused by adsorption of the drug to the tubing material and by spontaneous decomposition; the latter may be increased during hyperthermia [9]. Clearly, the elimination half-lives observed during limb perfusion

Table 1. Kinetics of elimination of melphalan from the perfusion system during isolation perfusion of the lower extremity

Patient no.	2	5	9	6	7	8	11	18	
Sex	M	M	M	F	F	F	F	F	Mean ± SE
Melphalan dosage (mg)	120	90	120	80	90	75	70	75	
$t_{1/2}$ (min)	34	26	44	38	33	28	20	28	32 ± 3
Cl (ml/min)	92	74	84	71	63	112	84	108	86 ± 6
V_D	0.37	0.31	0.44	0.49	0.33	0.61	0.35	0.59	0.4 ± 0.1
Tc leakage (%/min)	0.6	0.3	0.6	1.5	0.2	0.1	0.4	0.5	
Plasma flow (ml/min)[a]	23	6	15	30	4	–	5	11	
	11	6	11	30	4	2	8	9	

Data are individual values or arithmetic means ± SE; n.d., not determined. Melphalan was administered as a bolus of 10 mg/l limb volume. ^{99m}Tc-labeled erythrocytes were added at total dose of 1.95×10^7 Bq (0.5 mCi). $t_{1/2}$, elimination half-lives of the terminal phase; Cl, clearance (dose/AUC); V_D, initial volume of distribution of melphalan (Cl/k_{el}:k_{el}, elimination rate constant). Tc leakage was derived from the linear of Tc appearance in the peripheral blood.

[a] Plasma flow was calculated from volume of perfusate (upper row, derived from ^{99m}Tc distribution; lower row, derived from the hematocrit values) × Tc leakage × plasma fraction of perfusate after connection.

Table 2. Comparison of expected and observed melphalan concentrations in the systemic circulation

Patient no.	2	5	9	6	7	8	11	18	Mean ± SE
Cl_{total} (ml/min)	432	226	442	333	354	390	354	312	
Drug leakage (mg/min)	0.4	0.1	0.4	0.2	0.1	n.d.	0.1	0.2	
	0.2	0.1	0.5	0.2	0.1	0.1	0.2	0.1	
% of dose, 50 min	(12)	(5)	(19)	(12)	(5)	(7)	(10)	(10)	(10 ± 1)
% Tc leakage 50 min	24	14	20	63	15	4	29	17	23 ± 6
C_{syst} (μg/ml) Expected	0.9	0.6	0.9	0.7	0.2	n.d.	0.3	0.6	
	0.5	0.6	1.1	0.7	0.2	0.1	0.4	0.5	
Observed Minimal	0.4	n.d.	0.6	0.7	n.d.	0.2	0.5	n.d.	
Observed Maximal	0.3	n.d.	0.4	0.5	n.d.	0.1	0.3	n.d.	

Data are individual values or arithmetic means ± SE; n.d; not determined. Cl_{total}, individual total body clearance of melphalan derived from a mean Cl value of 5.21/(min × kg) × body weight [4]. Drug leakage, calculated plasma flow (upper and lower rows corresponding to upper and lower rows of data for plasma flow in Table 1) × average drug concentration in the perfusate ($C_{AV} = AUC/\tau$); % of dose, drug leakage extrapolated from the linear phase to 50 min perfusion time. Cyst expected, drug leakage/Cltotal; Cyst observed, melphalan concentrations in peripheral plasma observed during perfusion.

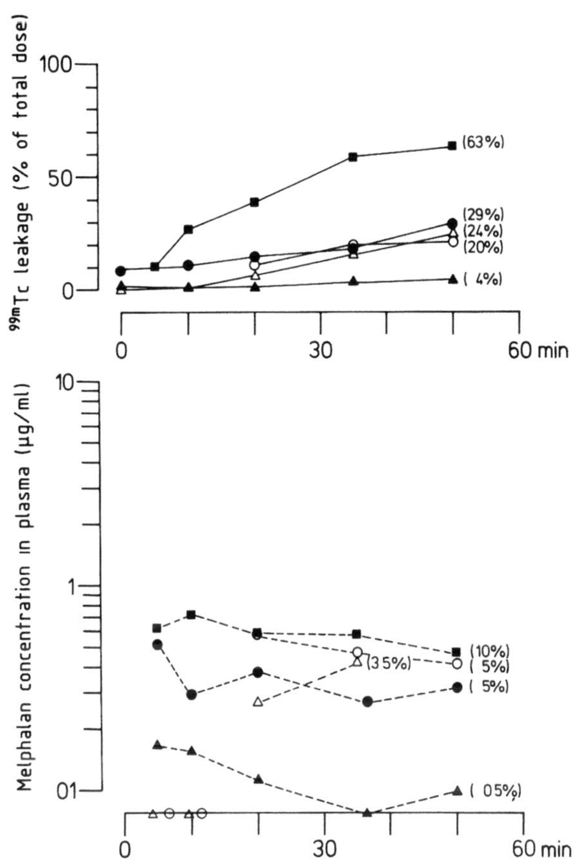

Fig. 1. Appearance of ^{99m}Tc-labeled erythrocytes in the systemic circulation (*upper panel*) and concentrations of melphalan in plasma (*lower panel*). *Values in parentheses*, percentage of concentrations in the perfusate at 50 min

cannot be fully explained by these processes. Therefore we attempted to measure the contribution of leakage of perfusion medium from the artificial circuit into the systemic circulation. ^{99m}Tc-labeled erythrocytes were added to the perfusion system to indicate leakage associated with flow. An almost linear increase in systemic Tc-derived radioactivity was observed, amounting to loss of 4%–63% of the total dose within 50 min (Fig. 1). Leakage of Tc radioactivity expressed as percentage of total dose lost per minute may be converted to the corresponding blood flow rate using the total volume of perfusate after connection. This volume was calculated by estimating the individual V_D of Tc-labeled erythrocytes. Alternatively, it was derived as a mean value from the differences in hematocrit values measured in another series of perfusions before and after connection according to [8]. The results obtained by the two methods agreed satisfactorily, indicating plasma flow rates ranging between 2 and 30 ml/min.

Concomitantly with the flow of ^{99m}Tc-labeled erythrocytes, a fraction of melphalan reaches the systemic circulation. Plasma concentrations ranged from 0.1

to 0.7 μg/ml throughout the perfusion period, and were thus within the range of concentrations established and maintained during systemic chemotherapy by multiple oral dosing [2, 13]. On the other hand, these systemic concentrations were low compared with the drug concentrations in the perfusion medium. The perfusate concentrations were 10- to 200-fold higher than the systemic values shown in the lower panel of Fig. 1. Thus melphalan leakage is much lower than Tc leakage, and the question arises of whether melphalan leakage can be correlated quantitatively with Tc-labeled erythrocyte kinetics so that it can be used as an indicator for systemic melphalan concentration during limb perfusion. Melphalan leakage can be interpreted as individually constant. In order to predict the amount of drug leakage, the average concentration of melphalan in the perfusate was derived from kinetic parameters. According to the basic concepts of infusion kinetics the range of expected systemic drug concentration was calculated from these data (Table 2). Comparison with the melphalan concentrations actually measured in the systemic circulation (depicted for clarity as the minimal and maximal observed values) showed that correct prediction of the overall drug leakage was possible (Table 2).

Discussion

It is generally accepted that in addition to wide excision of malignant melanoma an attack on the tumor cells by a chemotherapeutic approach in combination with hyperthermia will improve therapeutic success [3, 7, 10, 12]. If tumor localization is adequate, hyperthermic isolation perfusion with the alkylating agent melphalan becomes feasible, thereby concentrating the therapy on the melanoma-bearing tissue. The frequency of local toxic side effects such as damage to muscle tissue, edema formation, blistering of the skin, necrosis or thrombophlebitis can be kept low by preventing the temperature from exceeding 40 °C in the subcutaneous tissue [3, 11, 12].

The occurrence of systemic toxicity mediated by the fraction of dose reaching the systemic circulation can be minimized by functional isolation of the perfused tissue using a tight tourniquet. As already reported [6, 8], the leakage of perfusion medium from the artificial circuit into the systemic circulation cannot be prevented completely. Despite the use of standardized techniques during surgery, the extent of melphalan leakage showed marked interindividual differences. The melphalan concentrations occurring in the systemic circulation during perfusion are within the range established during systemic chemotherapy [1, 2, 5, 13], and are therefore of therapeutic relevance.

On the other hand a large concentration gradient existed between the artificial circuit and the systemic circulation. Thus, although leakage occurs, there is a rationale for establishing high concentrations of the cytostatic within the target tissue.

It is essential to estimate the leakage in each individual patient during the perfusion period in order to minimize the severity of systemic toxicity. As the measurement of melphalan concentration is time consuming, the possibility that Tc-labeled erythrocytes might serve as an indicator for the amount of drug leakage was investigated. In this study, there was good agreement between observed melphalan concentrations in the systemic circulation and those predicted by Tc leakage. Taking into consideration the basic pharmacokinetic relationships used here, the results indicate that melphalan leakage is mediated by blood transport which is described adequately by infusion kinetics. In consequence, only that fraction of melphalan present in the perfusion circuit and not the amount trapped in the tissue can be correlated with leakage of Tc-labeled erythrocytes.

In conclusion, our results have shown that leakage of Tc-labeled erythrocytes during isolation perfusion of the lower limb with the cytostatic drug melphalan may serve as an indicator for systemic concentrations of melphalan. As Tc-labeled erythrocytes can be measured during operation, this method potentially enables reliable assessment of major systemic exposure.

References

1. Ardiet C, Tranchand B, Biron P, Rebattu P, Philip T (1986) Pharmacokinetics of high-dose intravenous melphalan in children and adults with forced diuresis. Cancer Chemother Pharmacol 16:300–305
2. Bosanquet AG, Gilby ED (1982) Pharmacokinetics of oral and intravenous melphalan during routine treatment of multiple myeloma. Eur J Cancer Clin Oncol 18:355–362
3. Ghussen F, Nagel K, Groth W, Müller JM, Stützer H (1984) A prospective randomized study of regional extremity perfusions in patients with malignant melanoma. Ann Surg 200:764–768
4. Goodman LS, Gilman A (1985) The pharmacological basis of therapeutics, 7th edn. Macmillan, New York, pp 1694, 1725
5. Gouyette A, Hartmann O, Pico JL (1986) Pharmacokinetics of high-dose melphalan in children and adults. Cancer Chemother Pharmacol 16:184–189
6. Hafstrom L, Hugander A, Jonsson PE, Westling H, Ehrsson H (1984) Blood leakage and melphalan leakage from the perfusion circuit during regional hyperthermic perfusion for malignant melanoma. Cancer Treat Rep 68:867–872
7. Krementz ET, Carter RD, Sutherland CM, Muchmore JH (1987) Chemotherapy by regional perfusion for limb melanoma. Am Surg 53:133–140
8. Lejeune FJ, Ghanem EG (1987) A simple and accurate new method for cytostatics dosimetry in isolation perfusion of the limbs based on exchangeable blood volume determination. Cancer Res 47:639–643
9. Loos U, Musch E, Rauschecker H, Willenbrock C (1988) Melphalan kinetics in hyperthermic isolation perfusion of the extremities. Sixth Mediterranean congress of chemotherapy. Taormina, 22–27 May 1988 (abstr 439)
10. Martijn H, Schraffordt Koops H, Milton GW, Nap M, Oosterhuis JW, Shaw HM, Oldhoff J (1986) Comparison of two methods of treating primary malignant melanomas Clark IV and V, thickness 1.5 mm and greater, localized on the extremities. Cancer 57:1923–1930
11. Minor DR, Allen RE, Alberts D, Peng YM, Tardelli G, Hutchinson J (1985) A clinical and pharmacokinetic study of isolated limb perfusion with heat and melphalan for melanoma. Cancer 55:2638–2644
12. Rege VB, Leone AL, Soderberg CH, Coleman GV, Robidoux HJ, Fijman R, Brown J (1983) Hyperthermic adjuvant perfusion chemotherapy for stage I malignant melanoma of the extremity with literature review. Cancer 52:2033–2039
13. Taha IAK, Ahmad RA, Gray H, Roberts CI, Rogers HJ (1982) Plasma melphalan and prednisolone concentrations during oral therapy for multiple myeloma. Cancer Chemother Pharmacol 9:57–60
14. Woodhouse KW, Henderson DB (1981) High pressure liquid chromatographic method for the determination of melphalan in plasma. Proceedings of British Pharmacological Society, 16–18 Dec. Br J Clin Pharmacol 13(4):605 pp

Clinical and Histopathological Aspects of Hyperthermic Isolated Regional Perfusion of Soft Tissue Sarcomas of the Extremities

H.J. Hoekstra, W.M. Molenaar, H. Schraffordt Koops, and J. Oldhoff

Division of Surgical Oncology, Groningen University Hospital, P.O. Box 30001, 9700 RB Groningen, The Netherlands

Introduction

The treatment of a soft tissue sarcoma (STS) of an extremity depends on the location and size of the tumor, the histological diagnosis and tumor grade, the tumor stage, and the previous therapy. Limb salvage and prevention of local recurrence are the two major considerations in the treatment of a malignant STS of an extremity. After inadequate therapy, there is a grave risk of local recurrence, which generally occurs within two years [16]. This is why "unresectable" STS of an extremity have been treated preferably by amputation of the limb. Hyperthermic isolated regional perfusion was introduced into the treatment of STS of the extremity with the idea of increasing the resectability rate without increasing the risk of local recurrence [9]. The rationale of combined modality therapy is that with hyperthermic isolated regional perfusion the tumor and adjacent tissue can be treated with high doses of chemotherapeutic agents and that hyperthermia enhances the sensitivity of tumor cells to chemotherapy [3, 4, 19].

Patients and Methods

During the period 1965–1976 a total of 18 patients with STS of an extremity were treated by regional perfusion with cytostatics and local excision of the tumor. None of the patients received additional radiotherapy or chemotherapy. All patients treated during this period were analyzed in detail. The tumor histology was reexamined by one pathologist (WMM). The disease was classified according to the guidelines of the American Joint Committee on Cancer [1].

During the period 1965–1969 patients were perfused under hypothermic or normothermic conditions (temperature below or equal to 37°C). All perfusions performed since have been hyperthermic (39–40°C). Skin and muscle temperatures of upper and lower extremity were monitored using thermistor probes. For perfusion of the upper extremity the axillary artery and vein were cannulated after general heparinization (3.3 mg/kg body weight), for the lower extremity, the external iliac artery and vein. To prevent leakage of cytostatics to the systemic circulation, a tourniquet was placed round the shoulder or thigh. The limb was heated with the aid

R. Jakesz/H. Rainer (Eds.)
Progress in Regional Cancer Therapy

Table 1. Clinical data, histologic type, tumor stage, therapy, and follow-up

Patient no	Age (years)	Sex	Year of publication	Tumor site	Primary/ recurrent	Diagnosis	Metastases	Stage	Perfusion	Recurrence	Follow-up
1	41	F	1965	Thigh	Primary	Fibrosarcoma	—	IIIB	Melphalan	—	NED 23 years
2	19	M	1968	Forearm	Primary	Epithelioid sarcoma	Axilla, bicipital sulcus	IIIC	Melphalan	—	NED 20 years
3	49	M	1970	Thigh	Primary	Myxoid liposarcoma	—	IB	Melphalan	—	NED 18 years
4	59	F	1970	Thigh	Primary	MFH	Inguinal	IIIC	Melphalan	Lung/bone 11 months	DOD 11 months
5	32	F	1970	Wrist	Recurrent	Epithelioid sarcoma	Bicipital suscus	IIIC	Melphalan	Lung 24 months	DOD 35 months
6	20	F	1971	Elbow	Primary	Clear cell sarcoma	—	IIIB	Melphalan	Axilla 43 months	DOD 56 months
7	54	F	1971	Thigh	Primary	MFH	—	IIIB	Melphalan	—	NED 17 years
8	35	M	1971	Foot	Primary	Fibrosarcoma	—	IIIA	Melphalan	Liver 46 mo	DOD 52 mo
9	46	M	1972	Thigh	Recurrent	Liposarcoma	—	IA	Melphalan	—	NED 16 years
10	19	M	1972	Upper arm	Primary	Fibrosarcoma	—	IB	Melphalan	—	NED 16 years
11	31	F	1975	Thigh	Primary	Synovial sarcoma	—	IIIB	Melphalan/ dactinomycin	—	NED 13 years
12	17	M	1975	Knee	Recurrent	Synovial sarcoma	—	IIIB	Melphalan/ dactinomycin	—	NED 13 years
13	60	F	1975	Lower leg	Primary	MFH	—	IIIB	Melphalan/ dactinomycin	Scar 48 months	NED[a] 13 years
14	51	F	1975	Thigh	Recurrent	MFH	—	IIIA	Melphalan/ dactinomycin	Lung 48 months	NED[a] 13 years
15	62	M	1975	Forearm	Primary	MFH	—	IIIA	Melphalan/ dactinomycin	—	Died 8 months, lung carcinoma
16	64	F	1975	Thigh	Recurrent	MFH	—	IIIB	Melphalan/ dactinomycin	—	NED 13 years
17	64	F	1976	Thigh	Primary	MFH	—	IIIB	Melphalan/ dactinomycin	—	NED 12 years
18	48	F	1976	Thigh	Primary	Liposarcoma	—	IB	Melphalan/ dactinomycin	Abdomen 21 months	DOD 6 years

MFH, malignant fibrous histiocytoma; NED no evidence of disease; DOD, dead of disease.
[a] Resection recurrence.

of a heat exchanger in the oxygenator and locally with a warm-water mattress. The limb was perfused with the aid of a pump oxygenator. The perfusate contained 350 ml Isodex (Pharmacia AB, Sweden), 500 ml blood, and 30 ml 8.4% sodium bicarbonate and heparin. Melphalan (L-phenylalanine mustard) was added to the perfusate: 1–1.5 mg/kg body weight for the lower extremity, 0.5–0.7 mg/kg body weight for the upper extremity. From 1975 melphalan was combined with 0.5–1 mg dactinomycin (0.014 mg and 0.006 mg/kg body weight for the lower and upper extremity respectively). After 60 min perfusion the extremity was washed with a neutral fluid, the catheters removed, and the vessels closed and heparin antagonized with 1.65 mg protamine chloride/kg body weight. The perfusion technique was described previously in detail [18]. After completion of the perfusion the tumor was radically excised. In view of lymph node metastases, a lymph node dissection was performed. All patients with an upper extremity sarcoma underwent axillary lymph node dissection for technical reasons. In all patients fasciotomy of the limb was performed to prevent a compartment syndrome [17].

The clinical data, histologic type, tumor stage, therapy, and follow-up are presented in Table 1. In six patients the tumor resected after perfusion was compared to the late follow-up material of metastatic disease for morphological changes in relation to therapy. Fourteen tumors were classified grade III, four grade I; 11 were primary and seven recurrent STS. Three patients had lymph node metastasis. None of the patients received systemic adjuvant chemotherapy or external beam radiotherapy.

Results

In one patient (no. 5) the perfusion was discontinued after 15 min due to severe leakage of cytostatic to the systemic circulation. There was no peroperative or 30-day mortality and no vascular complications. The median follow-up was 16 years. The actuarial 5-year and 10-year survival rates were 76% and 69% respectively for high-grade STS and 100% and 75% respectively for low-grade STS (Fig. 1). A local recurrence was diagnosed in one patient (6%) and distant metastases in six patients (33%). The disease-free 5-year and 10-year survival rates were 71% and 57% respectively for high-grade STS and 75% for low-grade STS (Fig. 2).

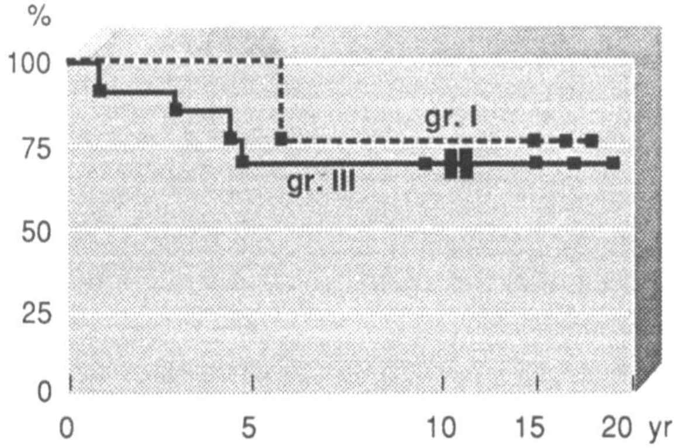

Fig. 1. Regional perfusion treatment for soft tissue sarcomas: actuarial survival

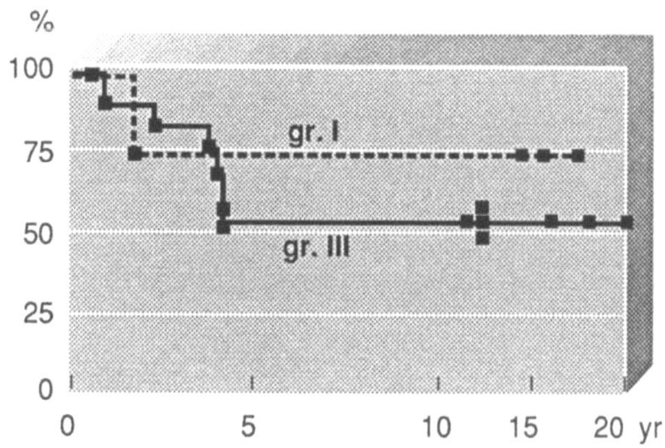

Fig. 2. Regional perfusion treatment for soft tissue sacromas: recurrence-free survival

The histology of the recurrent or metastatic tumor was similar to the respective primary tumors or revealed progression in the histologic malignancy and were previously described in detail [15].

Discussion

In the mid-1970s a switch was made in the treatment of STS to combined surgery and postoperative radiotherapy, based on the favorable results reported in the literature [21]. The results of isolated regional perfusion and surgery are generally comparable to those of surgery and postoperative radiotherapy [3, 8, 11, 12, 14, 20]. The local recurrence rate ranges from 6% to 25% with a 2-year survival rate of 69%–100% and a 5-year survival rate of 56%–76%. Generally 30%–40% of patients with high-grade STS will develop distant metastasis.

The morbidity of the isolated regional perfusion treatment with melphalan and dactinomycin is lower than that of the combined surgery and postoperative radiotherapy. Isolated regional perfusion with doxorubicin bears a high complication rate. In a small series of 14 patients, 36% underwent amputation due to doxorubicin-related complications, and in children a toxic effect on the epiphyseal growth plates of the long bones with epiphyseal fusion was found [2]. Isolated regional perfusion is also used in combination with a variety of post-treatment schedules, such as postoperative radiotherapy and intra-arterial chemotherapy [6]. It is also employed as an adjuvant treatment after primary surgical resection of an extremity sarcoma, without improving local control rates [13].

Another combined modality therapy in the treatment of STS is intra-arterial chemotherapy and preoperative radiotherapy, resection, and postoperative radiotherapy. This treatment schedule is especially used in the treatment of primarily "unresectable" high-grade STS of the extremity. The combination of intra-arterial chemotherapy and preoperative radiotherapy may produce shrinkage of the tumor. The results are promising, but morbidity is high compared to perfusion treatment [5, 10].

In our limited experience, perfusion treatment for STS appears to be highly effective. Isolated perfusion under physiological conditions with optimal dosage of cytostatic agents may increase the perfusion effect [7, 22, 23]. There is renewed

Table 2. Tumor recurrence and survival in patients with malignant soft tissue sarcomas of the extremities treated by isolated regional perfusion and surgery with or without chemotherapy and/or radiotherapy

Reference	Year	Number of patients	AJCC stage	Adjuvant chemo- and/or radio-therapy	Median follow-up (years)	Recurrence		Survival		
						Local	Distant	Two years	Five years	Ten years
McBride [14]	1974	90	I–IV	No	?	25%	?	69%	59%	45%
Stehlin et al. [20]	1975	37	I–IV	If indicated	?	16%	?	76%	62%	—
Ghussen and Nagel [8]	1984	15	I–III	No	2	7%	0%	100%	—	—
Lehti et al. [12]	1986	64	I–IV	If indicated	5	10%	?	88%	67%	—
Krementz [11]	1986	56	I–III	If indicated	?	21%	?	?	65%	65%
Filippo et al. [6]	1988	29	I–IV	No	?	24%	37%	75%	48%	48%
Hoekstra et al. [10]	1989	18	I–III	No	16	6%	33%	94%	76%	71%

interest in perfusion treatment for STS of the extremities. A new option might be hyperthermic isolated regional perfusion under optimal physiological conditions with optimal dosage of cytostatic agents, followed by delayed excision [3–6 weeks later), allowing shrinkage of the tumor and assessment of tumor response to chemotherapy. In view of our results and the findings reported in the literature, further investigations into the value of hyperthermic isolated regional perfusion in the treatment of STS of the extremity seem to be indicated.

References

1. Beahrs OH, Myers MH (eds) (1983) Manual for staging of cancer: soft tissues. American Joint Committee on Cancer, 2nd edn. Lippincott, Philadelphia, pp 111–115
2. Braat RP, Wieberdink J, van Slooten EA, Olthuis G (1983) Regional perfusion with Adriamycin in soft tissue sarcomas. In: Schwemmle K, Aignerk (eds) Vascular perfusion in cancer therapy. Springer, Berlin Heidelberg New York, Recent results in cancer research, vol 86, pp 260–263
3. Cavaliere R, Ciogatto EC, Giovanella BC et al. (1967) Selective heat sensitivity of cancer cells: biochemical and clinical studies. Cancer 20:1351–1381
4. Creech O Jr, Krementz ET, Ryan RF, Winblad JN (1958) Chemotherapy for cancer. Ann Surg 148:616–632
5. Eilber FR, Morton DL, Eckhardt J, Grant TT, Weisenburger T (1984) Limb salvage for skeletal and soft tissue sarcomas. Multidisciplinary preoperative therapy. Cancer 53:2579–2584
6. Filippo FD, Calabro AM, Cavallari A et al. (1988) The role of hyperthermic perfusion as a first step in the treatment of soft tissue sarcoma of the extremities. World J Surg 12: 332–339
7. Fontijne WPJ, Mook PH, Schraffordt Koops H, Oldhoff J, Wildevuur ChRH (1985) Improved tissue perfusion during pressure regulated hyperthermic regional perfusion: a clinical study. Cancer 3:278–284
8. Ghussen F, Nagel K (1984) Die regionale hypertherme Cytostatica perfusion als Alternative bei der Behandlung von malignen Weichgewebetumoren der Extremitäten. Chirurg 55:505–507
9. Hoekstra HJ, Schraffordt Koops H, Molenaar WM, Oldhoff J (1987) Results of isolated regional perfusion in the treatment of malignant soft tissue tumors of the extremities. Cancer 60:1703–1707
10. Hoekstra HJ, Schraffordt Koops H, Molenaar WM et al. (1989) A combination of intraarterial chemotherapy, pre- and postoperative radiotherapy and surgery as limb-saving treatment of primarily "unresectable" high grade soft tissue sarcomas of the extremities Cancer 63:59–62
11. Krementz ET (1986) Regional perfusion: current sophistication, what next? Cancer 3:416–432
12. Lehti PM, Moseley HS, Janoff K, Stevens K, Fletcher WS (1986) Improved survival for soft tissue sarcoma of the extremities by regional hyperthermic perfusion, local excision and radiation therapy. Surg Gynecol Obstet 162:149–152
13. Lejeune FJ, Lienard D, Ewalenko P (1988) Hyperthermic isolation perfusion of the limbs with cytostatics after surgical excision of sarcomas. World J Surg 12:345–348
14. McBride CM (1974) Sarcomas of the limbs: results of adjuvant chemotherapy using isolation perfusion. Arch Surg 109:304–308
15. Molenaar WM, Hoekstra HJ, Dam-Meiring A (1990) Histopathological aspects and DNA ploidy in soft tissue sarcomas treated with combined modality therapy. In preparation

16. Chang AE, Rosenberg SA, Glatstein EJ, Antham KH (1989) Sarcomas of soft tissues. In: DeVita VT, Hellman S, Rosenberg SA (eds) Cancer principles and practice of oncology, 3rd edn. Lippincott, Philadelphia, pp 1345–1398
17. Schraffordt Koops H (1972) Prevention of neural and muscular lesions during hyperthermic regional perfusion. Surg Gynecol Obstet 135:401–403
18. Schraffordt Koops H, Oldhoff J, Oosterhuis JW, Beekhuis H (1987) Isolated perfusion in malignant melanoma of the extremities. World J Surg 11:527–533
19. Stehlin JS Jr (1969) Hyperthermic perfusion with chemotherapy for cancers of the extremities. Surg Gynecol Obstet 129:305–308
20. Stehlin JS, Delpolyi PD, Giovanella BC, Guiterrez AE, Anderson RF (1975) Soft tissue sarcomas of the extremity: multidisciplinary therapy employing hyperthermic perfusion. Am J Surg 130:643–646
21. Suit HD, Russell WO, Martin RG (1975) Sarcoma of soft tissue: Clinical and histopathologic parameters and response to treatment. Cancer 35:1478–1483
22. van Os J, Schraffordt Koops H, Oldhoff J (1985) Dosimetry of cytostatics in hyperthermic regional isolated perfusion. Cancer 3:698–701
23. Wieberdink J, Benkhuizen C, Braat RP, van Slooten EA, Olthuis GAA (1982) Dosimetry in isolated perfusion of the limbs by assessment of perfused tissue volume and grading of toxic reaction. Eur J Cancer Clin Oncol 18:905–910

LASER THERAPY

Experimental Basis of CO_2 Laser Application in Tumor Surgery

A. Tuchmann, C. Armbruster, W. Blauensteiner, and S. Kriwanek

1. Chirurgische Abteilung, Rudolfstiftung, Juchgasse 25, 1030 Wien, Austria

Introduction

Lasers have been applied in a wide field of medicine and surgery: recently, experience in general surgery has been reported [1, 15]. Especially regarding tumor surgery, there was great hope among laser surgeons of achieving better results than with conventional means such as cold knife and electrocautery. This paper deals with the cutting type CO_2 laser, reporting on survival rate, local recurrence, and contact metastases in animal experiments

Animal Experiments: Methods and Results

Local Recurrence and Morality Due to the Tumor

In the 1970s Frishman et al. [3] and Peled et al. [10] compared the mortality of the scalpel, electrocautery, and CO_2 laser methods of tumor excision in mice which had been inoculated with 3LL fibrosarcoma [3]. The mortality rates (7% by laser, 23% by scalpel, 21% by electrocautery) confirm laser excision as the method of choice. Peled et al. [10] reported similar results in mice when the operation took place on the 5th day following tumor inoculation (Lewis lung carcinoma) mortality was 28% by laser, 75% by scalpel, and 45% by electrocautery. Mortality rates were identical when the tumors were excised on the 6th day after inoculation (73% by laser, 75% by scalpel).

Mahn et al. [5] compared local recurrence and mortality in mice after curative and palliative tumor excision in the Lewis lung carcinoma. In the case of curative resection the local recurrence rate was 12% for CO_2 laser and 23% for scalpel; mortality was 45% vs 66%. The differences became highly significant when tumor excision was non radical (palliative operation): local recurrence rate 36% (laser) vs 81% (scalpel); mortality 55% vs 100%.

Our own excision experiments [14] with Lewis lung carcinoma in C57Bl/6 mice yielded similar survival curves for CO_2 laser excision and conventional scalpel excision. However, there was a difference ($p < 0.005$, Breslow test) in local recurrence in favor of the laser method (Fig. 1). Distinguishing between different sizes of tumor

R. Jakesz/H Rainer (Eds)
Progress in Regional Cancer Therapy

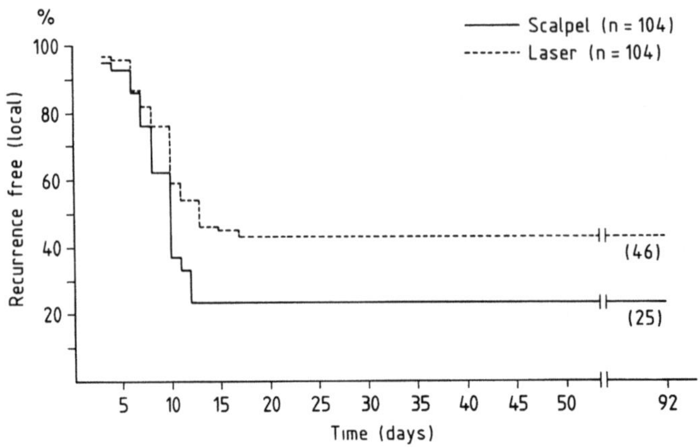

Fig. 1. Local recurrence: scalpel vs CO_2 laser excision [14]

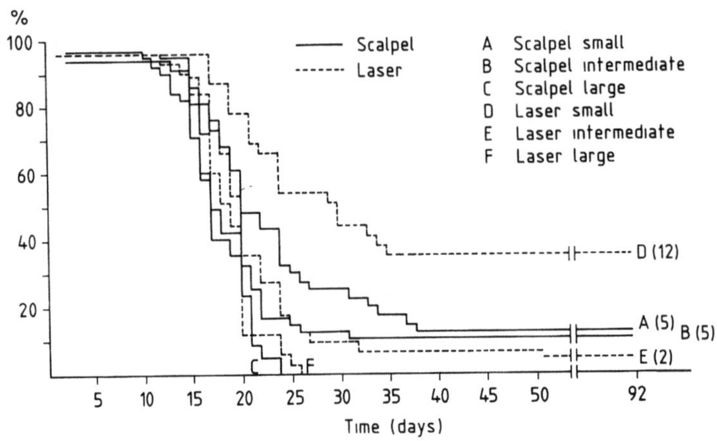

Fig. 2. Survival curves for different sizes of tumor [14]

excised by laser or scalpel, it transpired that the laser method yielded better survival rates only with small tumors (Fig. 2).

Lanzafame et al. [4] experimented with R 3230 AC mammary carcinoma in Fisher 344 rats. Local recurrence occurred in 5/15 rats treated by CO_2 laser and in 14/15 treated by scalpel. The disease-free interval was 26 days and 12 days respectively ($p < 0.001$).

Sealing of Lymph and Blood Vessels

The sealing of lymph and blood vessels was assessed differently. Pariente [8] experimented with the rabbit ear model and Evans blue. There were no particles of Evans blue opposite the laser incision. Blood vessels of up to 1.5 mm in diameter were sealed.

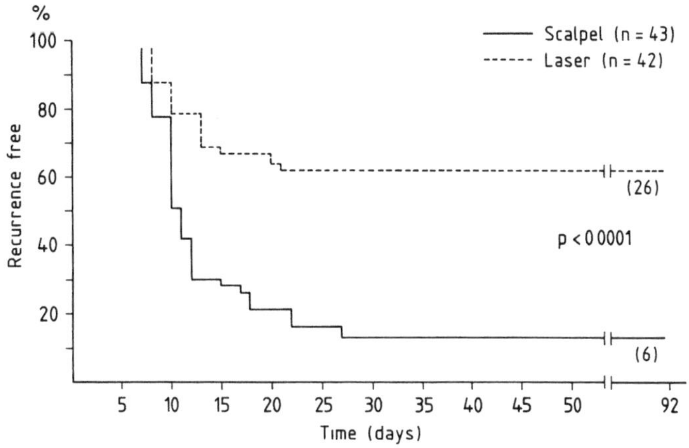

Fig. 3. Contact metastases: scalpel-produced vs CO_2 laser-produced tumor surface ($p < 0.0001$) [14]

Oosterhuis [6] found a decreased activity of ^{3}H-thymidine-labeled tumor cells in mouse iliac lymph nodes using a CO_2 laser instead of a cold knife (Cloudman S91 melanoma: On the other hand, Ehrenberger and Innitzer [2] reported seeing Evans blue beyond the laser incision because the laser seals lymph vessels only temporarily due to its carbonization zone. Plenk and coworkers [11] found particles of India ink in regional lymph nodes, confirming lack of sealing with the laser technique.

Contact Metastases

A smear of cells of Lewis lung carcinoma was swabbed onto the subcutaneous tissue of tumor-free C57Bl/6 mice. This tumor smear was taken from a tumor surface produced by cutting either with a scalpel or with a CO_2 laser [14]. Tumor growth rates were lower and host survival times were longer when laser was used ($p < 0.0001$; Fig. 3). Pavelka et al. [9] induced contact metastases in C57Bl/6 mice by means of tumor disks of defined thickness (Lewis lung carcinoma). Tumor growth was 100% with the scalpel method. When such disks were cut with a laser and implanted in tumor-free animals, the rate of growth depended on the thickness of the disk. No growth was seen at a thickness of 0.8 mm, but rates of 50% and 83% were seen at disk thicknesses of 1.26 mm and 1.32 mm respectively ($p < 0.001$).

Discussion and Conclusions

Up to now no specific anticancerous effect of laser has been reported. The effects of some lasers (noncontact Nd:YAG, contact Nd:YAG, CO_2) like those of electrocautery, are no more than thermic [12]. Nevertheless, malignant tumors can be destroyed by electro-coagulation; this method yielded complete remission in 16/64 rats (mammary tumor) [13]. Lower rates of local recurrence were reported in most studies whenever the CO_2 laser was used for tumor excision. Survival depends more on the interval between tumor inoculation and excision [10] and on tumor size [14] than on the method employed (CO_2 laser, scalpel). Contact metastases are avoided by using CO_2 lasers [9, 14]. A tumor disk of 0.8 mm thickness did not produce tumor growth because tumor cells at a distance of 0.4 mm from the laser cut are not viable [9]. Most likely there were no viable tumor cells in the waste products (debris and smoke) of the laser operation [7].

If one may extrapolate the results of animal experiments to tumor surgery in humans, the following conclusions appear to be relevant. CO_2 laser excision is superior to scalpel excision if the site of the incision is close to the tumor; in the event that the tumor is opened by the surgeon, contact metastases are less likely to develop.

However, when cutting through nontumorous tissue, as in the case of mastectomy, the CO_2 laser only lowers rates of postoperative pain and seroma rather than conveying any oncological benefit.

References

1. Dixon JA (1988) Current laser applications in general surgery. Ann Surg 207:355–372
2. Ehrenberger K, Innitzer J (1978) Die Wirkung des CO_2-Lasers auf Hautlymphgefäße. Wien Klin Wochenschr 90:307–309
3. Frishman A, Gassner S, Kaplan I, Ger R (1974) Excision of subcutaneous fibrosarcoma in mice. A comparative experimental study of various methods. Isr J Med Sci 10:637–641
4. Lanzafame RJ, Rogers DW, Naim JO, DeFranco CA, Ochej H, Hinshaw JR (1986) Reduction of local tumor recurrence by excision with the CO_2 laser. Lasers Surg Med 6:439–441
5. Mahn HR, Nowak C, Audring H, Liebetruth J, Lindenau KF (1982) Tierexperimenteller Vergleich der therapeutischen Effektivität einer Tumorexcision mittels Skalpell oder CO_2-Laser am subkutan implantierten Lewis-lung-Karzinom. Z Exp Chir 15:38–47
6. Oosterhuis JW (1978) Lymphatic migration after laser surgery. Lancet I:446–447
7. Oosterhuis JW, Verschueren RCJ, Eidergen R, Oldhoff J (1982) The viability of cells in the waste products of CO_2 laser evaporation of Cloudman mouse Melanomas. Cancer 49:61–67
8. Pariente R (1976) The Sharplan 791 laser in the treatment of skin tumors. In: Kaplan I (ed) Laser surgery I. Jerusalem Academic, Jerusalem, pp 31–35
9. Pavelka R, Köhler W, Neuhold N, Burian K (1987) Gibt es einen spezifischen Einfluß des CO_2-Laserchnittes auf das Tumorwachstum? Arch Otorhinolaryngol [Suppl II]:21–22
10. Peled I, Shohat B, Gassner S, Kaplan I (1976) Excision of epithelial tumors: CO_2 laser versus conventional methods. Cancer Lett 2:41–46
11. Plenk H jr, Kyrle P, Fischer PL (1981) Bringt der CO_2-Laserchnitt Vorteile? Wien Klin Wochenschr 93:230–235
12. Schroder T, Brackett K, Joffe SN (1987) An experimental study of the effects of electrocautery and various lasers on gastrointestinal tissue. Surgery 101:691–697
13. Strauss AA, Appel M, Saphir O (1962) Electrocoagulation of malignant tumors. Am J Surg 104:37–45
14. Tuchmann A, Bauer P, Plenk H jr, Braun O, Dinstl K (1986) Comparative study of conventional scalpel and CO_2-laser in experimental tumor surgery. Res Exp Med (Berl) 186:375–386
15. Wieman TJ (1986) Lasers and the surgeon. Am J Surg 151:493–500

Experience with CO_2 Laser in Tumor Surgery

K. Dinstl and A. Tuchmann

1. Chirurgische Abteilung, Krankenanstalt Rudolfstiftung, Juchgasse 25, 1030 Wien, Austria

Introduction

The CO_2 laser is used in general surgery for noncontact cutting of tissues. Its use in tumor surgery is based on speculation that it seals lymph vessels, thus preventing lymphogenous spread of tumor cells during the operation. This was first reported by Kaplan and Ger [3], but results of experimental investigations have been controversial. Our own experiments have demonstrated the following:

1. The incidence of tumor growth is much lower when wounds are exposed to CO_2 laser before swabbing tumor cells into them.
2. The local recurrence rate is lower when tumor excision is done by CO_2 laser.

We have used the CO_2 laser in 1600 operations since 1975. Most were done in patients with superficial tumors, including breast cancer in women and malignant tumors of the soft tissue and the skin.

In 1973 Kaplan and Ger [3] were the first to report the results of CO_2 laser surgery for breast cancer: Since then several clinical studies [1,2,4,6] have demonstrated positive effects of laser surgery on intraoperative blood loss and hematoma and seroma formation. However, no data exist on the local recurrence rate and long-term survival after laser therapy for breast cancer. Lanzafame [5] reported fewer local recurrences after laser therapy for breast cancer in rats. The follow-up of 449 patients operated on for breast cancer from 1975 to 1985 showed reduced incidence of recurrences only when radical mastectomy had been done (Table 1). The incidence of tumor recurrence depended on the procedure used, but it seems that the use of CO_2 laser in breast cancer surgery gives an advantage over conventional methods relating to local recurrence. The standardized axillary lymph node dissection could not be done by laser because laser dissection would endanger axillary vessels or nerves.

In order to assess the usefulness of CO_2 laser resection in breast cancer a randomized study was started in 1981.

Patients and Method

One hundred and forty-one women (mean age 56 years) have been operated upon since 1981. Seventy-six were treated by laser, 65 by scalpel resection. After ensuring

R. Jakesz/H Rainer (Eds.)
Progress in Regional Cancer Therapy

Table 1. Local recurrence after CO_2 laser operations for breast cancer

Resection	*n*	Recurrence
Lumpectomy	18	6 (33%)
Modified radical	15	6 (40%)
Radical	416	20 (4.8%)
	449	32 (7.1%)

comparability by age, clinical tumor stage, and pre- or postmenopausal state, assignment to the treatment groups was random. Radical mastectomy with axillary lymph node dissection was performed in all patients. The laser used was a CO_2 SHARPLAN. Skin incisions and axillary dissections were always carried out by conventional techniques.

Results

Microscopic examination of the surgical specimens demonstrated a similar distribution of histological tumor stages in both groups (Table 2). Hormone receptor analysis showed comparable results in both groups. The percentage of patients receiving chemotherapy was similar too (Table 3).

One hundred and thirty-six patients (96%) were followed up. The mean duration of follow-up was 37 months range 3–110 months). We found local recurrence rates of 8% after laser and 3% after conventional surgery (difference not significant). Mortality rates were similar (28% after laser, 24% after conventional therapy).

Kaplan–Meier evaluation of survival demonstrated a highly significant difference

Table 2. Controlled study of CO_2laser vs scalpel in breast cancer: tumor stage

	Clinical tumor stage (*n*)		Histological tumor stage			
	T1	T2	pT1	pT2	pT3	pT4
Laser group	39	37	29%	59%	8%	4%
Conventional group	33	32	27%	60%	10%	3%

Table 3. Controlled study of CO_2 laser vs scalpel in breast cancer: hormone receptors and chemotherapy

	Hormone receptors		Chemotherapy
	+	–	
Laser group	70%	30%	50%
Conventional group	64%	36%	47%

between the therapy groups [3]. Thus, CO_2 laser therapy does not seem to offer a significant advantage over conventional techniques in the treatment of breast cancer according to local recurrence and survival.

Undeniable, however, are the benefits of CO_2 laser in the excision of extensive tumors of the breast. Our experience in 39 patients with extensive tumors showed the following advantages of laser surgery over conventional procedures:

1. Less bleeding
2. Potential reduction of excision of skin to a minimum
3. Reduction of local recurrence
4. Less postoperative pain
5. Possibility of primary skin grafting in exulcerated or infected tumors

No definitive statement regarding survival time can be made, as the number of patients is too small to perform a prospective study.

Our findings in CO_2 laser surgery of soft tissue tumors and skin tumors are similar. There are no comparative studies, but the tendency toward lower recurrence rates is noteworthy.

Conclusions

In our experience, the advantages of CO_2 laser in the surgery of malignant tumors are as follows:

1. Operative: (a) cutting without pressure, (b) reduced bleeding, (c) less postoperative pain, (d) fewer wound infections (and seromas)
2. Oncologic: reduced local recurrence rate (?), but probably no influence on survival time.

The disadvantages are:

1. Longer operating time
2. Slower healing of skin incisions
3. Possibility of thermic lesions
4. Excessive smoke production
5. Indications limited for surgery of superficial tumors

References

1. Ansanelli VW (1986) CO_2 laser in cancer surgery of the breast: a comparative clinical study. Lasers Surg Med. 6(5):470
2. Dinstl K (1982) Die Operation des Mammakarzinoms mit dem CO_2-Laser. In: Verhandlungsbericht der Deutschen Gesellschaft für Laser-medizin e. V., Munich, p 65
3. Kaplan I, Ger R (1973) Partial mastectomy and mammaplasty performed with a CO_2 surgical laser. J Plast Surg 26:363
4. Kott J (1981) The CO_2 laser in mastectomy. A comparative study. In: Proceedings of 4th Congress of International Society for Laser Surgery, Tokyo (abstr 244)
5. Lanzafame RJ (1986) The effects of CO_2 laser excision on local tumor recurrence. Laser Surg Med 6:103
6. Wang YH (1987) Laser operation for breast cancer. Int Surg 72(4):208

Nd:YAG Laser Application in the Surgical Treatment of Cancer

H.-J. Meyer and R. Pichlmayr

Zentrum Chirurgie, Klinik für Abdominal- und Transplantationschirurgie, Medizinische Hochschule Hannover, Konstanty-Gutschow-Straße 8, 3000 Hannover 61, FRG

Introduction

The application of the destructive or even curative power of fire or other forms of heat has a long medical history: it was mentioned in the oldest textbook of surgery, the Edwin Smith papyrus (2800 B.C.). Now, nearly 5000 years later, the surgical potential of lasers is being explored [4, 8, 17].

The following provides a short overview of the current clinical applications of the Nd:YAG laser in the surgical treatment of cancer – 13 years after Kiefhaber's description of the first successful treatment of gastric bleeding [12].

Advantages of Laser Surgery of Cancer

Based on the primary thermal reactions as laser light impinges upon tissue, lasers bear some general advantages in surgery, including that of cancer; namely, precise control of the line of resection and the depth of penetration, coagulation to reduce blood loss, and the sealing of lymphatic vessels [4, 5, 18]. This last aspect, sealing of lymphatics by lasers in tumor surgery, is still under discussion, but recent experimental studies using CO_2 as well as Nd:YAG lasers, showed lesser migration through a laser barrier or reduced rates of local recurrence and implantation metastasis [24, 25]. Furthermore, in addition to the noncontact technique, laser light can nowadays be applied by means of a wide variety of sapphire or ceramic contact tips [6, 7]. These promising new developments should prompt investigations of CO_2 and Nd:YAG laser surgery in nearly every operative speciality – dermatology, urology, neurosurgery, pulmonology, gastroenterology, surgery of parenchymal organs [1–7, 12–14, 19, 20]. In some areas, such as neurosurgery or urology, so-called absolute indications for the use of the Nd:YAG laser have been established and prospective trials have been performed, for example on the Nd:YAG laser treatment of tumors of the urinary bladder: recurrence rates and median survival time were better with laser treatment, alone or combined with chemotherapy, than with the established transurethral resection technique [9].

Although such advantages of Nd:YAG laser application may exist in some specialities today and possibly in others, especially general and abdominal oncological surgery, in the near future, Nd:YAG laser surgery must be restricted to procedure selected cases only, with limited indications, mostly palliative, compared to other, conventional methods [5, 6, 18, 21].

Experimental Application of Nd:YAG Lasers in Surgery of the Liver

Although the perioperative mortality associated with liver resection has been reduced in recent years thanks to increased experience and standardization of the operative technique, severe complications such as recurrent bleeding, bile leakage, necrosis of liver tissue and liver failure still occur, even in the cirrhotic liver; not for nothing are there so many physical methods for cutting and/or coagulation [17, 18, 22, 23]. Therefore – based on experimental investigations with the CO_2 laser – in 1978 we started a trial of the effect of simultaneous cutting and hemostasis using different Nd:YAG lasers and combined CO_2/Nd:YAG laser systems. In the first series laboratory laser systems were used. Performing partial liver resection – the thickness of the resected lobe was about 2 cm – sufficient cutting coagulating efficiency was achieved. The depth of thermal damage or necrosis at the resection line ranged from 4.5 to 5.8 mm, with no statistically significant differences between different lasers; the average extent of tissue lesions as assessed by histomorphometric examination was 5.5 mm using these lasers, the same as after application of the infrared contact coagulator [17]. In a second experimental series a Medilas-2 Nd:YAG laser with a power output of 120 W at the end of the operative handpiece was used. To perform partial liver resections mean energy of 15 000 J was necessary; the depth of necrosis was about 5.8 mm. In a further experimental step the cutting and hemostatic potency of a Nd:YAG laser with a wavelength of 1.32 μm (designed by Dr. F. Frank, MBB, Munich) was tested. The power output of this laser was 6 or 24 W, resulting in a power density of 19 and 8.5 kW/cm^2 respectively. In these preliminary trials the quality of both cutting and hemostasis was impressive; the extent of necrosis at the resection line ranged from 2 to 4 mm. Histological investigation revealed that compared with Nd:YAG lasers with a wavelength of 1.06 μm, the zone of carbonization was very small, whereas the blister zone with empty cellular spaces was more pronounced. In the third area the tissue was severely altered with extensively condensed and shruken cells [18]. These experimental findings seem promising – independent of our own clinical experience with the Medilas-2 Nd:YAG laser – but other investigators, though reporting similar results, are less optimistic regarding the Nd:YAG laser, using the contact or the noncontact technique, in comparison with blunt dissection, the ultrasonic dissector (CUSA), or the suction knife. The best results were obtained using the CUSA or the suction knife; potential advantages of the noncontact laser were outweighed by the disadvantages, even in comparison with the contact laser technique [11, 22, 23].

Clinical Applications

The clinical applications of Nd:YAG lasers in the surgical treatment of cancer can be divided generally into open and endoscopic or ultrasound-guided techniques with or without tissue contact [4–6].

Based on the satisfactory initial experimental results, the Nd:YAG laser was used in open surgery of the liver. In comparison with other conventional or physical methods, however, the results were disappointing for lobe resection and for palliative resection of metastases in terms of cutting and coagulating efficacy and operating time [18]. More satisfactory results could be achieved with the contact technique. This was also the case in the pediatric surgery of parenchymal organs such as liver, spleen or pancreas [11, 15, 16]. Furthermore, our experience with vaporization of local recurrent tumors, though limited, has been disappointing; the result of the attempt to vaporize a perineal recurrence of a carcinoma of the rectum was unsatisfactory [18].

Nevertheless, remarkable progress has been achieved in the endoscopic or ultrasound-guided laser treatment of malignant tumors of the upper and lower gastrointestinal tract and the biliary tract. Typical indications for palliative laser surgery are bleeding and/or obstructive tumors of the gastrointestinal tract; the success rate is high, independent of whether treatment is purely palliative or whether it involves preoperative recanalization of a cancerous obstruction with the intention of proceeding to after-loading therapy or surgical resective procedures [2, 3, 7, 10, 12, 13, 19, 20].

Another interesting application is laser vaporization – endoscopically guided or via the percutaneous transhepatic approach – of obstructive tumors in the intrahepatic duct or the common bile duct [6].

Furthermore, multiple liver metastases can be destroyed exactly by means of ultrasound-guided and stereotactic techniques [8].

Conclusions

Reviewing the relevant literature and taking into account our own experimental findings and subjective feelings about the use of lasers in the surgical treatment of cancer, it becomes clear that this innovative therapeutic procedure is already a tried and tested method in fields such as urology, neurosurgery, and pulmonology [1, 4, 5, 9, 14]. Even in general surgery there is a small but stable range of indications – primarily using endoscopic guidance. With the aim of achieving "good medicine and surgery" [1], however, further technological advances and reductions of costs must be our priority. Ongoing experience with techniques such as the utilization of photosensitizers may alter patterns of acceptance or rejection of laser surgery with its destructive thermal effects [5, 6].

References

1. Aronoff BL (1983) Lasers in general surgery. World J Surg 7:681–683
2. Bader M, Dittler HJ, Ultsch B, Ries G, Siewert JR (1986) Palliative treatment of malignant stenoses of the upper gastrointestinal tract using a combination of laser and afterloading therapy. Endoscopy 18:27–31
3. Bown SG, Barr H, Matthewson K, Hawes R, Swain CP, Boulos PB (1986) Endoscopic treatment of inoperable colorectal cancers with the Nd:YAG laser. Br J Surg 73:949–952
4. Dinstl K, Fischer PL (1981) Der Laser: Grundlagen und klinische Anwendung. Springer, Berlin Heidelberg New York

5. Dixon MD (1984) Lasers in surgery. Current Probl Surg 9:3–65
6. Dixon JA (1988) Current laser applications in general surgery. Ann Surg 4:355–372
7. Ell C, Hochberger J, Lux G (1986) Clinical experience of non-contact and contact Nd:YAG laser therapy for inoperable malignant stenosis of the oesophagus and stomach. Lasers Med Sci 1:143–146
8. Godlewski G, Rouy S, Eledjam JJ (1986) Thermal and morphological effects of hepatic blood flow variations during liver resections with the Nd:YAG laser. Lasers Med Sci: 41–46
9. Hofstetter A, Schmeller N (1986) Application of the Nd:YAG laser in urology. Lasers Surg Med 2:98–100
10. Hohenberger W, Altendorf A, Hermanek P jr, Gall FP (1986) The laser in gastroenterology: malignant tumors in the lower gastrointestinal tract – therapeutic alternatives. Endoscopy 18:47–52
11. Joffe SN, Brackett KA, Sankar MY, Daikuzono N (1986) Liver resection with the Nd:YAG laser: a comparison of a new contact probe, the laser scalpel, with the conventional non-contact method. In: Waidelich W, Kiefhaber P (eds) Laser Optoelektronik in der Medizin. Springer, Berlin Heidelberg New York
12. Kiefhaber P (1987) Indications for endoscopic Neodymium: YAG laser treatment in the gastrointestinal tract. Twelve years' experience. Scand J Gastroenterol 22:53–63
13. Mathus-Vliegen EMH, Tytgat GN (1986) Laser ablation and palliation in colorectal malignancy. Results of a multicenter inquiry. Gastrointest Endosc 6:393–396
14. Mathus-Vliegen EMH, Tytgat GNJ (1986) Laser photocoagulation in the palliative treatment of upper digestive tract tumors. Cancer: 396–399
15. Meier H (1986) Experience of Neodym:YAG laser in pediatric surgery. Lasers Surg Med 1:10–16
16. Meier H, Dietl KH, Stöhr G, Willital GH (1986) Experience of Neodym:YAG laser in pediatric surgery. Lasers Surg Med 2:68–74
17. Meyer H-J (1981) Physikalische Methoden zum Schneiden und Koagulieren in der operativen Medizin. Habilitationsschrift, University of Hannover
18. Meyer H-J, Dinstl K (1988) Anwendung der Laser-Chirurgie and parenchymatösen Organen. Chirurg 59:68–75
19. Pietrafitta JJ, Richard M, Dwyer M (1986) Endoscopic laser therapy of malignant esophageal obstruction. Arch Surg 121:395–400
20. Russin DJ, Kaplan SR, Goldberg RI, Barkin JS (1986) Neodymium:YAG laser. A new palliative tool in the treatment of colorectal cancer. Arch Surg 121:1399–1403
21. Schildberg FW (1988) Laser in der Chirurgie – Aktueller Stand und Perspektiven (Kongreßbericht). Langenbecks Arch Chir [Suppl II]:533–542
22. Schröder T, Hasselgren PO, Brackett K, Joffe SN (1987) Techniques of liver resection. Arch Surg 122:1166–1171
23. Tranberg KG, Rigotti P, Brackett KA, Bjomsen HS, Fischer JE, Joffe SN (1986) Liver resection. A comparison using the Nd:YAG laser, an ultrasonic surgical aspirator, or blunt dissection. Am J Surg 151:368–373
24. Tuchmann A, Fischer PL, Bauer P, Plenk H Jr, Braun O (1986) Skalpell und CO_2-Laser im Tierexperiment. Eine Vergleichs-studie an Impftumoren der Maus. Langenbecks Arch Chir 368:125–136
25. Zimmermann I, Stern J, Frank F (1984) Interruption of lymphatic drainage by neodymium:YAG laser irradiation in rat urinary bladder. Lasers Surg Med 4:167–169

Neodymium:
YAG Laser Therapy in Gastroduodenal Cancer

J.R. Anderson and C.G. Morran

University Department of Surgery, Royal Infirmary,
Glasgow G31 2ER, United Kingdom

Introduction

Endoscopic laser therapy is of proven value in patients with bleeding peptic ulcers [1], and has been used in the management of oesophageal carcinoma [2] and colorectal cancer [3]. We have assessed the value of laser therapy in patients with gastroduodenal malignancies causing significant symptoms.

Patients and Methods

Over a 30-month period 52 patients (35 men and 17 women) with a mean age of 71 years (range 48–84) were treated. The indications for laser therapy were inoperability ($n = 22$) unfitness for laparotomy ($n = 17$) widespread metastases ($n = 11$) and refusal of surgery ($n = 2$). The tumor was located in the fundus in 16 patients (involving the cardia in 12), the proximal third of the stomach in nine (involving cardia in seven), the body in four, the distal half in six, and the whole stomach was involved in three patients (two with previous partial gastrectomies). Four tumours occurred in the second part of the duodenum; two of these arose from the pancreas (involving the medial wall of the duodenum) and two were recurrent renal cell carcinomas (involving the lateral wall). Forty-seven of the gastric tumours were adenocarcinomas and one was a fibrosarcoma. The predominant symptoms were dysphagia ($n = 19$), vomiting from gastric outlet obstruction ($n = 12$; partial obstruction in seven patients, total obstruction in five) and bleeding ($n = 33$). Of these latter 33 patients, 14 presented with melaena, nine with haematemesis and melaena and 10 with iron deficiency anaemia with positive faecal occult blood testing.

The laser system used was a Fibrelase 100 (Living Technology) set to deliver 60–100 W in pulses of 1–4 s. The laser fibre was passed down the biopsy channel of an Olympus GIFXQ gastroscope which had a nasogastric tube attached to it in order to vent the coaxial carbon dioxide. Patients received laser therapy at weekly intervals under sedation with intravenous diazepam and pethidine, and were allowed home the following day if their general condition and social circumstances allowed. When the presenting clinical condition was under control the patients

R. Jakesz/H Rainer (Eds)
Progress in Regional Cancer Therapy

underwent repeat endoscopy at intervals varying between 3 weeks and 3 months, depending on their response and clinical course.

Results

Our results are outlined in Table 1. Success in the management of dysphagia and gastric outlet obstruction was defined as the patient's ability to eat as he or she wished until the day of death or last review. The six patients with partial success in the dysphagia group all had initial restoration of normal or near normal swallowing, but the dysphagia returned in all six cases. In one, tumour regrowth proved impossible to control with laser therapy, and in the remaining five extrinsic compression with minimal or no exophytic tumour was found. All six patients underwent Celestin intubation at subsequent laparotomy. The only failure in the group with dysphagia was encountered in a man with linitis plastica in whom laser therapy was subsequently judged inappropriate.

All of the seven patients with partial gastric outlet obstruction (retaining fluids only, vomiting solids) returned to eating as they wished. Three of the five patients with total obstruction tolerated fluids without vomiting after laser therapy, but the treatment failed in the other two patients, in whom marked luminal angulation made access to some areas of the tumour impossible.

Control of bleeding was defined as successful if there was no overt bleeding and the haemoglobin was maintained until death or last review without evidence of occult bleeding. Control was successful in 28 patients and partially successful in three. In two of these latter patients the transfusion requirement was significantly reduced; the third, a woman of 74 years whose tumour was controlled for 89 weeks, was found 1 week prior to her death to have a haemoglobin of 7.9 g/dl, and we were unable to obtain stool specimens for occult blood testing. The cause of death was a myocardial infarction. The two failures to control bleeding occurred in patients who had extensive tumours to which access was severely restricted. Both of these patients died within 4 weeks.

One major complication occurred in a patient with a pancreatic carcinoma involving the second part of the duodenum who presented with melaena. She had a major haematemesis after her second laser session requiring transfusion with three units of blood. Her condition settled with conservative treatment, and she has not subsequently bled. Many patients experienced a transient epigastric burning

Table 1. Presentation and outcome

Symptom	No. of patients	No. of sessions (range)	Follow-up (weeks) Died (range)	Follow-up (weeks) Alive (range)	Outcome Success	Outcome Partial success	Outcome Failure
Dysphagia	19	3 (1–7)	21 (4–37)	39 (24–77)	12	6	1
Vomiting	12	3 (1–5)	11 (6–40)	47 (26–67)	7	3	2
Bleeding	33	2 (1–5)	14 (1–89)	38 (13–92)	28	3	2

sensation during the laser therapy, and two patients developed reflux oesophagitis which was easily controlled with cimetidine and antacids. Overall, control of symptoms was achieved in 36 of the 52 patients. Laser therapy was partially successful in a further 11, and treatment failed in five.

Discussion

The aim of palliative treatment is to relieve distressing symptoms and so improve the quality of the patient's remaining life and reduce the time spent in hospital. Our initial experience suggests that the greatest success was achieved in the control of bleeding if access was not restricted. Many patients with dysphagia were helped, and over half the patients with gastric outlet obstruction were significantly improved. In a recent study of 328 patients with gastric carcinoma from our hospital, 51 (16%) underwent no surgical treatment, 58 (18%) laparotomy alone and 59 (18%) palliative bypass or Celestin intubation [4]. In these patients (over 50% of those presenting with gastric cancer) laser therapy may have a role in management. Palliative laser therapy offers relief of symptoms to a significant number of patients with gastroduodenal malignancies unsuitable for surgery in whom the therapeutic options are otherwise limited.

Acknowledgements. We thank Staff Nurse Russell and the nurses of the Endoscopy Unit for their help with the patients. Mrs. W. Hughes typed the manuscript.

References

1. Swain CP, Kirkham JS, Salmon PR, Bown SG, Northfield TC (1986) Controlled trial of Nd:YAG laser photocoagulation in bleeding peptic ulcers. Lancet i:1113–1116
2. Krasner N, Barr H, Skidmore C, Morris AI (1987) Palliative laser therapy for malignant dysphagia. Gut 28:792–798
3. Bown SG, Barr H, Matthewson K, Hawes R, Swain CP, Clark CG, Boulos PB (1986) Endoscopic treatment of inoperable colorectal cancers with the Nd:YAG laser. Br J Surg 73:949–952
4. Cunningham D, Hole D, Taggart DJ, Soukop M, Carter DC, McArdle CS (1987) Evaluation of the prognostic factors in gastric cancer: the effect of chemotherapy on survival. Br J Surg 74:715–720

INNOVATIVE APPROACHES

The Use of Tumor-Infiltrating Lymphocytes in Cancer Therapy

B.S. Packard

Division of Cytokine Biology, Center for Biologics Evaluation and Research, U.S. Food and Drug Administration, Bethesda, MD 20892, USA

Introduction

The expansion in culture of lymphocytes directly from a tumor offers the possibility of generating a specific immune response to a malignancy. The idea that lymphocytes may be selected in vivo to recognize a tumor and then be expanded in the presence of the lymphokine interleukin-2 (IL-2) has led to the subject of this paper, namely, the large-scale production of tumor-infiltrating lymphocytes (TIL) for the treatment of human cancers.

Earlier studies from the Surgery Branch of the U.S. National Cancer Institute [1–3] as well as from other laboratories [4–7] indicated that lymphocytes from tumors of various histologies could be expanded in culture for several weeks in the presence of IL-2 with retention of lytic activity in vitro. Although much of the rationale for this approach to cancer treatment was based on the assayable lytic activity of the expanded lymphocytes, the effectiveness of this therapy may result to a significant degree from the in vivo amplification of infused cell populations and/or recruitment of immunocytes of the host.

In the present work data profiles of TIL from 13 patients with metastatic melanoma are presented. These patients were consecutively enrolled in the Surgery Branch protocol, and their data bases were completed between September, 1987 and June, 1988. The question of recognition of tumor by cultured lymphocytes was examined in detail by probing both the lytic and the proliferative specificities of cultured lymphocytes for autologous and allogeneic tumors of the same histology in vitro. In addition the ability of these lymphocytes to home in on tumor sites in vivo was studied.

Methods

Cell Growth Conditions

TIL were isolated and grown by the following procedure. Tumors were received directly from the operating room, placed in a sterile hood, cut such that no continuous surface extended beyond 5 mm, and then immediately placed in RPMI

R. Jakesz/H. Rainer (Eds.)
Progress in Regional Cancer Therapy

1640 containing collagenase type IV (0.1%), hyaluronidase type V (0.01%), and DNase type 1 (0.002%). After the suspension had been stirred overnight at room temperature, viable mononuclear and tumor cells were harvested after passage over Hypaque-Ficoll. Cells at the interface were collected, washed three times with HBSS, and placed in culture. All cultures throughout this project contained IL-2 (Cetus) at a concentration of 1×10^3 Cetus units/ml, except where indicated in the proliferation assays. Cultures were initiated under the following conditions: 5×10^5 total cells/ml were suspended in a medium of which 80% was RPMI 1640 containing 10% human serum or AIM-V (GIBCO), and 20% was autologous lymphokine-activated killer cell (LAK) supernatant. The latter was prepared by incubating 1×10^6 mononuclear peripheral blood cells either in RPMI medium containing 2% human serum or in AIM-V, both of which were supplemented with 1×10^6 U/ml of recombinant IL-2 (rIL-2) for 3–4 days. After 7 days, the cells were centrifuged and resuspended at a concentration of 2.5×10^5 lymphocytes/ml. Cultures were fed weekly by centrifuging, discarding old media, and converting the majority of cells to the medium in which proliferation was greater. In almost all cases the medium which supported superior cell growth was AIM-V. Cultures were maintained in LAK supernatant-containing medium until the latter was depleted. Cells were grown in plastic multi-well dishes if the total volume of the particular culture was less than 90 ml. For culture volumes which exceeded 90 ml cells were placed in Fenwal culture bags (Baxter Scientific).

At the time of infusion cells were harvested on CS3000 centrifuges; the product from each machine was a bag containing $0.2–1.5 \times 10^{11}$ TIL in 250–500 ml of 0.9% NaCl, 5% human albumin, and 3.75×10^4 U rIL-2/ml.

Phenotyping

All staining was carried out at 4°C for 30–60 min in HBSS containing 10% fetal calf serum and 0.02% NaN_3. Labeled antibodies listed in Table 3 were purchased from Becton–Dickinson, except 7G7, which was a gift from Dr. D. Nelson. The latter was directly labeled with 5-dichlorotriazinoaminofluorescein (DCTAF; Molecular Probes, Junction City, Oregon).

^{51}*Cr Release Assay*

Some 5×10^3 target cells loaded with Na_2CrO_4 plus effector cells at 100, 40, 10, and/or 25:1 effector : target ratios were plated in each well of a 96-well round-bottom plate and incubated for 4 h. The medium employed was RPMI 1640 containing 2% human serum. Spontaneous release was determined by the number of counts released from wells which contained only targets and maximum release by those containing targets plus 1% sodium dodecylsulfate. Cytotoxicity was calculated as

$$\%\ \text{lysis} = \frac{\text{experimental cpm} - \text{spontaneous cpm}}{\text{maximal cpm} - \text{spontaneous cpm}} \times 100.$$

All assays were carried out in triplicate. Statistical significance was determined using Student's t-test ($P < 0.05$, experimental lysis compared with spontaneous release control). Each assay contained fresh frozen autologous tumor cells, fresh frozen allogeneic melanoma cells, and Daudi and K562 cell lines as targets. A minimum of 50% lysis of Daudi cells by LAK cells served as the positive control for each experiment.

Proliferation Assay

TIL were resuspended in RPMI 1640 containing 10% type A human serum at a concentration of 2×10^5 cells per ml. Two hundred μl of this suspension was placed in each well of a 96-well flat-bottom plate. Twenty-five μl of a suspension containing irradiated (2×10^3 rads) 8×10^5 tumor cells per ml or 25 μl of medium for controls was placed in six separate wells for each TIL being assayed. Twenty-five μl of IL-2 in medium containing 1×10^5, 1×10^3, and 0 U/ml was added to two wells in each group of six. Six to eight days later lymphocytes were counted with a hemacytometer.

^{111}In Labeling of Cells

A fraction of a TIL culture to be infused, consisting of approximately 1×10^{10} cells, were harvested for radiolabeling. TIL were incubated with 500–800 μCi ^{111}In oxine for 15 min, during which time the suspension was rocked gently. After being washed twice with autologous plasma, the labeled cells were resuspended in normal saline, transferred to a transfusion bag, and infused immediately.

Results

Tables 1, 2, and 3 show data for culture periods, expansion indices, preculture cellular parameters, phenotyping, cytotoxicity, trafficking, and clinical responses.

Cytotoxicity Assay

Results from ^{51}Cr release assays (Table 3) were placed in one of the five classes: in class 0 cells had virtually no lytic activity, i.e., lysis of all targets tested was less than 5%; in class I only the autologous tumor was lysed; in class II the autologous and Daudi and/or K562 cell lines were lysed, with no lysis of allogeneic targets; in class III all targets were lysed with a preference for the autologous and Daudi and/or K562 cells over the allogeneic targets; and in class IV the TIL were lytic but showed no discrimination among any targets.

Only cells from the culture of patient 6 could clearly be placed in class 0. Cells from two patients were marginally lytic (< 10% lysis against the most lysable target). Thus, cells from cultures 4 and 8 (Fig. 1a) exhibited lytic activity borderline between classes 0 and I (lysis against the respective autologous tumors of 9% and 10%), with no statistically significant lytic activity against any other targets.

Table 1. Culture and preculture data

Patient	No. cells infused $\times 10^{-11}$	No. days in culture	Expansion index	% Tumor cells[a]	Tumor			
					%MHC I[b]	%MHC II[b]	%Leu2 pre[c]	%Leu3 pre[c]
1	2.5	28	4633	90	96	5	2	2
2	3.0	38 + 24	27100	93	90–95	10	3	5
3	2.5	33	5017	93	95	5	2	1
4	2.3	35	2423	72	NT	NT	NT	NT
5	1.3	40	588	55	85–90	60	12	8
6	1.9	43	44450	93	unsat.	5	3	4
7	7.5	28	2317	73	95	11	13	10
8	1.2	57	1802	36	48	37	13	29
9	3.5	30	4867	92	97	65	3	2
10	4.3	45	2443	81	94	38	3	3
11	3.0	39	> 1000	NT	95	1	1	3
12	2.9	34	32017	78	50, 80	2	6	5
13	3.5	49	> 800	> 95	NT	NT	NT	NT

NT, not tested, unsat., unsatisfactory.

[a] Percent tumor cells of total population obtained after enzyme treatment and Hypaque-ficoll gradient.

[b] Percent major histocompatibility antigens classes I and II on the tumor cells.

[c] Percent Leu2/CD8 and Leu3/CD4 of precultured lymphocytes.

Table 2. Phenotyping of expanded lymphocyte populations

Patient	% Leu4	% Leu2	% Leu3	% Leu7	% Leu19	% LeuM3	% HLA-DR	% Tac	% 7G7
1	97	83	12	10	3	2	84	42	51
2	98	82	20	23	7	3	97	47	50
3	100	29	74	11		1	96	34	47
4	83	93	10	25	3	0	97	19	41
5	99	98	< 3	3	2	3	98	21	31
6	97	*19	> 90	16	1	4	99	12	31
7	98	98	< 3	16	18	0	98	2	4
8	93	87	3	14	5	1	95	9	19
9	99	93	3		3		95	7	27
10	76	73	1[illegible]	23	37	1	90	10	1
11	69	59	34	20	8	0	96?	12	9?
12	95	80	14	15	17	4	98?	21	41
13	96	89	3		9	1	94	16?	19

Table 3. Cytotocity, specific proliferation, in vivo trafficking, and clinical response

Patient	Cytotoxicity	Specific proliferation: + Tumor	Specific proliferation: Specificity	Specific proliferation: -IL-2	Trafficking	Response
1	II	+	–	+ without tumor	+	PR
2	II	+	–	+ without tumor	+	PR
3	I→II	–	NA	–	+	NR
4	0→I	+	–	–	+	PR
5	I	+	+	+ auto tumor	+	NR
6	0	–	NA	–	–	PR
7	I	+	–	–	NT	PR
8	0→I	+	–	–	NT	PR + prog.
9	I	+	+	+ auto tumor	+	NR
10	II	+	+	+ auto tumor	+	NR
11	III	+	–	+ #10 tumor	+	MR
12	III	+	+	–	+	PR
13	I→II	+	+	+ auto tumor	NT	NT

PR, partial response (decrease of at least 50/ of the sum of the cross-sectional areas of all tumor deposits and no progression of disease after therapy); MR, marginal response (25%–50% decrease and no progression).

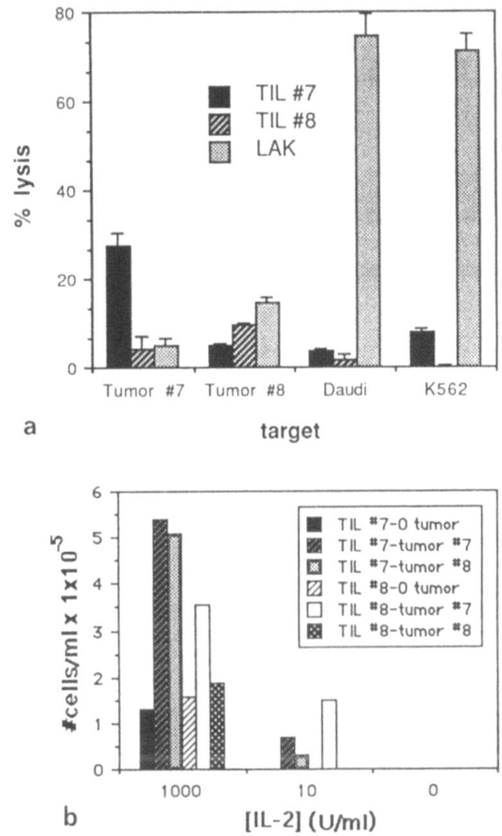

Fig. 1a, b. Criss-cross in vitro recognition assays between TIL from patients 7 and 8. **a** ^{51}Cr release assay; **b** proliferation assay. Conditions described in text

Cultures from patients 5, 7, and 9 were placed in class I because they exhibited strong lytic activity against their autologous targets (53% ± 3%, 27% ± 3%, and 57% ± 2%, respectively) and were virtually nonlytic against allogeneic, Daudi, and K562 cells, whereas cultures 3 and 13 showed preferences for but not exclusivity toward their autologous targets.

Cells from patients 1 and 2 lysed their respective autologous targets and Daudi cells with no significant lysis above background of any allogeneic targets; these were therefore, placed in class II. TIL 10 also fell into this group, as the autologous and the two cultured lines served as statistically significant targets, with the allogeneic not being lysed (Fig. 2a).

Culture 12, which contained cells that exhibited ca. 20% lysis against the autologous target, ca. 35% against one allogeneic target, and less than 10% against two other allogeneic and Daudi targets, was placed in class III. Culture 11 was also placed in this class, as the autologous tumor and Daudi cells provided the most effective targets, and allogeneic cells were lysed less efficiently.

Proliferation Assay

Results from proliferation assays are presented in Table 3. For cells in 11 of the 13 cultures (1, 2, 4, 5, and 7–13) addition of irradiated melanoma cells induced an

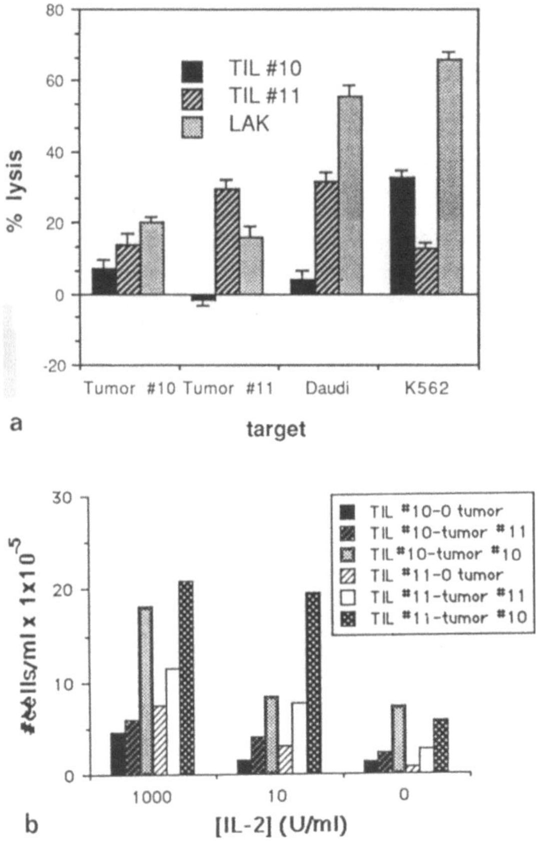

Fig. 2 a, b. Criss-cross in vitro recognition assays between TIL from patients 10 and 11. **a** ^{51}Cr release assay; **b** proliferation assay. Conditions described in text

increase (> 50%) in the number of lymphocytes when counted after 6 to 8 days. Five of these 11 cultures (5, 9, 10, 12, and 13) showed an increase in proliferative activity only in response to the presence of the autologous tumor, while enhancement of the other six was observed on addition of only allogeneic stimulators (1, 8, and 11) or allogeneic as well as autologous stimulators (2, 4, and 7).

The question of whether IL-2 was essential for proliferation was addressed by growing cells in the absence of this lymphokine either with or without tumor added back. For two cultures (1 and 2) the number of cells at least doubled in the absence of both IL-2 and added tumor. Cells in four cultures (5, 9, 10 and 13) grew in the absence of IL-2 and the presence of autologous tumor. Cells of culture 11 proliferated in the absence of IL-2 and the presence of tumor 10; however, no growth was observed in the absence of IL-2 and the presence of autologous tumor for this culture (Fig. 2b). All other cultures required IL-2 in both the presence and the absence of added tumor (Fig. 1b).

Discussion

In this study TIL from 13 patients with metastatic melanoma were cultured in the presence of IL-2 for periods ranging between 26 and 57 days. At the end of culture the ability of cells to recognize the respective autologous tumor was assayed by cytotoxicity and proliferation assays in vitro and by trafficking of ^{111}In-labeled cells in vivo. No single characteristic or profile describes the cells from all cultures; rather, there appears to be a spectrum which encompasses all the cultures with respect to phenotypic, lytic, proliferative, and in vivo homing activities. Furthermore, patients whose cells represent all regions of this in vitro spectrum induced clinical responses on reinfusion and treatment with IL-2 (Table 3).

The majority ($>68\%$) of cells from all cultures were T lymphocytes (Leu4/CD3-positive). In 11 of the 13 cultures (1, 2, 4, 5, 7–13) the cytotoxic/suppressor (Leu2/CD8) phenotype predominated. The question of whether the cultured TIL could lyse fresh frozen autologous tumor targets in a 4-h ^{51}Cr release assay was thus considered. Although low in some cultures ($<10\%$ in cultures 8 and 10), autologous lytic activity was statistically significant in all cultures except culture 6.

Cells from culture 6 represent one extreme of this spectrum, i.e. virtually all cells bore the helper/inducer (Leu3/CD4) antigen with 19% double labeling for Leu2 and Leu3; these lymphocytes did not lyse any of the targets tested. Following infusion the sum of the cross-sectional areas of all tumor deposits in this patient decreased by more than 50%, and no disease progression was observed.

Most cultures (12 of the 13), however, contained at least a statistically finite degree ($>7\%$) of lytic activity. Cells from three cultures (10, 11, and 12) were able to lyse both fresh frozen autologous and allogeneic targets, while ten (1, 2, 3, 4, 5, 7, 8, 9, 10, and 13) lysed predominantly only the former.

Having analyzed the lytic abilities with respect to lysis of fresh frozen melanoma targets, the proliferative characteristics of these cultures were next examined. The issue of proliferative specificity, i.e. whether or not addition of fresh frozen irradiated tumor cells enhanced the rate of proliferation, was explored. Proliferation of cells from the one nonlytic (grade 0) culture (6) was not affected by the addition of tumor. Both of the cultures capable of lysing allogeneic as well as autologous targets (11 and 12) showed an enhancement in proliferation upon addition of tumor cells with 12 responding to its autologous stimulator and 11 showing an increase in TIL number in the presence of an allogeneic tumor (10) but not the autologous tumor. Of the ten TIL cultures that exhibited some degree of lytic specificity for their autologous targets, nine (1, 2, 3, 4, 5, 7, 8, 9, 10, and 13) demonstrated increased proliferation in the presence of added tumor – four (5, 9, 10, and 13) in the presence of autologous tumor only, three (2, 4, 7) in the presence of either autologous or allogeneic stimulators, and two (1 and 8) with only allogeneic cells. Except for culture 12, the proliferative enhancement of all TIL that responded to autologous stimulators only (5, 9, 10, and 13) was independent of IL-2, i.e., all TIL except culture 12 that showed an increase in proliferation in the presence of autologous but not allogeneic tumor did so whether or not IL-2 was present. None of the cultures which responded to allogeneic stimulators showed this enhancement in the absence of IL-2. It might also be noted that in this work, contrary to some reports, suppression of growth was never observed upon addition of tumor.

As might be predicted, all TIL that exhibited some form of recognition in vitro were able to recognize tumor in vivo. Whether specific recognition is a prerequisite for homing is unclear, as other explanations such as inflammation and increased drainage around tumor sites are feasible. However, the observed in vivo trafficking correlated at the very least with the apparent recognition capabilities these cells exhibited in in vitro assays.

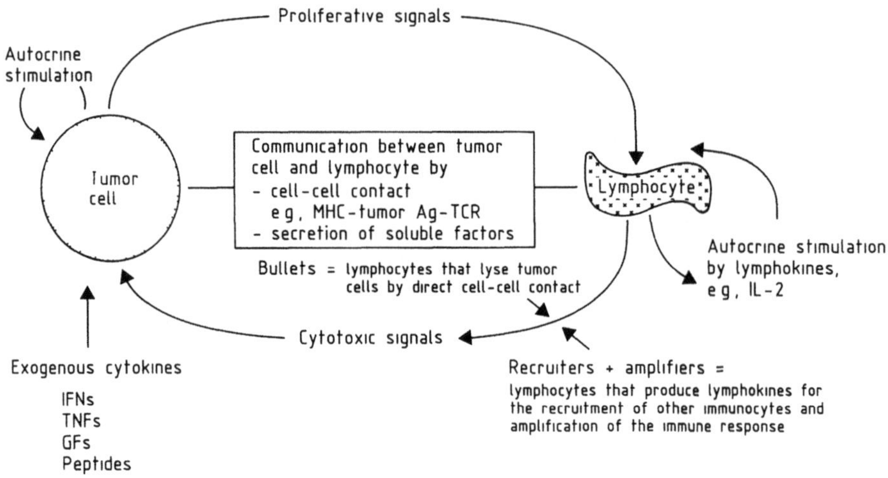

Fig. 3. Potential mechanisms for interaction between lymphocytes and tumor cells

The ability of in vitro assays to predict in vivo responses is a point of major concern and interest. Although tests of recognition in vitro would seem to provide reasonable criteria for predicting in vivo response a priori, other factors may in fact dominate in in vivo environments. For example, if one believed that a pure cytotoxic population with specific, high cytolytic activity were the cell type of choice in this therapy, then one would have predicted that patients 5, 7, and 9 would have responded, in that all three cultures were phenotypically and functionally pure cytotoxic T cells (CTL), i.e., Leu2/CD8-positive with both high and specific activity lytic. Patient 7 underwent a reduction in tumor mass of greater than 50%; unfortunately, disease in patients 5 and 9 progressed after treatment. Interestingly, of these three cultures only cells from patient 7 made a detectable amount of mRNA for tumor necrosis factor (TNF); conceivably, CTL require TNF for lysis. The most dramatic responses were observed in patients 1, 2, 4, 6, 7, and 12, most of whom did not exhibit remarkable lytic activity.

Although believed to originate clonally, tumors are known to evolve into heterogeneous collections of cells. It is possible that the population of TIL that grows in vitro is a function of the strongest antigenic and/or proliferative stimulus present in culture; however, tumors in vivo may be composed of cells with much greater heterogeneity, and thus recognition by infused cells might be limited. Requirements for growth such as IL-2 dependence might be an additional indication of the recognition capabilities. Thus, the most efficient TIL in vivo may turn out to be those cellular populations that can integrate many functions, such as direct cell-cell killing, amplification of infusate populations, and recruitment of host cells (Fig. 3), as opposed to those possessing narrower functional capabilities.

References

1. Yron I, Wood TA, Spiess P, Rosenberg SA (1980) In vitro growth of murine T cells V. The isolation and growth of lymphoid cells infiltrating syngeneic solid tumors. J Immunol 125:238–245
2. Rosenberg SA, Spiess P, Lafreniere R (1986) A new approach to the adoptive immunotherapy of cancer with tumor-infiltrating lymphocytes. Science 223:1318–1321
3. Topalian S, Solomon D, Avis FP, Chang AE, Freerksen DL, Linehan WM, Lotze MT, Robertson CN, Seipp CA, Simon P, Simpson CG, Rosenberg SA (1988) Immunotherapy of patients with advanced cancer using tumor infiltrating lymphocytes and recombinant interleukin-2: a pilot study. J Clin Oncol 6:839–853
4. Itoh K, Tilden AB, Balch CM (1986) Interleukin-2 activation of cytotoxic T-lymphocytes infiltrating into human metastatic melanomas. Cancer Res 46:3011–3017
5. Rabinowich H, Cohen R, Bruderman I, Steiner Z, Klajman A (1987) Functional analysis of mononuclear cells infiltrating into tumors: lysis of autologous human tumor cells by cultured infiltrating lymphocytes. Cancer Res 47:173–177
6. Miescher S, Whiteside TL, Moretta L, Von Fliedner V (1987) Clonal and frequency analyses of tumor-infiltrating T lymphocytes from human solid tumors. J Immunol 138:4004–4011
7. Kradin RL, Boyle LA, Preffer FI, Callahan RJ, Barlai-Kovach M, Strauss HW, Dubinett S, Kurnick JT (1987) Tumor-derived interleukin-2 dependent lymphocytes in adoptive immunotherapy of lung cancer. Cancer Immunol Immunother 24:76–85

Adoptive Immunotherapy for Renal Adenocarcinoma: Use of Oxidizing Mitogen-Treated Mononuclear Leukocytes and Continuous Infusion of Interleukin-2

K.H. Stenzel, J. Wang, A. Walle, M. Suthanthiran, R.T. Silver, and A. Novogrodsky

The Rogosin Institute and the New York Hospital–Cornell Medical Center, 505 E. 70th Street, New York, NY 10021, USA

Introduction

Infusion of recombinant interleukin-2 (rIL-2) in combination with autologous peripheral blood mononuclear cells (PBM) treated with rIL-2 can induce regression of tumors in some patients with metastatic renal adenocarcinoma or melanoma. Initial response rates in metastatic renal adenocarcinoma of 16%–33% were reported [1, 5].

We found that the oxidizing mitogens induce IL-2 receptors on PBM and sensitize them to the effects of IL-2 [6]. We considered the possibility that treatment of PBM with an oxidizing mitogen and IL-2 would result in enhanced antitumor properties and provide cells that would be effective in adoptive immunotherapy in conjunction with lower, less toxic doses of IL-2 than had hitherto been used. The oxidizing mitogens have several unique properties that make them especially attractive for clinical studies. First, the cells need only be exposed to these agents for 15–20 min, and the oxidizing mitogen may then be completely removed. Second, oxidizing mitogentreated cells can induce activation in untreated cells, thus raising the possibility of inducing additional cell stimulation in vivo. In this review we will summarize basic properties of the oxidizing mitogens, preclinical studies, a clinical study involving patients with renal adenocarcinoma, and immunologic alterations induced by adoptive immunotherapy in man.

Basic Properties of the Oxidizing Mitogens

Two oxidizing mitogens have been discovered; sodium periodate (IO_4^-) [3], and sequential treatment with neuraminidase and galactose oxidase (NAGO) [4]. IO_4^- generates aldehyde groups on cell surface sialic acid residues, and the aldehyde is essential for induction of blastogenesis and cytotoxicity. Reduction of aldehyde groups within the first several hours aborts cell activation, but after 18–24 h the cells are committed and the aldehyde is no longer required. Removal of sialyl residues with neuraminidase exposes guluctose residues that are the penultimate sugars in many cell surface carbohydrate trees. Treatment of the desialylated cells with galactose oxidase results in mitogenic response. Similar to the response induced by

R. Jakesz/H Rainer (Eds)
Progress in Regional Cancer Therapy

IO_4^-, it is dependent on aldehydes generated, in this case, on galectosyl groups. Activation of the cell by direct treatment is known as direct activation, to differentiate it from another property of these cells known as indirect activation. Blastogenesis can be induced in untreated PBM by exposing them to oxidizing mitogen-treated and irradiated cells. This indirect activation is dependent on aldehyde groups on the surface of the stimulating cells [2].

The oxidizing mitogens activate both T lymphocytes and natural killer (NK) cells. They are strictly dependent on accessory cells for T cell activation. Both IO_4^- and NAGO induce increased numbers and an increased density of IL-2 receptors (Table 1).

Combined treatment of PBM with the oxidizing mitogens and IL-2 results in enhanced cytotoxicity (Table 2). The cells manifest lymphokine-activated killer (LAK) activity, since they are cytotoxic for NK-resistant cells, such as fresh tumor cells and solid tumor cell lines. IO_4^- is a weak mitogen and a weak inducer of LAK activity; NAGO, however, is potent in both these activities. While IL-2 does not significantly enhance LAK activity of NAGO-treated cells, the combination of IO_4^- and IL-2 is synergistic and results in cells with the highest level of cytotoxicity among the various combinations of IL-2 and the oxidizing mitogens that we assessed.

Table 1. Induction of receptors (anti-Tac) for IL-2 in cells treated with the oxidizing mitogens and IL-2

Additions	% Cells with IL-2 receptors	Mean channel fluorescence
None	9.4 ± 3.1	41.7 ± 11.3
IL-2 (1000 units/ml)	19.2 ± 3.5	95.3 ± 1.7
IO_4^-	39.6 ± 4.3	115 ± 10.9
IO_4^- + IL-2 (1000 units/ml)	47.0 + 1.3	126 ± 1.0
NAGO	74.9 ± 10.5	145 ± 7.5
NAGO + IL-2 (1000 units/ml)	78.3 ± 0.4	146 ± 1.5
(Adapted from [6])		

Table 2. LAK activity of PBM treated with the oxidizing mitogens and IL-2

	% Specific ^{51}Cr release (SEM)	
Mitogen	Without IL-2	With IL-2
None	1.5 ± 1.8	22.0 ± 9.5
IO_4^-	10.5 ⊥ 5.7	46.8 ± 8.2
NAGO	35.2 ± 9.0	44.2 ± 7.5
(Adapted from [6])		

Cells mediating killing of the renal adenocarcinoma cell line consisted predominantly of cells expressing the NKH1A phenotype. This conclusion was reached in studies designed to remove different cell populations by incubation with complement and a monoclonal antibody directed against a specific cell surface structure, followed or preceded by activation with IO_4^- and IL-2. LAK activity of the remaining cells was then determined. Removal of T cells had little effect, whereas removal of NK cells by incubation with an antibody directed against NKHIA and complement removed over 90% of the activity. The procedure markedly reduced LAK activity when cells were treated either before or after activation.

Preclinical Studies

A variety of preclinical studies were done to assess the anti-tumor properties of cells activated with the oxidizing mitogens. The human renal adenocarcinoma cell line, SK-RC-29, grows rapidly when injected subcutaneously in nude mice. We mixed human PBM, activated with either NAGO or IO_4^-, with SK-RC-29 in varying effector: target (E:T) cell ratios and immediately injected the mixtures subcutaneously in nude mice (a modified Winn assay). Untreated PBM had no effect on tumor growth at the highest E:T cell ratio tested, 50:1. NAGO-treated cells completely eliminated tumor growth at E:T ratios as low as 1:1. IO_4^--treated cells also prevented tumor growth at the 50:1 and 10:1 ratios. Tumors did appear at 1:1 ratios, but their appearance was markedly delayed [6]. We next investigated the ability of splenocytes activated by the oxidizing mitogens to inhibit established B16-F10 pulmonary metastases in C57BL mice. Tumor cells were injected IV on day 0, and splenocytes (10^8), cultured for 48 h following NAGO or IO_4^- treatment, were administered on day 3. Two weeks later the animals were killed and pulmonary metastases counted. Both NAGO- and IO_4^--treated splenocytes mediated a decrease in the number of pulmonary metastases compared with animals receiving no cells, or receiving untreated cells cultured for 48 h.

Clinical Studies

Initial feasibility and toxicity studies of oxidizing mitogen-treated autologous lymphocytes were carried out in five patients with stage IV renal adenocarcinoma. The toxicity encountered was minimal and consisted of fever and chills beginning 30–90 min following intravenous infusion of cells. There was no objective tumor response in these patients.

Based on: (1) our preclinical studies; (2) the initial feasibility study; (3) the induction of IL-2 receptors by IO_4^-; (4) the demonstrated synergy between IO_4^- and IL-2 in generating activated killer cells; and (5) the report of Rosenberg et al. [5] indicating that the combination of activated killer cells and systemic administration of IL-2 was much more effective than cells alone, we developed a protocol combining IO_4^-/IL-2-activated cells and systemic administration of IL-2. We chose to administer IL-2 as a continuous infusion at lower dosages than used by Rosenberg et al. to both maintain a constant level of IL-2 for a prolonged period and to minimize toxicity. We are currently completing a phase II study to determine efficacy and toxicity of this approach. Following this, we will conduct a phase III study to compare results in patients treated with IO_4^-/IL-2-activated cells with those in patients receiving cells activated with IL-2 alone, keeping all other aspects of the protocol the same.

We have completed therapy in 31 patients as of June 1988. Criteria for patient entry into the study include: histologically confirmed metastatic renal adenocarcinoma that is clearly progressive; measurable disease; age 21–70; ambulatory with ECOG of 0 or 1; adequate organ function; absence of brain metastases; and no other anti-tumor therapy concurrently or in the past month. Signed informed consent was obtained from all patients before entry into the study.

PBM ($5-10 \times 10^9$) were removed by leukapheresis 3 times per week (Monday, Wednesday, Friday), isolated by Ficoll-Hypaque density gradient centrifugation, and treated with sodium periodate (2mM) at 0 °C for 30 min. The cells were then cultured at a density of 1.5×10^6/ml in 500-ml disposable culture flasks in RPMI 1640 medium containing 2.5% autologous serum and 500 U/ml rIL-2 (Cetus). More recently, a closed system was introduced using the Travenol CS 3000. The cells were harvested after 48–72 h by centrifugation, washed in low-pyrogen phosphate-buffered saline, and suspended in 50 ml lactated Ringer's solution for reinfusion. A sample of cells was sent for overnight microbial culture the day prior to harvest and another for long-term culture on the day of harvest. Pyrogen assays were done by the Limulus lysate method. Cells were reinfused following the next leukapheresis procedure. rIL-2 was diluted in 500 ml 5% dextrose and water and given as a continuous infusion for 5 days/week at a dose of 10000–50000 U/kg/24 hr. For the first 15 patients, a regimen of leukapheresis 3 times a week and continuous IL-2 infusion was begun the 1st week, continued for 3 weeks, and then repeated after a 3-week rest period. Since relatively few cells were recovered during the 1st week, after the first 15 patients we began leukapheresis in the 2nd week. Imaging studies were done prior to and at intervals following completion of the study protocol to determine extent of disease. Clinical evaluations and biochemical studies were done to determine toxicity, and several in vitro cell-mediated responses were evaluated to determine alterations in immune function.

Of the 31 patients entered into the study by June 1988, 25 have measureable lesions and are evaluable at the time of writing. Four patients did not complete the protocol, and two had disease that was not measurable. Applying stringent criteria, and following independent review by several radiologists, to date two patients have a complete response (CR) and three show a partial response (PR). Thus the overall response rate (CR + PR) was 20%. Significant responses were observed in lung, bone, liver, soft tissue, adrenal, and contralateral kidney. An additional 20% of the patients had minor or mixed responses.

Toxicity was significant in most patients. Major problems were hypotension, nausea, diarrhea, and fluid accumulation. There were two deaths: both patients had far advanced disease and one had massive pulmonary metastases. The results of the initial phase of this study were recently published [7].

We and others noted that responses were short-lived and recurrences developed in 4–8 months. In an attempt to prolong responses we instituted a maintenance regimen consisting of α-interferon 3×10^6 units 3 times a week and 2 days of continuous IL-2 infusion once a month coupled with one leukapheresis and reinfusion of activated cells. The results of this regimen have been most encouraging, with markedly enhanced patient survival.

Immunologic Alterations

We investigated the effect of continuous IL-2 infusions and intermittent administration of IO_4^-/IL-2-activated cells on PBM populations, and on NK and LAK activity as well as antibody-dependent cellular cytotoxicity (ADCC), mitogen responsiveness, and spontaneous blastogenesis.

There was a significant and sustained increase in peripheral blood cells bearing NK markers, NKH-1A and Leull. This was first noted after the weekend following 5 days of IL-2 infusion alone, and then was sustained during the ensuing 2 weeks of treatment. When patients were readmitted after a 3-week interval, cells bearing these antigens remained increased and there was no further significant increment. $T3^+$ cells decreased during the second cycle of treatment. There was no consistent increase in IL-2 receptor $(Tac)^+$ cells, but individual patients had marked fluctuations in these cells during the course of treatment.

One of the most striking findings was rapid induction of LAK activity following brief treatment with IL-2 in vitro. The experimental paradigm is as follows. PBM are isolated from patients' blood by Ficoll-Hypaque centrifugation and tested for cytotoxicity in short-term ^{51}Cr release assays using SK-RC-29 as target cells. The 3-h assays are done in the presence and absence of IL-2. We found that this brief, concurrent exposure to IL-2 induced significant LAK activity as determined by cytotoxicity for the NK resistant target, SK-RC-29. This phenomenon was not observed during the 1st week of IL-2 infusion, but was manifest after the 2-day rest period following the first week of therapy. Thereafter, the activity remained high for the treatment period.

NK activity also increased. This occurred during the first 3-week cycle of treatment and NK activity remained elevated for several weeks after cessation of treatment.

ADCC activity was increased in the patients we studied with renal adenocarcinoma prior to treatment, and values remained slightly higher than controls throughout the course of therapy. Con A and PHA stimulation was marginally lower than controls and remained low during the two cycles of treatment. Spontaneous blastogenesis, a measure of circulating cells entering S phase, was only slightly and insignificantly increased over control values.

Discussion

Treatment with low-dose continuous infusion of IL-2 and intermittent administration of autologous cells activated by combined treatment with IO_4^- and IL-2 results in regression of metastases of renal adenocarcinoma in some patients. Since this is a phase II study the individual contribution of each element in the protocol cannot be determined. In other studies, IL-2 alone has not been sufficient to induce tumor regression at the dose levels we are using. Activated cells alone were insufficient in previous studies we and others conducted. There is ample experimental evidence that the two modalities, IL-2 and cells, are synergistic in animal models.

A more compelling question is whether the mitogen, IO_4^-, is having any effect or whether we would see the same degree of regression without this modification. This question will be resolved in phase III studies that will soon be initiated.

Most of our responding patients have had partial or mixed responses rather than complete responses. Nevertheless, the response may be sustained if maintenance therapy with α-interferon and monthly IL-2 and activated cells is initiated. While complete response is the goal of clinical oncology, it has, unfortunately, been an evanescent goal in most cases of solid tumor metastases. The concept of maintenance of partial, mixed or minimal responses for long periods of time may be reasonable, at least in the case of renal adenocarcinoma. The natural history of this disease indicates that in some instances lesions do remain stable for long periods of time. This presumably results from a host-tumor relationship favoring control of tumor growth. Perhaps such a state can be induced in patients by the judicious application of a variety of biologic response modifiers.

References

1. Fisher RI, Coltman CA, Doroshow JH et al. (1988) Matastatic renal cancer treated with interleukin-2 and lymphokine-activated killer cells. Ann Intern Med 108:518–523
2. Lipkowitz S, Rubin AL, Stenzel KH, Novogrodsky A (1983) Cellular and growth factor requirements for activation of human T lymphocytes by neuraminidase and galactose oxidase-treated lymphoid cells. J Immunol 130:2702
3. Novogrodsky A, Katchalski E (1972) Membrane site modified on induction of the transformation of lymphocytes by periodate. Proc Natl Acad Sci USA 69:3207
4. Novogrodsky A, Katchalski E (1973) Induction of lymphocyte transformation by sequential treatment with neuraminidase and galactose oxidase. Proc Natl Acad Sci USA 70:1824
5. Rosenberg SA, Lotze MT, Muul LM et al. (1987) A progress report on the treatment of 157 patients with advanced canced using lymphokine-activated killer cells and interleukin-2 or high-dose interleukin 2 alone. N Engl J Med 316:889
6. Wang J, Suthanthiran M, Walle A, Lagman M, Schwartz R, Murthi V, Novogrodsky A, Stenzel KH (1986) Anti-tumor properties of lymphocytes activated by the oxidizing mitogens. J Immunol 136:4735
7. Wang J, Walle A, Gordon B, Novogrodsky A, Suthanthiran M, Rubin AL, Morrison H, Silver RT, Stenzel KH (1987) Adoptive immunotherapy for stage IV renal cell carcinoma: a novel protocol utilizing periodate and interleukin-2-activated autologous leukocytes and continuous infusions of low-dose interleukin-2. Am J Med 83:1016

Processing of Antigen-Antibody Complexes at the Level of the Tumor Cell

S. Matzku, W. Tilgen, and H. Bihl

Institut für Radiologie und Pathophysiologie, Deutsches Krebsforschungszentrum, Postfach 101949, 6900 Heidelberg, FRG

Introduction

After incubation with antigen-positive tumor cells, a bound monoclonal antibody (MAb) may stay at the cell surface or be subjected to a process of modulation, which may lead either to internalization or to shedding of the immune complex [2,7]. These alternatives are important for tumor targeting, since internalization can bring a MAb conjugate to its intracellular site of action (e.g., immunotoxins), or result in the cumulative storage of a radionuclide (e.g., heavy metal nuclides), or lead to degradation of the MAb and release of the radionuclide (e.g., tyrosine-coupled iodine). Shedding, on the other hand, will impede long-lasting accumulation of the MAb conjugate. We report on experiments designed to categorize and understand post-binding phenomena. Although the experiments have been carried out with radioiodinated MAb, most of the conclusions apply, with due modifications, to other types of MAb conjugates as well.

Characterization of Antitumor MAbs

We have routinely analyzed the kinetics of binding to tissue-cultured tumor cells, and we determined internalization by the technically simple pH 2.8 desorption procedure [7]. Externally bound MAb are desorbed by the acid buffer treatment, while internalized MAb remain with the cell pellet. Of 26 MAb recognizing tumor-associated (differentiation) antigens, 14 showed little or no internalization, five showed partial internalization, five showed predominant internalization, and two showed binding behavior compatible with immune complex shedding (Table 1). Alternative methods of detecting internalization include radioimmunoelectron microscopy [14] and immunoelectron microscopy with gold-labeled MAb [4], both of which provide ultrastructural information regarding the route of entry into the cell, and FACS analysis, which records release from fluorescence quenching after internalization of MAb-dye conjugates [6]. Although comprehensive comparative analyses have not yet been carried out, results obtained with these methods and with the pH 2.8 desorption technique appear to be fairly consistent.

R. Jakesz/H. Rainer (Eds.)
Progress in Regional Cancer Therapy

Table 1. Characterization of internalization behavior of various MAb tested by the pH 2.8 desorption method

Mab	Tumor type	Antigen	Source
Predominant internalization (> 75%)[a]			
M.2.7.6	Melanoma	gp?	A
HD6	Lymphoma	CD22	B
42/6	Lymphoma	Tf-receptor	C
HEA 19	Colorectal	CEA/NCA	D
C1.6	Rat sarcoma	gp 145/195	E
Partial internalization (≈ 50%)[a]			
M.2.9.4	Melanoma	gp 100	A
HD39	Lymphoma	CD22	B
HEA 81	Colorectal	CEA/NCA	D
#35	Colorectal	CEA	F
MOv17	Ovarian	gp38	G
Very low internalization (< 20%)[b]			
L10, 96.5	Melanoma	gp95	H, I
225.28	Melanoma	Proteoglycan 250–450 KD	K
KG 6–56	Melanoma	Proteoglycan 250–450 kD	A
M.2.10.15	Melanoma	gp200	A
HD28	Lymphoma	CD37	B
HD37[c]	Lymphoma	CD19	B
HD50	Lymphoma	CD23	B
C1-P83	Colorectal	CEA	L
BW431/26	Colorectal	CEA	M
F023C5	Colorectal	CEA	N
MLuC2	Mammary	gp75	G
MOv19	Ovarian	gp38	G
C4.4	Rat sarcoma	gp86	E
A2.4	Rat sarcoma	gp42–195	E
"Shedding"[d]			
R24	Melanoma	Glycolipid GD3	H
M.2.2.4	Melanoma	Glycolipid	A

[a] Fraction of total binding internalized at 37°C.
[b] Some of the MAb showed no internalization at all.
[c] In some experiments, HD37 showed partial internalization.
[d] In our system, shedding is defined by higher binding levels at 0°C then at 37°C.
Sources of MAbs: *A*, C. Sorg, Münster; *B*, B. Dörken, Heidelberg; *C*, I.S. Trowbridge, San Diego; *D*, G. Moldenhauer, Heidelberg; *E*, S. Matzku, Heidelberg; *F*, J.P. Mach, Lausanne; *G*, M. Colnaghi, Milan; *H*, W.G. Dippold, Mainz; *I*. I. Hellström, Seattle; *K*, S. Ferrone, Valhalla; *L*, H. Kalthoff, Hamburg; *M*, Behringwerke, Marburg; *N*, Sorin, Saluggia.

Antibody Internalization in Different Tumor Systems

Some interesting aspects have emerged from the results summarized in Table 1.

1. From our limited experience, no clear-cut correlation between internalization potential and tumor type can be postulated.
2. In some tumor systems it has been possible to raise MAb directed against distinct determinants of a given tumor-associated antigen. In Table 1 this applies to MAb against CD22, CEA, and gp38. With these reagents striking differences in internalization behavior were observed, in that fractional internalization varied significantly from one MAb (determinant) to the other. This could be interpreted as meaning that internalization depends on the site on the antigen molecule at which a given MAb actually binds. However, the issue is not absolutely settled because some of the antigenic determinants in question are expressed on a family of related antigens rather than on a single antigen molecule. Thus, if the tumor cell expresses more than one type of molecule bearing the determinants (e.g., CEA and normal cross-reacting antigens), neither the identity of the internalized molecule nor the extent of its internalization will be known. Furthermore, antibodies may become functionally monovalent as soon as the nuclide or any other substituent becomes covalently linked within the combining site. When there are more than two acceptor sites per IgG molecule, substitution will occur at random. This will result in a mixture of differently substituted molecules. According to binding studies with Fab fragments [7], the monovalent species within the mixture will have lost the potential of internalization. In this case differences in internalization, though still of practical importance, would simply result from an artifact introduced by the conjugation procedure. Finally, the formal proof is lacking that the pH 2.8 treatment is in fact sufficient for desorbing bound antibody irrespective of binding affinity in every single instance.
3. A further source of concern is the parallelism of internalization in vitro versus in vivo. Studies of antibody binding in various systems have revealed differences in both directions, i.e., internalization took place in vitro but not in vivo, or vice versa [2,3]. Direct evaluation of internalization in vivo is complicated by the fact that MAb uptake into most solid tissues is restricted by limited accessibility and that internalization can only be evaluated in an indirect way, e.g., by comparing retention and excretion of radioactivity after injection of differently radioiodinated antibodies [13]. We have analyzed in detail the situation encountered with MAb 12–15A directed against a surface molecule on the murine T lymphoma variant ESb-Mp [8]. This MAb showed moderate internalization in vitro both in lymphoma cells and in normal spleen cells. Yet biodistribution in vivo was dominated by a rapid and saturable binding to spleen and lymph node tissue, followed by rapid clearance and excretion of radioiodine. ESb-Mp lymphoma tissue, on the other hand, retained the labeled MAb for prolonged periods of time. This difference, together with the preferential saturation/modulation of binding sites on normal lymphatic tissue, could be exploited in a targeting procedure of lymphoma tissue which was operationally selective; preinjection of graded doses of unlabeled 12–15A (IgG or fragments) followed by the labeled MAb was found to result in a shift of preferential uptake from normal spleen, lymph nodes, and bone marrow into lymphoma tissue.

4. It is of interest to note that rapid internalization was induced in vitro when MAb bound to the surface of tumor cells were cross-linked with anti-immunoglobulin antibody [9,10]. The effect was achieved with all MAb listed in the "very low internalization" group in Table 1, a representative example being shown in Fig. 1. Thus anti-Ig treatment, and possibly other cross-linking events as well offer a means of pushing internalization to completeness even in systems which do not show spontaneous internalization. Whether the route of anti-Ig-induced internalization is the same as the route of spontaneous internalization cannot be decided in a general way. The effect may gain practical importance in ex vivo treatments of cell suspensions or in protocols that include elimination of circulating MAb by treatment with anti-IgG antibody, provided that the tissue concentration of anti-Ig ever reaches a substantial level.

Release of MAbs from the Target Cell

The fate of a MAb conjugate after binding and internalization has been studied by loading target cells with radioiodinated MAb at 37 °C, removing unbound MAb in a

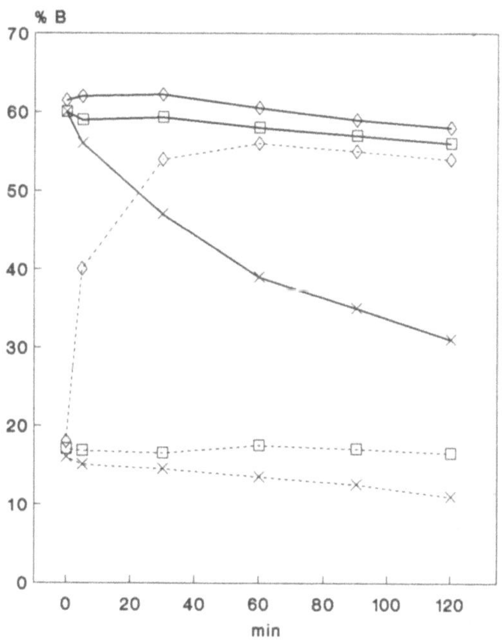

Fig. 1. Internalization and release of ^{125}I-labeled MAb 225.28 after binding to MeWo melanoma cells [11]. After a 2-h period of uptake at 37 °C, cells were transferred into fresh media containing control IgG (□), unlabeled 225.28 (×), or antimouse IgG (◇) at concentrations of 4 μg/ml. *Unbroken lines*, total cell-bound activity; *dashed lines*, internalized activity as measured after pH 2.8 treatment of cells. The antibody was barely internalized during the uptake period, but anti-IgG induced complete internalization within 30 min. Release of bound MAb was greatly enhanced by an excess of cold MAb in the media. MAb 225.28 was donated by S. Ferrone

washing step, and transferring cells into fresh media containing different unlabeled antibodies. When cells were then kept at 0 °C, virtually no release of radioactivity was observed [7]. When cells were kept at 37 °C, release took place at a low or high rate in the absence or presence, respectively, of a high concentration of the unlabeled MAb corresponding to the labeled MAb used during uptake (Fig. 1). Excess unlabeled MAb was found to accelerate release not only of the externally bound labeled MAb but also of the internalized portion [9,10], provided divalent IgG was used rather than monovalent Fab. Released radioactivity was bound to intact antibody, while the small amount of radioiodine released after anti-Ig-driven internalization was bound to degraded material. These results were obtained with almost every MAb tested, with the exception of some of the antilymphoma MAb.

Tumor Targeting with MAbs Binding to Extra-Cellular Depots of Antigen

When the results of clinical studies are critically evaluated, it is surprising to see that in general success was achieved with MAb directed against secreted antigens [11]. This emphasizes the role of disturbance of polarity of (protein) secretion observed in many carcinoma tissues. Unlike normal epithelia, in which transport processes are strictly oriented toward the luminal side, many types of carcinoma cells have lost polarity, secreting indiscriminately so that extracellular pools of antigen and, finally, positive levels of circulating antigen may be detected. When this type of tumor cell was examined in culture using MAb RA-96 that recognized a secreted mucin, a complete lack of MAb binding to the cell surface was observed (H. Kalthoff et al. to be published). But binding occurred after permeabilization of cell membranes, when intracellular antigen is accessible. Nevertheless, high uptake levels were achieved in vivo [10]. Autoradiographic evidence indicates that extracellular reservoirs of the antigen coincide with sites of pronounced MAb accumulation and retention [1,5,11,12]. This may be one reason, favorable accessibility of some types of carcinomas possibly being another, why among (immunoscintigraphic) targeting studies those which used MAb against secreted carcinoma-associated antigens proved to be relatively successful. However, undifferentiated tumors often show a complete loss of secretory potential. In this case, the antigen is only expressed intracellularly, which is less than favorable for MAb binding and retention in the tumor.

Acknowledgements. This work was supported by the Tumor Center Heidelberg-Mannheim. The groups listed below Table 1 are thanked for generously supplying MAb.

References

1. Buchegger F, Haskell CM, Schreyer M, Scazziga BR, Randin S, Carrel S, Mach JP (1983) Radiolabeled fragments of monoclonal antibodies against carcinoembryonic antigen for localization of human colon carcinoma grafted into nude mice. J Exp Med 158:413–427
2. Chatenoud L, Bach JF (1984) Antigenic modulation—a major mechanism of antibody action. Immunol Today 5:20–25

3. Chatenoud L, Baudrihaye MF, Kreis H, Goldstein G, Schindler J, Bach JF (1982) Human in vivo antigenic modulation induced by the anti-T cell OKT3 monoclonal antibody. Eur J Immunol 12:979–982
4. Della Torre G, Canevari S, Orlandi R, Colnaghi MI (1987) Internalization of a monoclonal antibody against human breast cancer by immunoelectron microscopy. Br J Cancer 55:357–359
5. Epenetos AA, Britton KE Mather S, Shepherd J, Granowska M, Taylor-Papadimitriou J, Nimmon CC, Durbin H, Hawkins LA, Malpas JS, Bodmer WF (1982) Targeting of iodine-123-labelled tumour-associated monoclonal antibodies to ovarian, breast, and gastrointestinal tumors. Lancet:999–1004
6. Garnett MC, Baldwin RW (1986) Endocytosis of a monoclonal antibody recognising a cell surface glycoprotein antigen visualised using fluorescent conjugates. Eur J Cell Biol 41:214–218
7. Matzku S, Bröcker EB, Brüggen J, Dippold WG, Tilgen W (1986) Modes of binding and internalization of monoclonal anti-melanoma antibodies to human melanoma cell lines. Cancer Res 46:3848–3854
8. Matzku S, Kirchgessner H, Schirrmacher V (1988) Antibody targeting to the murine lymphoma ESb-Mp: increased accumulation due to reduced internalization into lymphoma cells as compared to normal lymphoid cells. Int J Cancer 41:108–114
9. Matzku S, Kirchgeßner H, Bröcker EB, Tilgen W (1988a) Manipulation of melanoma targeting with monoclonal antibodies: influences of internalization and release. Eur J Cancer Clin Oncol 24:S75–S80
10. Matzku S, Tilgen W, Kalthoff H, Schmiegel W, Bröcker EB (1988b) Dynamics of antibody transport and internalization. Int J Cancer [suppl 2]:11–14
11. Matzku S, Tilgen W, Bihl H, Schwechheimer K, Kalthoff H, Schmiegel W (1988c) Tumor imaging: role of the target antigen. In: Gabius HJ, Nagel GA (eds) Lectins and glycoconjugates in oncology. Springer, Berlin Heidelberg New York, pp 67–76
12. Moshakis V, Ormerod MG, Westwood JH, Imrie S, Neville AM (1982) The site of binding of anti-CEA antibodies to tumour CEA in vivo: an immunocytochemical and autoradiografic approach. Br J Cancer 46:18–21
13. Pittman RC, Carew TE, Glass CK, Green SR, Taylor CA, Attie AD (1983) A radioiodinated, intracellularly trapped ligand for determining the sites of plasma protein degradation in vivo. Biochem J 212:791–800
14. Tilgen W, Matzku S, Kaufmann I, Engstner M, Brüggen J, Dippold W, Petzold D (1987) Modulation of melanoma-associated antigens by monoclonal antibodies as visualized by radioimmunoelectron microscopy and radioantibody binding assay. Arch Dermatol Res 279:S116–S126

Regional Immunotherapy and Chemotherapy in Lung Cancer

O. Kokron, M. Micksche, F. Olbert, and A. Schlegl

5. Medizinische Abteilung, Lainz Krankenhaus, Wolkersbergenstraße 1, 1130 Wien, Austria

This overview summarizes the results of various methods of regional immunotherapy and chemotherapy for lung cancer. There are different techniques, some still in development, others already obsolete. Their relative clinical merits must be assessed. Since immunotherapy and chemotherapy are fundamentally different methods, they are discussed separately.

Regional Immunotherapy

In recent years more insight into locoregional defense mechanisms of lung cancer has been gained by studying the functional activity of tumor-infiltrating, lymph node- and malignant effusion-derived lymphocytes and macrophages. A common finding has been that the cytotoxic activity of these cells against autologous and allogeneic as well as fresh and cultured tumor targets was significantly depressed. Preincubation of the effector cells with biological response modifiers (BRM) of bacterial origin, such as Bacille Calmette Guerin (BCG), *Corynebacterium parvum*, and the streptococcal preparation OK 432 has significantly augmentated cytotoxicity in vitro. Therefore it has been assumed that locoregional therapy with BRM can stimulate local and systemic immune reactions in lung cancer patients. This therapy might result in a direct and also, via the cytokine cascade, an indirect stimulation of cytotoxic reactions in the vicinity of the tumor, thereby contributing to tumor cell lysis.

Methods and Routes of Administration

In animal models it has been repeatedly demonstrated that therapy with bacterial BRM is most effective when administered in the vicinity of the tumor, i.e., intra- and perilesionally or in the presence of malignant intracavitary effusion. In the human situation, and especially in lung cancer, the lack of direct access to the tumor has been considered a limiting factor for regionally directed immunotherapy. One attempt to circumvent this has been the use of aerosols to deliver the agent at the tumor site within the bronchoalveolar system. The development of improved

R. Jakesz/H Rainer (Eds.)
Progress in Regional Cancer Therapy

Table 1. Methods and routes for regional immunotherapy

1. Topical administration: aerosol
2. Intralesional
a) Bronchoscopic
b) Transthoracic
3. Intravascular
a) Intralymphatic
b) Intra-arterial
4. Intrapleural

fiberscopic and imaging methods has made it feasible to inject BRM directly into the tumor via the endobronchial and transthoracic routes [2, 22]. In addition, attempts have recently been made to deliver BRM to the tumor site by means of intra-arterial and/or intralymphatic injection. [13]. The route of application most frequently used so far has been intrapleural injection especially in malignant pleural effusions. Using this route the agent is distributed within the pleural cavity, where it can stimulate lymphocytes and macrophages present in the effusion fluid and lymphatic vessels [12, 23] (Table 1).

Therapeutic Setting

Initially locoregional immunotherapy was used only in far-advanced lung cancer (non-small cell). The major objective was to develop an alternative, active method which could be used when conventional treatment modalities had reached their limits. Furthermore, studies of the preoperative intratumoral injection of BRM were designed; the aim was to stimulate local defence mechanisms preoperatively in order to achieve a better postoperative disease outcome. Finally based on the observation that postoperative empyema results in a better prognosis and improvement of survival, local immunotherapy has been used as adjuvant therapy following surgery for lung cancer [12]. Initial studies have been mainly performed with bacterial BRM such as BCG, *C. parvum*, *Nocardia rubra* and OK 432. These agents have been administered by aerosol in pilot studies with no significant influence on the outcome of the disease [13]. Preoperative intratumoral injection of BCG by endoscopic methods has shown that this agent can increase effector cell number and function. For this purpose effector cells have been isolated from surgical specimens and tested in cytotoxicity assays. Based on the already mentioned positive correlation between post-operative sepsis and survival in lung cancer, a pilot study for adjuvant therapy in patients with non-small cell lung cancer was initiated. Patients in the immediate post-operative phase received a single injection of BCG via a catheter into the resection site [2]. The results of this study pointed to a beneficial effects of the therapy. In the wake of this report several investigations using BCG and/or *C. parvum* as therapeutic agent for locoregional adjuvant treatment of non-small cell lung cancer were initiated with the aim of improving the postoperative prognosis. However neither McKneally et al. [12] nor the American and European (Ludwig) lung cancer study groups [9, 11] could demonstrate any significant beneficial effect of this therapy in either the short or the long term. A harmful effect on disease outcome has even been documented. In our own studies in patients with malignant pleural effusion, intrapleural injection of OK 432 resulted in a complete resolution of effusion fluid in three of 12 cases; seven patients had a significant reduction in fluid volume and two showed no change. A significant decrease in the proportion of malignant cells in the effusion fluid was also documented. Additionally, significant augmentation of natural killer cell activity and autologous cytotoxicity of effusion-derived effector cells was found in patients classified as responders. These results, suggest that the immunomodulation observed after intrapleural injection of OK 432 contributes to the beneficial clinical effects. Other studies using BCG and *C. parvum* for intrapleural therapy of malignant effusion have shown some effectiveness on the part of these agents.

Further studies using recombinant cytokines such as interferon, interleukin-2, and granulocyte-macrophage colony-stimulating factor are in progress with the intention of stimulating locoregional defense mechanisms via the intrapleural route in patients with malignant effusions.

Regional Chemotherapy in Lung Cancer

As shown in Table 2, several techniques are available for regional drug delivery in lung cancer patients. The purpose behind these methods is to achieve higher drug concentrations at the tumor site with less toxicity to the host.

Topical endobronchial administration as aerosol chemotherapy with poorly soluble drugs has been used for carcinomas with extensive bronchial and/or tracheal spread, or for carcinoma in situ, when surgery or radiotherapy might be contraindicated. Others have used bronchoscopic infusion with bleomycin [17] or pepleomycin adsorbed on activated charcoal [14]. The advantage of topical administraton is the achievement of a high local concentration of drug with little or no associated systemic toxicity. Experimental results in mice have been promising [6], but no clinical benefit has been demonstrated so far.

Table 2. Methods and routes for regional chemotherapy

1. Topical administration
   a) Aerosol
   b) Intrabronchial instillation
2. Intralesional
   a) Bronchoscopic, intratumoral
   b) Transthoracic, instratumoral
3. Intravascular
   a) Intralymphatic
   b) Intra-arterial
      via bronchial artery
      via pulmonary artery
4. Intraoperative regional instillation
5. Intrapleural
6. Intrapericardial

Intralesional administration is achieved either by bronchoscopy or transthoracally. Bronchoscopic intratumoral injection of cytostatics has been used in advanced central type lung cancer involving the tracheal bifurcation or the trachea itself, with bronchial obturation or obstructive pneumonia, and in some instances as an adjuvant therapy following endoscopic recanalization [25]. Clinical benefit of this method is palliative. With the advances of endoscopic laser therapy [18] and photo-radiotherapy [5], intralesional bronchoscopic chemotherapy has lost some of its attraction. Transthoracic intratumoral injection of drugs into large peripheral tumors under radiologic guidance is a rather problematic method.

Intralymphatic chemotherapy has been considered by many authors as an adjuvant treatment after surgery in cases of potential or proven lymphatic spread. Anticancer drugs such as emulsified bleomycin or 5-fluorouracil have been injected into the lymphatics of the visceral pleura and/or into the subcarinal lymph nodes at thoracotomy. The expectation is to lower the incidence of recurrences in the mediastinal lymph nodes. Clinical effectiveness has not so far been proven.

Intra-arterial infusion of cytostatics is probably the most promising method of locoregional chemotherapy for lung cancer. There are two rationales behind the superiority of this approach: First, this technique can deliver a high drug concentration to a localized tumor, resulting in a higher tissue level of the drug and producing a greater tumor kill; this depends on the nature of the dose-response relationship of the particular type of lung cancer involved. Second, a large amount of the drug will be removed during the first passage through the capillary bed of the target region, thereby lowering the systemic toxicity. The ideal situation for intra-arterial chemotherapy is the following: (a) the tumor is sensitive to the agent and is limited to the infused region; (b) the catheterized artery can be carefully selected for low flow rate and small numbers of anastomoses; (c) the drug acts directly, with high first-pass extraction by the target region, a short half-life, high total body clearance, and a cell kill proportional to the peak level. Finally, angiography must be carried out before these rather difficult catheterizations. The possible routes are (1) via a segment of the aorta from which the bronchial arteries arise (the historic route), (2) via the bronchial artery or another nutrient vessel, and (3) via the pulmonary artery system (venous catheter infusion or isolated lung perfusion) [17].

These therapies have so far attracted the attention of only a few dedicated physicians [19]. We can report our experience of intra-arterial chemotherapy in a group of 55 patients with lung cancer. In six of these 55, catheterization of a bronchial artery was not feasible technically. The remaining 49 patients comprised 37 men and 12 women, aged 24-71 years (median years 54). The following tumor types were observed; 15 small cell, two large cell, 12 epidermoid, 16 adenocarcinomas, two alveolar cell carcinomas, and two primary pulmonary sarcomas. No patient had distant metastases, and all growths were confined to the hemithorax. There of 49 patients had previously been subjected to chemotherapy, and two had undergone irradiation. In eight cases the catheter was introduced via the pulmonary artery, in 39 via the bronchial artery, in one via an intercostal artery, and in one via the internal thoracic artery. As shown in Table 3 no objective response could be achieved by infusion via the pulmonary artery, or, via the intercostal or the internal thoracic artery. There was one minor response via the internal thoracic artery. Via the bronchial artery, one complete and six partial responses were observed with different drugs and administration protocols. The characteristics of patients

Table 3. Intra-arterial chemotherapy in lung tumors: cytostatic drugs and tumor response

Route	Drug(s)	Dosage (mg)	*n*	Response		
				CR	PR	MR
Pulmonary artery	VM 26	150–200	3	—	—	1
	Cisplatin	90–110	2	—	—	—
	ADM	80	1	—	—	—
	Bleomycin	15	1	—	—	—
	Ifosfamide	1000	1	—	—	—
Bronchial artery	Cisplatin	50–100	9	—	4	1
	DTIC	500–1000	8	—	1	—
	ADM	50–100	4	—	—	1
	Bleomycin	15	4	—	—	1
	VP 16	200	2	—	—	—
	VM 26	200	2	—	1	—
	Mitoxantrone	20–30	2	—	—	—
	ADM + VM 26	50/100	1	1	—	—
	ADM + VP 16	80/200	1	—	—	1
	5-FU + VM 26	1000/100	1	—	—	—
	DDP + VP 16	50/100	2	—	—	—
	Other combinations		3	—	—	—
Internal thoracic artery	VCR + ADM + DTIC	1/80/500	1	—	—	1
Intercostal artery	VM 26 + 5-FU + DTIC	50/500/200	1	—	—	—

VP 16, etoposide; VM 26, teniposide; VCR, Vincristine; ADM, doxorubicin; 5FU, 5-fluorouracil; DDP, cisplation; CR, complete remission; PR, partial remission; MR, minor response.

Table 4. Characteristics of patients with tumor response

Patient	Tumor type	Tumor vascularization	Drugs	Number of infusions	Response
1	Adeno carcinoma	Poor	ADM + VM 26	2	CR
2	Small cell	Poor	VM 26	3	PR
3	Large cell	Very poor	DDP	1	PR
4	Adeno carcinoma	Rich	DTIC	3	PR
5	Alveolar	Poor	DDP	1	PR
6	Epidermoid	Poor	DDP	2	PR
7	Epidermoid	Poor	DDP	1	PR

showing a tumor response are given in Table 4. The duration of response was 1–7 months, with a median value of 2 months. The survival time of these patients from the commencement of therapy ranged from 27 to 565 days (median: 146 days). Side effects included chest pain in 21 patients, nausea in 20, raised temperature in 10, cough in five, hemoptysis in three, pleurodynia in two, arterial thrombosis in one, and thromboembolism in another; in one patient regional necrosis (aortic wall and esophagus) occurred 1 month after infusion, and the patient died of erosional bleeding. In conclusion, relatively good responses could bc obtained using our dosage schedules by intra-arterial chemotherapy via the bronchial artery, but these responses were of short duration. The superiority of intra-arterial over intravenous chemotherapy is not conclusively established. More ingenious pharmacologic models and clinical trails are needed, including more information on the possibilities and the risks of such treatment [8]. Theoretical aspects are discussed elsewhere [3, 4, 9, 20, 21].

Intraoperative regional instillation of drugs as an adjuvant treatment mode now has only historical importance.

Intrapleural and intrapericardial chemotherapy have to be considered as local treatments of lung cancer metastases, and are therefore outside our terms of references here. A large variety of drugs, either tumoricidal agents or local irritants, are effective against malignant effusions [1, 14, 16]. In our opinion intrapericardial chemotherapy is rarely indicated. Intrapleural chemotherapy [15] can be used when other measures, which include drainage, systemic chemotherapy, or the injection of a sclerosing agent such as quinacrine or tetracycline, fail [24].

Conclusion

Whereas phase I and phase II studies with intratumoral and intrapleural immunotherapy in lung cancer showed promising results, phase III comparative studies have shown no clinical benefit. Some techniques of regional chemotherapy for example bronchoscopic intralesional, intrapleural, and intrapericardial delivery, can achieve palliative effects but the value of others is unclear. The most promising form of treatment seems to be intra-arterial chemotherapy, although the data currently available have still not conclusively demonstrated a superiority over systemic chemotherapy.

References

1. Bölckskei P, Haydn G, Magnussen H (1981) Die Behandlung maligner Pleuraergüsse mit dem Gewebekleber Histoacryl. Prax Pneumol 35:941–943
2. Carmack Holmes E, Ramming, KP, Bein ME, Coulson WF, Callery C (1979) Intralesional BCG immunotherapy of pulmonary tumors. J Thorac Cardiovasc Surg 77:362–368
3. Chen HS, Cross JF (1980) Intra-arterial infusion of anticancer drugs: theoretic aspects of drug delivery and review of responses. Cancer Treat Rep 64:31–40
4. Collins JM (1984) Pharmacokinetic rationale for intraarterial therapy. In: Howell SB (ed) Intra-arterial and intracavitary cancer chemotherapy. Nijhoff, Boston, pp 1–10
5. Hayata Y, Harubumi K, Ono J et al. (1986) Effects of photodynamic therapy in lung cancer with particular reference to early stage cases. In: Hansen HH (ed) Lung cancer. Nijhoff, Boston, pp 221–232
6. Heyes J, Catheral EJ (1974) Aerosol chemotherapy of lung neoplasia. Nature 247: 485–487
7. Johnston M, Minchen R, Bumm P (1988) Isolated lung perfusion with high dose chemotherapy: early clinical experience. Lung Cancer (J) 4 [Suppl]: 5.04

8. Kokron O, Olbert F (1983) Intra-arterial infusion therapy for pulmonary tumours. In: Schwemmle K, Aigner K (eds) Vascular perfusion in cancer therapy. Springer, Berlin Heidelberg New York, pp 128–136
9. Ludwig Lung Cancer Cooperative Group (1982) Intrapleural *Corynebacterium parvum* as adjuvant therapy in operable bronchogenic non-small cell Carcinoma. In: Terry WD Rosenberg SA (eds) Immunotherapy of human cancer. Elsevier, Amsterdam. pp 111–115
10. Masuda H, Takagi K, Kikuchi K, Ogata T (1988) A study of the pharmacokinetics and tissue levels of cisplatin by bronchial artery infusion. Lung Cancer (J) 4 [Suppl]: 9.2.09
11. Mc Leod DT, Calverley PM, Millar JW, Horne NW (1985) Further experience of *Corynebacterium parvum* in malignant pleural effusion. Thorax 40:515–518
12. McKneally MF, Mauer CM, Alley RD, Kausel HW, Older TM, Foster ED, Lininger L (1979) Regional immunotherapy of lung cancer using intrapleural BCG: summary of a four year randomized study. In: Muggia F, Rozencweig M (eds) Lung cancer. Raven, New York, pp 471–475
13. Mitsui K, Sohara Y, Endo K, Suzuki Y, Kobayashi S, Nakada T (1982) Passive cellular immunotherapy against lung cancer by bronchial artery infusion with allogenic leukocytes. Third World Conference on Lung Cancer, Tokyo, 1982.(abstr P-63)
14. Nakabayashi T, Saito T, Koroku T, Yasuda S, Nagahama F, Ekimoto H, Yamashita Y, Matsuda A (1982) Local treatment of lung cancer with pepleomycin adsorbed on activated charcoal (PEP–AC). Third World Conference of Lung Cancer, Tokyo, 1982. (abstr 173)
15. Ostrowski MJ (1986) An assessment of the long-term results of controlling the reaccumulation of malignant effusions using intracavitary bleomycin. Cancer 57: 721–727
16. Salzer G, Müller H (1978) Die lokale Behandlung maligner Pleuraergüsse mit dem Mistelpräparat Iscador. Prax Pneumol 32:721–729
17. Sekiguchi N, Nishikawa M, Ariwa R (1982) Local intrabronchial instillation therapy in advanced central type lung cancer. Third World Conference on Lung Cancer, Tokyo, 1982. (abstr P–56)
18. Steppling H (1988) Endobronchiale Lasertherapie. Dtsch Med Wochenschr 113:1194–1197
19. Svanberg L, Hellekant C (1977) Combined therapy with bleomycin and selective intra-arterial infusion of mitomycin C in lung cancer. Jpn J, Antibiot 30 [Supply]:57–69
20. Swistel AJ, Bading JR, Raaf JH (1984) Intra-arterial versus intravenous Adriamycin in the rabbit VX–2 tumour system. Cancer 53:1397–1404
21. Watanabe Y, Shimizu J, Yoshida M, Murakami S, Kobayashi H, Komoto F, Iwa T, Kitagawa M (1988) Reappraisal of bronchial arterial infusion therapy for advanced hilar lung cancer. Lung Cancer (J) 4 [Suppl]:6.3.12
22. Yamashita T, Okunaka Y, Kagawa K, Bando H, Tsubura E (1982) Intratumoral injections of *Nocardia rubra*-cell wall skeleton as immunotherapy for lung cancer. Third World Conference on Lung Cancer, Tokyo, 1982. (abstr P–64)
23. Yasumoto K, Tanaka K, Ichinose Y, Yaita H, Hara N, Ohta M, Miyazaki K, Nakahashi H, Motohiro A, Furukawa T, Yoshida T, Inokuchi K (1982) Effect of intrapleural *Nocardia rubra* CWS in patients with lung cancer. In: Third World Conf on Lung Cancer, Tokyo, 1982. (abstr 197)
24. Zaloznik AJ, McStephen M, Oswald G, Captain D, Langin M (1983) Intrapleural Tetracycline in malignant pleural effusions. Cancer 51:752–755
25. Zwintz E, Olbert F (1977) Die endobronchiale Tumorausräumung beim inoperablen Bronchuskarzinon. Prax Pneumol 31:805–815

MIX
Papier aus verantwortungsvollen Quellen
Paper from responsible sources
FSC® C105338

If you have any concerns about our products,
you can contact us on
ProductSafety@springernature.com

In case Publisher is established outside the EU,
the EU authorized representative is:
Springer Nature Customer Service Center GmbH
Europaplatz 3, 69115 Heidelberg, Germany

Printed by Libri Plureos GmbH
in Hamburg, Germany